Isolator Technology

Applications in the Pharmaceutical and Biotechnology Industries

Edited by
Carmen M. Wagner
James E. Akers

Interpharm Press, Inc.
Buffalo Grove, IL

Invitation to Authors

Interpharm Press publishes books focused upon applied technology and regulatory affairs impacting Healthcare Manufacturers worldwide. If you are considering writing or contributing to a book applicable to the pharmaceutical, biotechnology, medical device, diagnostic, cosmetic, or veterinary medicine manufacturing industries, please contact our Director of Publications.

Social Responsibility Programs

Reforestation

Interpharm Press is concerned about the impact of the worldwide loss of trees upon both the environment and the availability of new drug sources. Therefore, Interpharm supports global reforestation and commits to replant trees sufficient to replace those used to meet the paper needs to print its books.

Pharmakos-2000

Through its Pharmakos-2000 program, Interpharm Press fosters the teaching of pharmaceutical technology. Under this program, complimentary copies of selected Interpharm titles are regularly sent to every College and School of Pharmacy worldwide. It is hoped that these books will be useful references to faculty and students in advancing the practice of pharmaceutical technology.

10 9 8 7 6 5 4 3

ISBN: 0-935184-78-3
Copyright © 1995 by Interpharm Press, Inc. All rights reserved.

All rights reserved. This book is protected by copyright. No part of it may be reproduced, stored in a retrieval system, or transmitted in any form or by any means, electronic, mechanical, photocopying, recording, or otherwise, without written permission from the publisher. Printed in the United States of America.

Where a product trademark, registration mark or other protected mark is made in the text, ownership of the mark remains with the lawful owner of the mark. No claim, intentional or otherwise, is made by reference to any such marks in this book.

While every effort has been made by Interpharm Press, Inc., to ensure the accuracy of the information contained in this book, this organization accepts no responsibility for errors or omissions.

Interpharm Press, Inc.
1358 Busch Parkway
Buffalo Grove, IL 60089, USA
Phone: + 1 + 708 + 459-8480
Fax: + 1 + 708 + 459-6644

Contents

Foreword — xv

Introduction — xvii

SECTION I. TECHNOLOGY OVERVIEW

1. **Current Challenges to Isolation Technology** — 3
   Carmen M. Wagner

   The Emergence of Advanced Aseptic Processing Isolators — 4
   Protective Barrier Systems—Definitions — 5
   　Barriers and Isolators—Conceptual Differences
   Isolator Design — 8
   Functional Requirements of Isolators — 11
   　Application Requirements
   　Containment
   　Pressure Requirements
   　Isolator Function Requirements
   Materials of Construction — 17
   Key Operational Features — 18
   　Ventilation/Filtration
   　Manipulation
   　Visibility
   　Materials Transfer

	Special Challenges to Designers and Users of Isolators	26
	Regulatory Compliance	
	European GMP	
	Guidelines	
	Material Transfer	
	Validation/Sterilization	
	Sterilization	
	Monitoring	
	Siting of Isolators	
	The Future of Isolation Technology	33
	References	35
2.	**Isolator Technology: Regulatory Issues and Performance Expectations**	**37**
	James E. Akers	
	A Glossary of Terms Commonly Used in Describing Advanced Aseptic Processing Technology	38
	Isolation Technology: Key Regulatory Issues	44
	Sterility Assurance	
	Summary	59
	Recommended Readings	60
3.	**Regulatory Aspects of Isolation/Barrier Technology**	**63**
	James C. Lyda	
	The Technology Today	64
	Who Are the Regulators?	64
	The First Problem—Definitions	65
	Definitions—FDA	
	Definitions—MCA	
	What Has Been Approved?	68
	Issue—The Background Environment	69

Issue—Monitoring of the Internal Isolator Environment	69
Issue—Aseptic Processing vs. Terminal Sterilization	70
Issue—Media Fills: Value and Interpretation	71
Issue—Weak Links in Isolation Systems	71
Isolator Standards—USP	72
Aseptic Processing Standard—ISO	72
Cleanroom Standards—ISO	73
The FDA and European International Standards Policies	73
Conclusions	74
References	74

4. British and European Experience with Isolator Technology 77

Gordon F. Farquharson

Historical Perspective	77
Market Stimulus to Use Isolators	78
Typical Applications	79
Radioactive Hazard Containment Cabinets	
Microbiological Safety Cabinets	
Laboratory Flexible Film Isolators	
Sterility Testing Isolators	
Potent Compound Dispensing Isolators	
Powder Handling System Isolators	
Small Scale Clean or Aseptic Processing Isolators	
Large Scale Clean or Aseptic Processing in Isolator Networks	
Development of Standards and Monographs	83
Definitions	
Specification of Requirements by European Documents	
European Regulatory Approach	90
The Environment Surrounding Isolators	91

5. Developing a Barrier/Isolator Implementation Plan — 97
Didier Meyer

Defining the Application — 98
  Positive Pressure Isolators
  Negative Pressure Isolators for Nonsterile Operations

Throughput Requirements — 102
  Manual Operations
  Automated Operations

Customizing Isolator Design — 103
  Quality Control (QC) Laboratory—Sterility Testing Systems
  Production Environment
  Other Possible Applications

Engineering Considerations — 109
  Existing Facilities
  Newly Designed and Built Facilities

Equipment Considerations — 112
  Modifying Existing Equipment to Accept an Isolator
  Modifications for Compatibility with Sterilization

Coordination of Vendor Efforts — 113
  Preshipment Equipment Specifications
  Assembly and Debugging
  Implementation Time Frames—Lead Times

Budget Considerations — 115
  Facility Costs
  Equipment Cost
  Operational Cost

Documentation — 118

Operator Training — 119

Monitoring — 120

Regulatory Compliance — 120

Conclusion — 121

References — 121

SECTION II. TECHNOLOGY IMPLEMENTATION

6. Engineering and Project Management Issues for a Hydrogen Peroxide Sterilized Filling System 125
Leslie M. Edwards
James R. Rickloff

Communications and Project Management 126

Retrofitting Existing Equipment vs. Purchasing New Equipment 130

System Design Considerations 135
Material Selection
Gas Distribution
Air Handling Requirements
Door, Seal, and Equipment Interface Designs
Transfer Systems
Automation/Control Systems
Control System and Parametric Documentation
Aeration Strategies and Considerations

Conclusions and Future Trends in Isolator Design and Sterilization 147

7. Modern Trends in Isolator Sterilization 149
James R. Rickloff
Leslie M. Edwards

Terminology of Antimicrobial Action 150

Antimicrobial Agents Used in Isolators 150
Peracetic Acid
Chlorine Dioxide
Hydrogen Peroxide
Other Methods

Material Compatibility 164

Safety and Environmental Regulations 167

References 169

8. Microbiological Monitoring and Control in Isolator Systems   173
Michael C. Carroll

Air Monitoring	174
Special Concerns for Isolator Systems	
Surface Monitoring	180
Process Validation	181
External Environment	182
Sterility Hold	184
Sterility Testing Isolators	
Production/Manufacturing Barriers	
Conclusion	186
References	187

9. Introduction to the Validation of Sterile Processing Using Isolation Technology   189
Richard M. Johnson

Materials Sterilization	192
Primary Packaging	
Product	
Gases	
Isolation Technology	193
Isolator Design	
References	194

10. Guideline to the Validation of Isolation Technology   197
Richard M. Johnson

Isolator Integrity	197
Isolator Sterilization	198
Isolator Validation	199

> Installation Qualification
> Operational Qualification
> Performance Qualification

References   202

11. Points to Consider in the Use of Sterility Testing Isolators   205

Richard T. Wood

Sterility Test Limitations   206

Isolator Technology   208
> *Advantages of an Isolator Laboratory*
> *Disadvantages of an Isolator Laboratory*

Designing an Isolator Laboratory   211
> *Location*
> *Size*
> *Material Flow*
> *Integrated Systems*
> *Utilities*
> *Methods of Sterilization*
> *Monitoring Instruments*
> *Environmental Monitoring*
> *Test Incubators*
> *Validation*

Conclusions   227

References   228

SECTION III. APPLICATIONS: THE INDUSTRY EXPERIENCE AND PERSPECTIVE

12. Barrier Isolation Technology: A Systems Approach   231

Jack P. Lysfjord
Paul J. Haas
Hans L. Melgaard
Irving J. Pflug

The System   240

Filler Design	240
The Barrier Isolator	243
Materials Selection and Compatibility	
Interface Issues	
Handling of Freeze-Dried Products	
Particulate Control Considerations	
Barrier Isolator Internal Condition Control and Monitoring	
Clean-in-Place of Barrier Isolators	262
Sterilization of Barrier Isolators	263
Atmospheric Steam/Hydrogen Peroxide Sterilization System	
Validation Considerations	271
Overview	272
Recommended Readings	277

13. The History and Future of Barrier Isolation Technology at Merck & Co., West Point, PA — 281

Michael E. Porter
Leslie M. Edwards

14. Use of Isolation Technology for Production of a Sterile Anti-Cancer Drug — 283

Paul Martin

Objectives	283
To Protect the People	
To Ensure Product Sterility	
To Protect the Environment	
Meeting the Objectives	286
The Facilities	
Environment Classification	

	Validation of Isolators—Sterility	289
	Methodology	
	Monitoring	
	Conclusion	291

15. Aseptic Filling in a Rigid Isolator at Evans Medical — 293

Julian Wilkins

	Project Requirements	295
	The Traditional Approach	295
	Isolator Network	296
	Detailed Development	296
	Ergonomic Modelling	297
	Separated Operations	297
	Control and Instrumentation	299
	Building Integration	299
	Reduced Work Volume	300

16. Isolation Technology for Sterility Testing at Burroughs Wellcome, Greenville, NC — 303

John Shirtz

17. Experience in the Design and Use of Isolator Systems for Sterility Testing — 309

James E. Akers
James P. Agalloco
Colleen M. Kennedy

	Specific Validation Testing	314
	Sterilization	314

Sterilization Cycle Development		315
Temperature Mapping		316
Determination of VHP Concentration		317
Biological Indicator Challenge Studies		318
Other Validation Issues		319
Conclusion		321
Recommended Readings		321

18. Isolation Technology: A Consultant's Perspective — 323

James Agalloco

History	324
Definitions	324
Advantages	326
Limitations and Obstacles	327
Application	327
Sterility Testing	
Filling	
Manufacturing	
Clinical Manufacturing	
Manual Procedures	
Sterilization	329
Regulatory Perspectives	330
Other Subjects	331
Retrofitting Isolation Technology to Existing Facilities	
Environmental Monitoring	
Process Validation	
Conclusion	333
References	334

19. **Isolation Technology Issues from an Engineering Company Viewpoint**   335
Dimitri P. Wirchansky

SECTION IV. RESOURCES

Glossary   343

Appendix. List of Resources   357

    Barrier/Isolator Manufacturers   357

    Filling Machine Manufacturers   359

    Validation Support and Consulting Services   361

    Engineering Companies and Consulting Services   362

    Sterilization Equipment   364

    Manufacturers of Accessory Equipment or Services   364

    Association, Institutes, and Laboratories— Information Resources   366

Name/Company Index   369

Subject Index   374

Foreword

This book was conceived at a Parenteral Drug Association (PDA) meeting in Philadelphia, where I moderated one of the first PDA roundtable discussions on Isolation Technology. As the co-founder and chair of the Isolation Technology Users Group (ITUG), now part of the PDA, I had been asked many times to provide information on the literature available on current issues associated with isolators. Assembling the information was always a challenge because most of the current knowledge was either available solely in unofficial publications (such as company literature), as unpublished observations, or in a few papers that had more recently addressed applications of isolators to sterility testing, production, and hospital applications. Many ITUG members continued to express their frustration with the lack of easy access to information discussed at ITUG and other meetings.

During early discussions about the book, many people from industry, PDA, and the International Society for Pharmaceutical Engineering (ISPE) highly recommended that I pursue the task. Like me, they believed that there was a need to make public the information that some of us had been accumulating for the last few years. They agreed that it was useful to share the experiences with those who need to know, but do not have a chance to attend meetings or courses on this topic.

Dr. Jim Akers, a past president of PDA and an early supported of isolation technology, agreed to join me as a co-editor. Many other experts from industry, from the two leading isolator technology supporting associations (PDA and ISPE), and from other professional organizations agreed to author chapters or updated summaries. Their participation added an important dimension to this book. I appreciate their effort and commitment.

This book was created to answer the perceived need for information. Our authoring team attempted to provide a fairly complete overview of the current applications of isolation technology in the United States and Europe, while incorporating as much basic information as the current knowledge allowed. This is not a complete reference or how-to book, but it does contain helpful information on important issues, such as terminology, design and engineering considerations, project management tools for successful implementation, sterilization methods, validation strategies, and real-life examples of how users are benefiting from this technology.

This is the first attempt to compile information that specifically addresses this emerging advanced aseptic processing technology. We enjoyed working on this book, and learned a lot along the way. We hope you will too.

Carmen M. Wagner

INTRODUCTION

Isolator Technology: Applications in the Pharmaceutical and Biotechnology Industries addresses the benefits and challenges of isolation technology. It reviews the status of isolator applications in the United States and Europe, including project management, engineering and design issues, regulatory compliance, sterilization, validation, and examples of applications. Until now, the information gathered in this text has been inaccessible to many industry professionals, at least in a written format. This is the first attempt to bring this information together in a comprehensive and organized way.

The book format is rather unconventional because it deals with a topic that is still evolving and is controversial. As may be expected, this book presents conflicting opinions, and perhaps some inconsistency in terminology. This was unavoidable because we wanted to preserve the integrity of each author's experience. Author experience has included meetings with the U.S. FDA, presentations at conferences and professional meetings, course instruction, and participation in the development of standards. Their knowledge and experience have been converted into 19 informative chapters that cover the most important issues associated with the implementation and use of isolation systems.

The isolators discussed in this book offer the highest degree of isolation and protection currently available against contamination. An isolator may be defined as an object that isolates or provides complete separation between people and product to maintain a germ-free environment. They are like clean rooms that have been shrunk to encompass only the area which must be controlled. They are "facilities" designed to prevent human-borne contamination and promote a germ-free environment that ensures sterility of aseptic processes.

Isolators have already impacted the quality of many facilities involved in pharmaceutical manufacturing. Their excellent performance in the sterility testing laboratory and manufacturing of sterile and potent products affirms their effectiveness. Operational savings and process control are just two more benefits that promise to make isolators an integral part of pharmaceutical manufacturing facilities in the near future.

While attention has been primarily focused on isolator applications for control of sterility, several chapters in this book are also relevant for those interested in containment applications. Pharmaceutical professionals, hospital pharmacists, and others in the health, agricultural, or biotechnology industries will find this to be an informative reference.

This book is organized into Sections I, II, III, and an Appendix. Section I, Technology Overview, includes basic information. Section II, Technology Implementation, presents detailed information on system implementation, sterilization, and validation. Section III, Applications: The Industry Experience and Perspective, contains real-life examples of applications in sterility testing and production settings. The Appendix introduces the reader to vendors who currently support this technology.

The first chapter in Section I, "Current Challenges to Isolation Technology," is about the history and evolution of events that marked the evolution of the systems that we know today. It proceeds with a discussion about the differences between barriers and isolators and the associated levels of protection against contamination. The author emphasizes the importance of clarifying the meaning of these two terms to facilitate the communication between users and regulatory agencies. This opinion is further supported by several other authors who address the terminology issues. This chapter also introduces concepts of isolator design, sterilization, validation, material transfer, monitoring, and regulatory compliance. These topics are covered in more detail in later chapters.

Chapter 2, "Isolator Technology: Regulatory Issues and Performance Expectations," provides a critical evaluation of five key regulatory issues that have attracted a lot of attention in virtually every meeting on isolation technology. It starts with a glossary of terms, and continues with a discussion of sterility assurance issues, the equivalence of isolator performance to terminal sterilization, siting requirements for isolators, the use of isolators for containment and environmental monitoring and control within isolators. The author comments that despite the extensive discussions of these topics, the issues remain unresolved and still need attention. Chapter 3, "Regulatory Aspects of Isolation/Barrier Technology," provides an excellent update of how regulatory agencies in the U.S. and Europe regard the implementation of isolators in pharmaceutical applications.

Chapter 4, "British and European Experience with Isolator Technology," provides a historical perspective of the evolution of isolator systems in Europe. A glossary of terms is also included here, again emphasizing clarification of terminology. The chapter also includes a thorough presentation on regulatory issues in Europe. The last chapter in Section I, "Developing a Barrier/Isolator Implementation Plan," includes information on how to plan and implement the use of isolation systems, with an emphasis on the systems approach and vendor participation in the planning process. It stresses the importance of carefully defining the application and the user's needs to ensure successful completion of the project. It addresses issues related to customization of design and retrofitting versus new building. The author emphasizes the importance of accounting for all phases in the implementation plan, from design to validation and start-up, particularly in the production environment.

Chapter 6, "Engineering and Project Management Issues for a Hydrogen Peroxide Filling System," begins Section II. It describes how to manage the design and engineering of isolator systems, emphasizing the need to form an expert, multifunctional team. According to the author, the team approach helps ensure the compatibility of isolator equipment and choice of sterilization method—all validated to meet the user's needs. Even though the concepts of teamwork and systems approach aren't new, they are essential for the successful implementation of isolator technology, primarily in the production environment. Vendor integration needs to happen early in the life of the project, and vendors must communicate among themselves and with the user to ensure the successful completion of the project. Chapter 7, "Modern Trends in Isolator Sterilization," reviews the sterilization technologies available for barrier systems. The comments center on vaporized hydrogen peroxide (VHP) sterilization because this is the commercially available method most widely used in the United States. It is also gaining acceptance in Europe, where several other methods, including peracetic acid, have been preferred.

In the final chapters of Section II, Michael Carroll, Richard Johnson, and Richard Wood provide guidance for the validation of isolation systems, including information on microbiological monitoring and control and overall points to consider for validation of aseptic processing. Up to now, companies have used existing conventional methodologies to monitor and control isolators. Only time will tell what new technologies will replace the existing methods.

Section III provides real-life examples of isolator applications in the sterility testing laboratory and production environments. The first two chapters in this section describe the systems approach used by members of the Barrier Users Group (BUG) to design filling machines within isolators. "Barrier Isolation Technology: A Systems Approach" offers an important account of how these professionals have approached this complex and challenging task. "The History and Future of Isolation Technology at Merck & Co." describes their experiences with the technology, including experimentation with an aseptic filling prototype being tested in a noncontrolled, nonclassified environment.

While as of this writing these applications have not yet been implemented, the close interaction between these organizations and the FDA could have a significant impact on how the regulatory agencies proceed with the development of validation standards, acceptance criteria, and classification of the environment outside the isolator.

The remaining chapters are good illustrations of the individualized approach that companies are taking towards the implementation of isolation technology. From pharmaceutical companies to consultants to engineering companies, we bring you a taste of how the industry sees the impact of isolation technology on the control of aseptic processing manufacturing. "Use of Isolation Technology for Production of a Sterile Anti-Cancer Drug" at Aquitaine Pharma (API) describes experiences of the first company using isolation technology for aseptic processing and containment to be successfully inspected by the U.S. FDA. The FDA approved API's shipment of Nevalbine to the United States for patient consumption in

1994. API's experience should be of interest to those considering the implementation of isolation for the control of sterile cytotoxic products. "Aseptic Filling in a Rigid Isolator at Evans Medical" summarizes information on the implementation of barrier isolators for the filling of syringes for vaccine production. Evans is the second company to be satisfactorily inspected by the U.S. FDA. "Isolation Technology for Sterility testing at Burroughs Wellcome Co." (BW) includes experiences with isolation technology at BW, from sterility testing to its limited use in the production environment. Consultants' perspectives are provided by Agalloco, Akers, and Kennedy in two different papers. An engineering company's perspective is related by Dimitri Wirchansky, a long-time supporter of this technology. He describes what they see as remaining issues to be addressed. Section III is not intended to represent all, or even most, of the companies using isolation technology but it gives a flavor of the kinds of choices currently available and the applications already in the market.

The "List of Resources," in the Appendix, provides lists of barrier and isolator manufacturers, and production machine manufacturers working with isolation systems. It also includes lists of validation services, manufacturers of accessory equipment, and associations dedicated to this topic and a useful glossary.

A special note of gratitude goes to the authors who helped make this book a reality. Their commitment, dedication, and patience is much appreciated. Special appreciation also to all our colleagues and associates who directly or indirectly helped us sustain our courage and determination to carry the dream to final form. We also want to recognize the assistance and encouragement that we received from Amy Davis and the editorial staff at Interpharm. Without their support we could not have managed such a demanding task. Last, but not least, special thanks are also extended to our spouses, Brian Wagner and Colleen Kennedy, for their endurance and patience as we worked to bring the material together and put the final touches to the book.

Carmen M. Wagner
James E. Akers
June 1995

Section I
Technology Overview

1
Current Challenges to Isolation Technology

Carmen M. Wagner
Lederle-Praxis Biologicals
Sanford, NC

The isolation concept is not new, but significant improvements in isolator design have warranted a new wave of attention. These improved systems called isolators can effectively prevent microbial contamination and maintain containment. Isolators prevent human-borne contamination, allow the sterile transfer of materials in and out of the work area, can maintain the sterilized state, and offer design flexibility to accommodate user requirements. This makes isolators an attractive alternative to improve control of aseptic manufacturing of heat-sensitive products.

This book attempts to bring together and clarify the issues associated with the use of isolators in pharmaceutical applications, in particular those used in aseptic product manufacturing. This introductory chapter addresses some of the challenges facing the user. It provides an overview of the field of isolation technology, starting with its history and the events that marked the evolution of the systems we know today. Next, it provides some food for thought on how to bring some systematization to the distinction between barriers and isolators. The remainder of the chapter covers topics related to the design and challenges facing the user of isolation technology.

THE EMERGENCE OF ADVANCED ASEPTIC PROCESSING ISOLATORS

Since the discovery of microbes, researchers have tried using the most current technology to ensure the exclusion of contamination from products and from the work area. The first isolators were used to rear germ-free animals, and were reported in the 1800s. By the 1940s these systems had been sufficiently developed to permit continuous maintenance of animals within the sterile space (Reyniers and Trexler 1943, 114–143).

Early isolators were rather difficult to use and maintain. They consisted of steam sterilized metal tanks with glass side ports and arm length rubber gloves, with simple double-door, pass-through locks for the transfer of materials in and out of the enclosure. A more versatile and easy-to-use flexible isolator was described by Trexler (1957). These workspaces were protected by a flexible, transparent plastic envelope that could be chemically treated. The sterile transfer of materials relied solely on manual wiping with disinfectants or autoclaving.

Since 1954 flexible isolators have been widely used to rear germ-free animals. However, they did not become attractive to the pharmaceutical industry until the 1960s when isolator design was modified to include improved air handling equipment, capabilities for sterilization-in-place, and sterile commodities transfer through the double-porte de transfert etanche (DPTE) patented by la Calhene in France. With the availability of the DPTE, tight, sealable, and reliable sterile transfers were possible, and isolators became a viable option to those interested in aseptic processing and cytotoxic containment. The DPTE is, in the author's opinion, a milestone in the evolution of advanced aseptic processing isolators.

PROTECTIVE BARRIER SYSTEMS—DEFINITIONS

Different terms have been used to describe the types of facilities used as alternatives to conventional human scale clean rooms. They include minienvironments, localized control environments, barriers, isolators, barrier isolators, and partial barriers. These terms have often been used as synonyms. However, these terms do not describe systems of equal levels of containment or sterility assurance, and their indiscriminate use is the source of much confusion in discussions revolving around isolation technology. The differences among these terms may be subtle but they are significant when attempting to create regulations and standards that will govern them. It is important for the success of this technology to clarify the terminology associated with it. The ideas presented in this book are meant to stimulate thought and discussion ultimately bringing the definitions issue to closure. Without clarity, it will be hard to lessen the confusion that exists regarding isolation technology and its associated concepts. It will also be hard to move forward with this technology with meaningful speed.

Barriers and Isolators—Conceptual Differences

For didactic purposes the general term *Protective Barrier Systems (PBSs)* can help define the group of systems that can be used to help exclude contamination from the product and work area. These systems help maintain containment or sterility. *PBSs* can be divided into two broad categories: barriers and isolators. The difference lies in the degree of isolation and level of protection provided to the product, process, and environment (Table 1.1).

In the context of this book the terms *barrier* and *isolator* are defined as follows:

Barrier—any physical obstacle to contamination.

As described in the *Webster New Collegiate dictionary* (1981),

> A material object or set of objects that separates, demarcates or serves as a barricade.

Or, as described in the *American Heritage Desk Dictionary* (1981),

Table 1.1. Key Concepts of Barriers and Isolators

Barriers

- May be personal protective equipment for cabinets, glove boxes, etc.
- May allow some contact of personnel with operation

Barrier equipment

- Does not have sterile transfer systems
- Is not capable of maintaining sterility, even if treated with agents such as formaldehyde, peracetic acid, VHP or other agents used to sterilize isolators
- Can be equipped with HEPA-filtered air
- Can have laminar (or unidirectional) air flow
- Can allow contaminants to penetrate core work area
- Can exchange air with the adjacent outside environment

Isolators

- Closed environments
- Full containment and sterility
- Reduction of size of controlled space
- Separation and protection of product and personnel
- Isolation from human-borne contamination
- Capable of maintaining sterile state
- Easily customized to fit user's requirements
- Like a clean room that has shrunk to a more controllable size

A... structure built to hold back or obstruct movement or passage... Anything that separates or holds apart.

One could complete these sentences by adding:

... obstruct the movement or passage of contamination
... Anything that separates or holds apart contamination.

Barriers offer lower degrees of isolation and protection than isolators. Protection apparatus, curtains in the clean room, biosafety cabinets, goggles, gloves, and face shields are examples of barriers. **Barriers** *are not* equipped with controlled rapid transfer ports, and allow some personnel-product contact. They cannot be sterilized and are usually not leaktight. According to this definition, many systems now called isolators would fit more appropriately within the category of barriers.

Isolator—an object that isolates or provides complete separation between areas.

As described in the *American Heritage Desk Dictionary* (1981),

Isolate means to separate from a group or whole; to set apart. From the Latin *insulatus*—meaning converted into an island.

Isolators offer the highest degree of separation and protection against contamination. In the context of this book, isolators are facilities that restrict access and provide complete segregation of people and product to maintain a germ-free or contained environment. They do not allow personnel and product contact, and can use pressure differentials to ensure containment and sterility. Isolators employ specially designed transfer ports to transfer materials in and out without compromising the integrity of the enclosure.

Isolators can also be described as shrunken clean rooms that encompass only the area which must be controlled. These are facilities designed to prevent human-borne contamination and promote a germ-free environment that ensures sterility of aseptic processes. They form an enclosed environment that exchanges air with the outside environment through HEPA or equivalent filters, or through controlled ports.

Barriers and isolators can be further subdivided into more specific categories based on levels of protection (see Figure 1.1), specific features, and applications. For example, partial barriers are open systems that offer the lowest level of protection (level 1, Table 1.2). They are used for applications that do not require complete separation of operation and personnel, and do not call for sterile or contained transfers. On the other hand, closed isolators offer the highest level of protection and containment (level 4, Table 1.2). They can be used for handling highly potent compounds and for operations that aim at

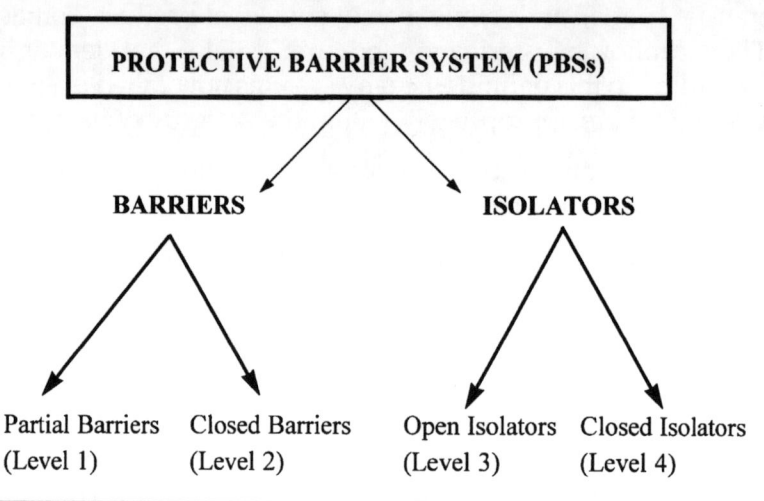

Figure 1.1. Protective Barrier Systems according to the definitions included in this book, and according to the Levels of Protection defined in Table 1.2.

the highest control of sterility. In this book, we concentrate on issues of sterility.

Other chapters in this book also address the issue of terminology. James Akers further defines the different types of isolators and barriers. Gordon Farquharson includes some of the definitions developed by the United Kingdom working group responsible for the *Guide on Isolators of Pharmaceutical Applications* (1994). James Agalloco adds some insight to the distinctions between barriers and isolators as well. Only time, and a lot of thought, will tell how clearly we will be able to refine these concepts. The consequence of hasty definitions will be the creation of ill-defined and unsuitable standards.

ISOLATOR DESIGN

This chapter centers on information related to basic design and structure of isolators based on application and function. Other chapters cover information on design engineering, project management, and project implementation of isolation systems.

Table 1.2. Levels of Protection—Contamination Control Continuum

Level	Type of PBS	Level of Protection	Impact on Work Area	Examples
1	Partial barrier	Minimum protection. The lowest level of protection against contamination.	No sterile transfer capability available. Sterility of work area **cannot** be ensured during performance of activity. People are not completely isolated from operation.	Personal protective equipment, curtains, conventional clean rooms
2	Closed barrier	Limited opening and handling. Better level of protection than level 1.	No sterile transfer capability available. Sterility of work area **cannot** be ensured during performance of activity. People are not completely isolated from operation. Closed barriers are usually decontaminated or sanitized, not sterilized.	Hospital isolators, restrictive access barriers, glove boxes

Continued on next page.

Continued from previous page.

Level	Type of PBS	Level of Protection	Impact on Work Area	Examples
3	Open isolator	Highly isolated process and transfer.	Sterility of work area **can** be maintained during performance of activity. Overpressure helps ensure the integrity of work area in spite of "mouse holes" or other such openings. Transfer of material in and out through special transfer devices.	Production isolators with small openings for exiting of vials
4	Closed isolator	Totally contained process and transfer. The highest level of protection available.	Closed systems. Sterility of work area **can** be maintained during performance of work, and does not rely on overpressure. Transfer of materials in and out through special transfer devices.	Closed, leaktight isolators used for batch production, QC testing, and containment applications

To realize maximum benefit from isolator systems, it is necessary to start with an appropriate design. The design should conform to some basic parameters but should not be restrictive. Ergonomics, regulatory requirements, ease of maintenance, cleanability, and automation capabilities are general considerations that should be part of the conceptual design phase. It is critical to understand the regulatory expectations that need to be met.

From a structural standpoint, isolator design should consider, at a minimum, the visibility, lighting, humidity, electrical safety, temperature, and pressure requirements. The designer should keep in mind the application, special process needs, and any facility constraints. The system design may aim at protecting the work area within the isolator, the environment outside the isolator, or both.

The remainder of this chapter will cover the following information

- Functional requirements of isolators
- Materials of construction
- Key operational features of isolators
- Special challenges to designers and users of isolators

FUNCTIONAL REQUIREMENTS OF ISOLATORS

During the design phase it is important to define the isolator application, function, and pressure requirements. These requirements are outlined in Figure 1.2 and are further discussed below.

Application Requirements

The application should be clearly defined as early as possible to direct the proper design of the system. Different applications may have unique requirements and may dictate the degree of customization needed. Applications are divided into two major categories: aseptic processing applications and containment. These are defined below.

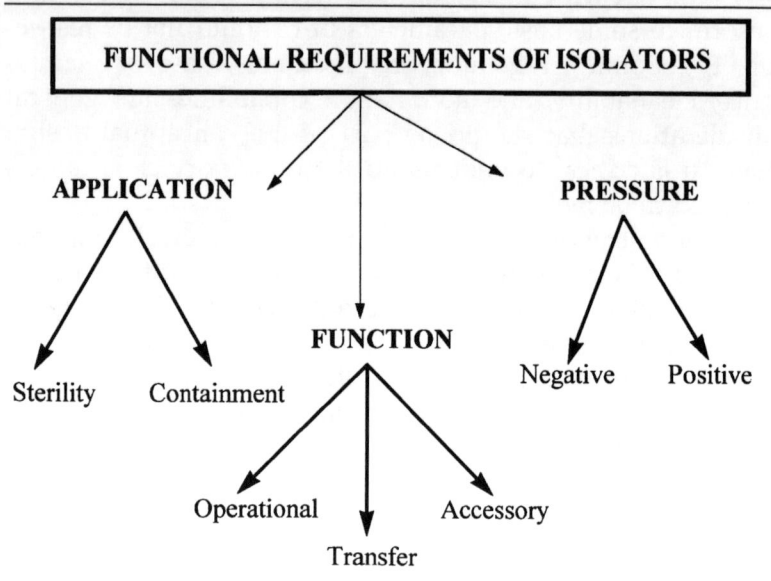

Figure 1.2. Isolator requirements.

Aseptic Processing Applications

In the aseptic processing category, sterility testing remains, by far, the largest application both in Europe and in the United States (U.S.). The U.S. FDA's initiative to eliminate retest of lots that fail first stage sterility testing may continue to encourage the use of isolators for this application (FDA 1987). Isolators are broadly accepted for sterility testing and may be currently regarded as state-of-the art for the Quality Control laboratory. The use of isolators in the production setting is less evident, but it is starting to take hold.

Designing Aseptic Processing Isolators

Aseptic processing isolators may be used in the quality control laboratory or in production. The design of these systems is intimately associated with the design of the sterilization process that will render the isolator sterile. Design considerations must take into account the compatibility of the sterilant with the isolator and the equipment, and with facility and process needs (see Figure 1.3).

Most quality control laboratory systems are off-the-shelf and require little, if any, customization (see Figures 1.4 and 1.5). The most common configuration includes one workstation isolator with two half-suits, one or two transfer isolators, and one sterilizer. An autoclave may or may not be connected to the isolation system. Sample incubation may or may not be done in isolation. These isolators are usually made of PVC and use turbulent air flow. Systems are usually sited in a standard, unclassified laboratory space with no requirements for special gowning for testing personnel. Some of these units have been in existence for five years or longer and have excellent performance records. To date, failures that have been reported at meetings or course discussions have been attributed to glove pinhole leaks or other breaks of integrity within the enclosure, such as during the transfer of nonsterile materials.

Figure 1.3. How a system's design can affect sterilization. (Courtesy of James R. Rickloff, Advanced Barrier Concepts, Cary, NC)

Design Feature	Sterilant Issues
Materials of construction	Material compatibility, residues, aerate time
Air circulation	Sterilize & aerate time, catalytic converter
Temperature limits	Concentration, sterilize time
Internal volume	Sterilant consumption, cycle time
HVAC	Enclosure conditioning prior to sterilization, catalytic converter
Outside exhaust	Aerate time, emissions
Complex surfaces	Penetration, sterilize time
Component entry	Penetration into packaging, sterilize and aerate times, sterilant consumption
Cleanability	Penetration, drying, cycle time

Note: Retrofitting existing equipment may not lead to the most efficient SIP (H_2O_2) cycle.

Figure 1.4. Example of sterility testing systems. (Courtesy of Isotech Designs, Montreal, Canada)

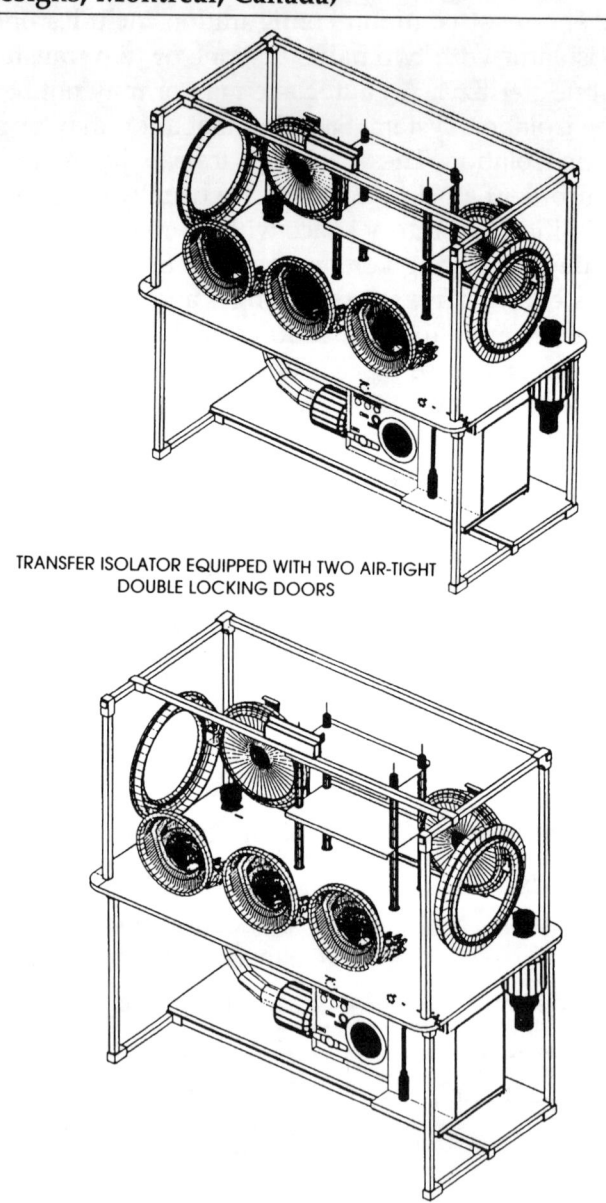

TRANSFER ISOLATOR EQUIPPED WITH TWO AIR-TIGHT DOUBLE LOCKING DOORS

ISOLATOR FOR STERILITY TESTING

Courtesy of Isotech Designs, Montreal, Canada

Figure 1.5. Example of sterility testing system with autoclave connection. (Courtesy of la Calhene)

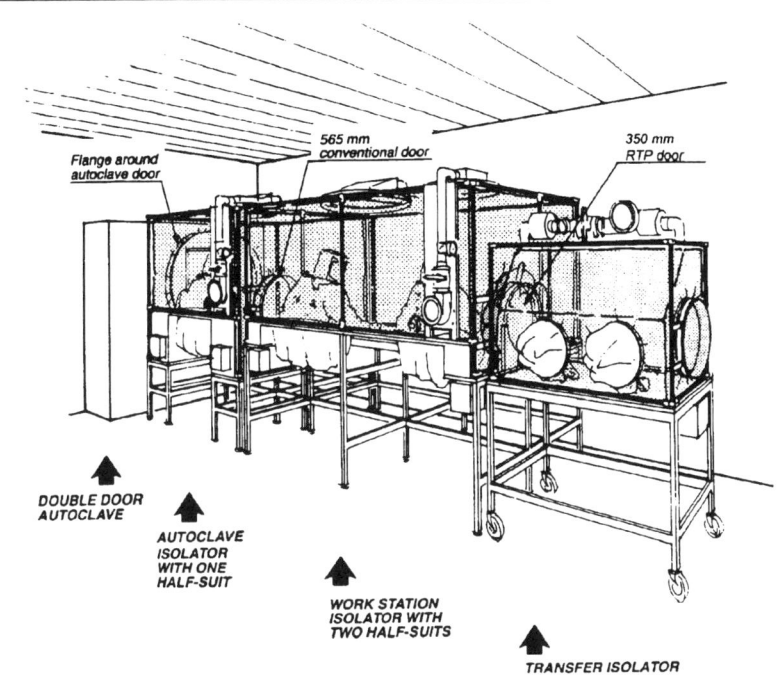

The design of manufacturing isolators is more challenging and often requires customization. The application will often dictate which special features need to be considered as part of the customized design. As described in Les Edward's chapter, the successful design of manufacturing systems is also dependent upon the quality of the communication, cooperation, and education of the various equipment vendors. Vendors who may be involved are suppliers of filling equipment, isolators, other accessory machines, and sterilization equipment. It is essential to start communication as early as possible, and continue it throughout the life of the project.

Isolators can be customized to fit different production applications. Isolators used in aseptic manufacturing may be made of rigid or flexible construction materials, may have turbulent or unidirectional air flow, and may be closed systems or depend on differential pressure to help maintain containment or sterility. Rigid isolators may be made of glass, stainless steel, or rigid plastic construction materials. Flexible isolators have canopies usually made of transparent PVC, built with airtight seams and supported by a tubular metal framework. In general, systems used for high speed filling processes are made of rigid materials, but some production applications have been successfully made with flexible materials. Rigid materials may be more durable, but flexible systems are lightweight, can be less costly, and provide greater visibility of the work area inside the canopy.

Additional design issues are addressed throughout the book, from different perspectives. In particular the chapters by Les Edwards, Richard Wood, and Jack Lysfjord have detailed information on this topic (see also Table 1.3).

Containment

Isolation technology is increasingly being applied to containment applications. The main goal in this application is to protect personnel from exposure to potentially biohazardous substances. This book does not cover in detail the design of isolators for containment, but the same basic principles discussed in most chapters apply to the containment issues as well.

Pressure Requirements

Differential pressure can be used to help isolators maintain sterility or containment. For example, isolators used in aseptic

Table 1.3. Isolators—Key Design Features

- Made of flexible or rigid material
- Easily customized to fit user's needs
- Can use HEPA or ULPA air filtration
- Can use automated controls
- Can use overpressurization for leaktightness control
- Can use unidirectional or turbulent airflow
- Can use RTPs

processing can be designed to include positive pressure to help maintain the sterile state. Isolators used in the production of cytotoxic materials can be equipped with negative pressure to ensure containment of hazardous material within the enclosure. In addition, some operations require systems that must maintain sterility while also ensuring containment. The pressure differential between the work area and the outside environment should be such that it prevents contaminants from leaving the work area, if negative pressure is used, or from entering the work area, if positive pressure is used to ensure sterility. It is advisable to continuously monitor the pressure and to install an alarm to detect pressurization failures.

Isolator Function Requirements

Isolator requirements can be defined by the function assigned to a given unit. Thus, isolators can be classified as operational units, transfer units, or accessory units according to the intended use. Accessory units can be further categorized into sterilization isolators, autoclave isolators, interface isolators, mobile isolators, and so on depending on their function. The basic principles of isolation still apply to all categories. Keep in mind that this terminology may differ in the literature.

MATERIALS OF CONSTRUCTION

Isolators are usually made of PVC or rigid plastics, stainless steel, or glass. Quality control laboratory units, used for sterility testing, are often made of PVC with a thickness that varies from 0.3 mm to 0.5 mm. The PVC seams are formed to yield smooth, uniform surfaces, usually by treatment with high-frequency sound waves. All canopy seams and connections to doors, platines, filter housings, and other such surfaces should be designed to achieve airtight conditions to guarantee sterility and containment. It is recommended that PVC canopies be kept between approximately 5 and 80°C, since PVC tends to crack below 5 and soften above 80°C.

In production settings, glass and stainless steel isolators are more commonly used. The requirements of production environments are better served with these types of construction materials. There are, however, flexible canopies in use with acceptable performance records.

KEY OPERATIONAL FEATURES

Most concerns about aseptic processing have originated from the necessity for human interaction with the process and the potential for human-borne contamination. People are considered to be the largest source of contamination in aseptic manufacturing (Whyte et al. 1982; Whyte 1991). Thus, most of the effort to control aseptic processing has centered around isolating people from the process. In isolation technology, the separation of personnel from the process is accomplished by implementing the design of key operational features as shown in Figure 1.6. Proper design of the ventilation and filtration, manipulation, visibility, and materials transfer systems ensure the proper performance of the isolator. A successful system carefully integrates these features with the process to allow the interaction of operators with the inside of the isolator without compromising the integrity of the enclosure.

Ventilation/Filtration

The leaktightness of the enclosure isolates the sterile product from the operator and from the outside environment. Air enters and exits the isolator by passing through one or more HEPA or ULPA filters. Double filters are often used for extra protection, especially when the enclosure is claimed to have a 10^{-6} SAL.

Air input may be laminar flow or turbulent flow. In some cases, the air is recirculated into the background environment through HEPA filters. The air change rate should be sufficient to maintain the required environment grade during use. High flow rates may be necessary in certain applications, but in many cases, if there are no concerns with particulates and the enclosure is maintained sterile, a rate as low as 20 volume changes per hour could be acceptable.

The air change rate and the air flow should be monitored continuously, preferably with an alarmed system. All exhausted air should be HEPA filtered. Half-suits also should

Figure 1.6. Key operational features of isolators. (Courtesy of la Calhene)

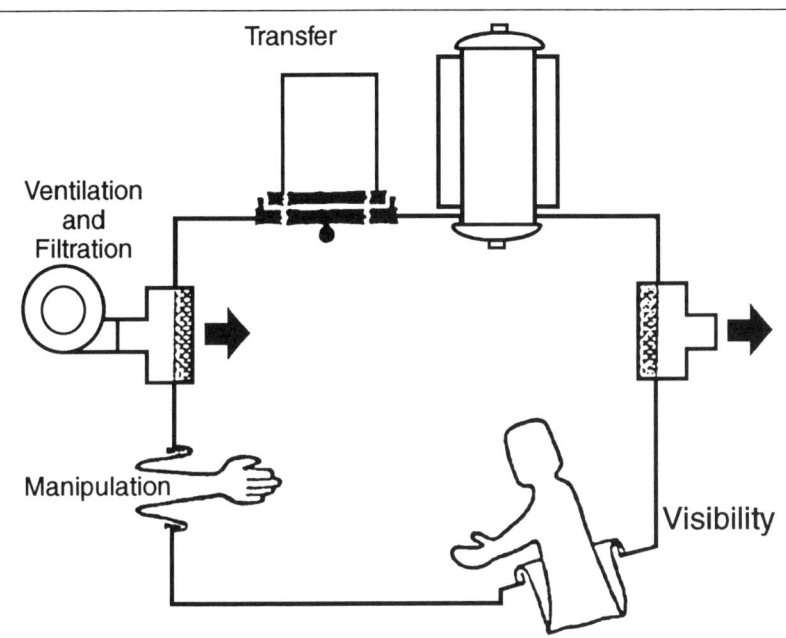

have individual HEPA filter units that can be individually adjusted for operator comfort.

An isolator should be designed so that all filters can be integrity tested in place. Dioctyl phthalate (DOP) aerosol challenge tests can be used to test the integrity and efficiency of filters, but the reagent DOP is rarely used today because of its classification as a carcinogen. More often other particle generating substances are used, such as Shell Ondina (Europe), mineral oil, Emery 3000, and others.

Manipulation

Manipulation is usually accomplished through the aid of gloves/sleeves, half-suits, or full-suits.

Gloves

All isolators have glove port systems to facilitate manipulation of operations in isolation. The glove/sleeve systems permit the introduction of operator hands and forearms into the enclosure, even though the operator remains outside the isolator without direct contact with the work area. Gloves are probably the weakest link in the use of isolation systems.

The glove system may include a sleeve and glove arrangement or a gauntlet and can be made of different materials. Different types and sizes of gloves are available in the market to suit individual user needs. Latex and neoprene are the materials most commonly used to manufacture the gloves. Neoprene gloves are more resistant to cuts and damage by sharps than latex gloves. However, for both gloves, care must be taken to avoid the handling of sharp instruments, sharp fingernails, or use of jewelry.

Half-Suits

Half-suits allow the introduction of the entire upper body into the protected work area while isolating the operator from the operation. Half-suits offer more reaching capabilities than the glove/sleeve systems and facilitate the handling of heavier or bulkier equipment. Half-suits are double-walled and have their own breathing apparatus to offer individual comfort to users. Individualized variable controls are available to offer flexibility to adjust the airflow to suit user needs. Half-suits are usually made of nylon-lined PVC (see Figure 1.7).

Full-Suits

Full-suits are used more often in the nuclear industry. They are less common in pharmaceutical applications than half-suits, but their popularity may increase as production applications become more available. Users gain another level of flexibility since full-suits provide unlimited movement within the enclosure. They are available and are a viable option if the application calls for handling heavy equipment or operations such as loading and unloading lyophilizers, or handling large autoclaves. Keep in mind, however, that there are lyophilizers being used without the help of full-suits.

Visibility

Since the operator is removed from the enclosed work area, visibility becomes an important factor in the design. Proper

Figure 1.7. Half-suit schematic. (Courtesy of la Calhene)

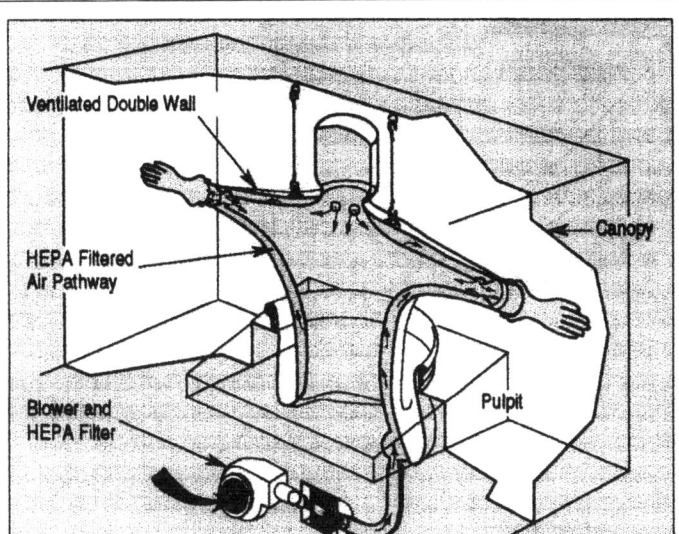

visibility is essential for worker safety and effectiveness. In the case of rigid isolators, visibility is more of an issue, primarily during the ergonomic assessment of the design. In flexible isolators, the canopies are made of clear PVC and offer a wide range of visibility.

Materials Transfer

The heart of the isolation system is the transfer port. Material and component transfer are key factors in the control of the isolator integrity; transfer devices are a key component to ensure sterile and contained transfers. Transfer devices are available in many different configurations and from several manufacturers. They can offer different degrees of isolator protection against contamination during the transfer of materials. To qualify as an effective transfer device, the transfer must be effected through a sealed and contained system without compromising the sterility and containment of the work area. In this author's opinion, the so-called jam-pots, conventional air-locks, and other such systems are not acceptable for use in closed isolators. The Double Porte de Transfert Etanche (DPTE) was patented by la Calhene in 1960, in France. It was a milestone in the development of today's isolator. Since then, many similar devices have been developed and are now known as Rapid Transfer Ports (RTPs). The DPTE and other RTPs are discussed below.

Double Porte de Transfert Etanche (DPTE)

DPTEs allow the rapid transfer of sterile materials from one field to another, without compromising the sterility of the work area, and in many cases ensuring the protection of workers from exposure to hazardous substances. The basic principle of the DPTE lies in the integration of four basic components that provide a tight seal and effect a tight connection. These are the door, the flange, the container door, and the container itself. When these are properly connected, the non-sterile surfaces are sealed together and are kept from contaminating the sterile areas. An improved device introduced more recently, the DPTE-S, has an extra safety feature ensuring that the door cannot be opened unless a container with lid is properly connected; the container may not be removed if the double door is not shut. Figure 1.8 illustrates how this seal and connection take place.

The four mechanical subassemblies are made of either polyethylene or stainless steel. They are engineered to a very high degree of precision and are subjected to extensive quality control testing by the manufacturer before release. The seals are designed and engineered carefully to ensure maintenance of containment and sterility. Seals can be made of PVC or stainless steel. The selection of seal material depends on the application. To help sealing, silicone grease or rubber can be used for transfer devices that require exposure to steam or other heat sources.

The DPTE can be mounted on other transfer containers to provide secure transfer of materials. The CQ Trans Plus® and the automatic transfer valve (ATV) (in the final design stages) are examples of such systems.

CQ Trans Plus®

The CQ Trans Plus® is a specially designed and automated adaptation of the simple DPTE system. It is highly effective for

Figure 1.8. The DPTE—its function and features. (Courtesy of la Calhene)

3 steps to have two enclosures in communication without any break in the containment:

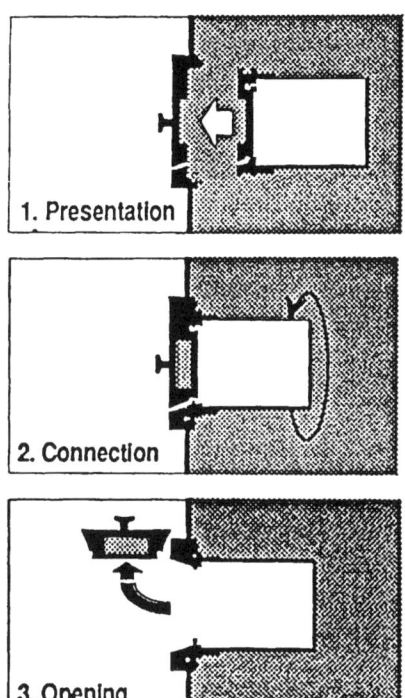

DPTE specifications

Model	Nominal diameter (mm)	Useful diameter (mm)	Wall drilling (mm)	Overall diameter (mm)	Hinge capability
105	105	95	152	182	no
270	270	250	348	388	yes
350	350	330	428	480	yes

the transfer of sterile and cytotoxic powders, and is easy to validate and monitor. Some of the advantages of the CQ Trans Plus® include the following:

- Totally enclosed sterilizable housing
- Adaptability to existing installations
- Proven technology, ensuring containment of cytotoxic materials
- Standard components

Automatic Transfer Valve (ATV)

ATVs can be used to transfer sterile and cytotoxic materials without breaking sterility or containment. They can be used for stoppers or other small components and for transfer of powders. The system includes a sealed box made of stainless steel with a window for viewing, a thermal sensor, capabilities for steam sterilization and liquid cleaning, and movable panels to facilitate equipment maintenance. The main design features of ATVs include the following:

- Sealed chute for the transfer of powders, assuming a double containment during the transfer
- Ability to rotate the alpha door instead of the container
- All pneumatic actuators located outside the sealed box
- Easy cleanability by liquid spray or immersion and rinsing
- Temperature resistance equal or greater than 150°C

Many devices similar to the DPTE have been developed and are available in the U.S. and Europe. Some of these are illustrated below.

The Passport™

The Passport™ is a type of RTP developed by Isolation Technologies in the United States. The flange is made of type 316 stainless steel in various sizes, and the system adapts well to mechanical, pneumatic, or vacuum operation. The double door system connects bags, canisters, or other enclosures. The design eliminates most moving parts and is easy to maintain and clean (see Figure 1.9). The system presents the following features:

- Simultaneously functions as both seal and locking mechanism

Figure 1.9. The Passport™ rapid transfer port.

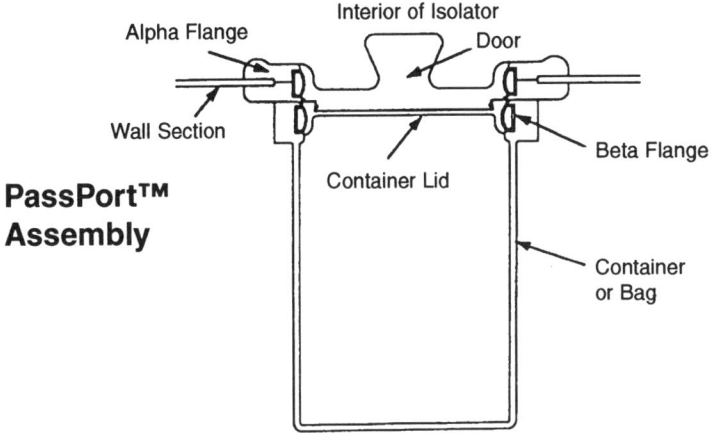

PassPort™ Assembly

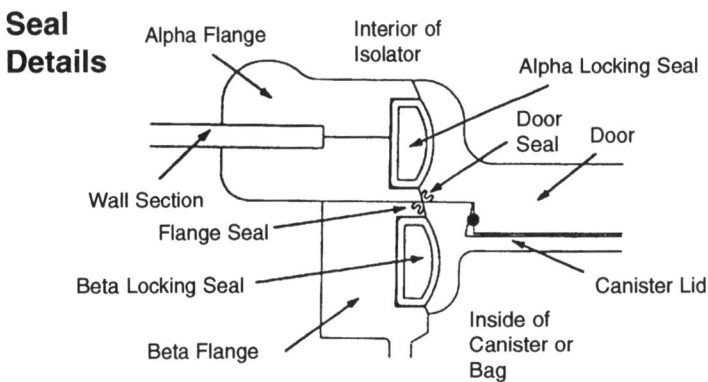

Seal Details

- Alpha flange and door seal mounted to the enclosure
- Beta flange and seal attached to the second enclosure, product container, or bag
- Rotation of container not necessary to effect connection and mating

High Containment Port (HCT)

The HCT is an RTP designed and patented by Total Process Containment, in the United Kingdom. The HCT port consists of two elements: the active and the passive ports. The active port provides flexibility to the system; it is the part that can be manipulated. The passive port cannot be opened once the active port is connected. The passive port connects to bags, canisters, bottles, or other isolators. The active port is comprised of a frame and a door.

SPECIAL CHALLENGES TO DESIGNERS AND USERS OF ISOLATORS

There is no doubt that progress has been made in understanding isolation technology and its applications. However, it is also obvious that several challenges remain and the delay in resolving them is responsible, in part, for the hesitation that companies have shown in implementing isolators in their facilities. These challenges have been discussed at every ITUG meeting to date, without final resolution. A brief discussion of these follows.

Regulatory Compliance

Regulatory officials worldwide are becoming familiar with isolation technology. In the U.S. the Center for Biological Evaluation and Research (CBER) and the Center for Drug Evaluation and Research (CDER) have inspected several facilities using isolation technology in the QC laboratory for sterility testing. To date, however, no aseptic product has been approved in the U.S. for filling in isolators. Since October 1993 (FDA 1993), the FDA has publicly expressed its support for applications of isolators in aseptic processing; however, progress in this area has been slower than many have expected. At this time there is only one pilot plant facility set up and validated to fill aseptic products in isolators. This facility was retrofitted to include isolation systems and VHP sterilization. It was designed, built, and validated in about two years. Since it is a clinical production facility it does not require FDA approval for use.

The inspections of the United States sterility testing facilities have generated some FDA 483s, but most of the issues have been basic compliance issues, and not specifc to the use of isolators. The observations listed in Table 1.4 have been collected from conversations with FDA officials and users.

The FDA has affirmed that it does not want to impede progress in the improvement of aseptic manufacturing facilities. The FDA agrees that the use of isolators to protect filling lines is a desirable concept. To date, however, no guidelines or standards are available in the United States. The only guidance expected in the near future is from the U.S. Pharmacopeia (USP). Table 1.5 includes information on the USP documents expected to contain information on isolation technology, and which are currently under review.

Europe has been the leader in isolation technology. In Europe the current isolator design has been used in pharmaceutical companies since the 1970s. Several working groups have been formed to address the development of standards and guidelines. The European GMP also includes a brief comment on isolation technology. These are further detailed below.

Table 1.4. U.S. FDA Inspections—Observations (FDA 483s)

- SOPs not being followed
- HEPA filter certification not completed as scheduled
- Preventative maintenance issues
- Records for glove failure investigation not available
- Issues regarding training of laboratory staff
- No records for sterilization of enclosures. (Difficult to verify if validation recommendations are being followed.)

Table 1.5. USP Documents to Address Isolation Technology

- Proposed General Information Chapter (1116)
- Sterility Testing Chapter
- Monograph on Biological Indicators for VHP sterilization
- Update of chapter on Sterilization and Sterility Assurance

European GMP

"Guide to GMP for Medicinal Products"—Manufacture of sterile medicinal products, from the rules governing medicinal products in the European Community, volume IV, page 71, January 1992. The guide states:

> The utilization of absolute barrier technology and automated systems to minimize human intervention in processing areas can produce significant advantages in assurance of sterility of manufactured products.
>
> When such techniques are used, the recommendations in these supplementary guidelines, particularly those relating to air quality and monitoring, still apply, with appropriate interpretation of the terms "work station" and "environment."

Guidelines

Isolators for Pharmaceutical Applications—This document applies to the United Kingdom but the working group considers it to be a possible reference for adoption by the British Standards Institute (BSI) and EC CEN and/or ISO committees. The first edition was published in 1993 by the Regional Quality Control Sub-Committee of Regional Pharmaceutical Officers (RQCS). It was entitled "The Design and Monitoring of Isolators—A Specification for Pharmaceutical Applications." The information was derived from discussions of a working group (24 members) which included representation primarily from isolator manufacturers (11), regional pharmacists (8), and the Medicines Control Agency (MCA) inspectorate (1). A few pharmaceutical industry representatives (4) were also part of the group. This document addressed primarily the systems used in pharmacies in the UK. The intention was to review the document after two years of use, with an update planned for 1996. However, changes in this field have been so rapid that it necessitated a new, extensively updated, revision sooner than expected. Hence the new revision in 1994 edited by Gerard Lee, from the Northwest Regional Health Authority in Liverpool, and Brian Midcalf, from St. James University Hospital in Leeds, for the UK Pharmaceutical Isolator Group (Lee and Midcalf 1994).

Regulatory issues are further addressed by James Lyda and James Akers in later chapters in this book.

Material Transfer

Material transfer remains one of the biggest challenges for the implementation of isolation technology in manufacturing applications. In sterility testing, because of the small scale and contained nature of the operation, it is easier to control the sterile transfer of materials, reagents, and samples, thus more easily maintaining the sterility of the enclosure. In the case of large scale aseptic operations, it is harder to prevent the existence of openings and harder to convince the regulatory authorities that the system is completely contained.

In aseptic systems, to maintain the sterility of the working areas, it is essential that all components, materials, and equipment be sterilized before being introduced into the working area. Issues with materials transfer are further covered in the Industry Experience section and in other chapters, particularly Jack Lysfjord's and Gordon Farquharson's.

Validation/Sterilization

As depicted in Figure 1.10, the success of these systems depends on the integration of three main components: the isolator, the materials/equipment used (applications), and the sterilization method. These must be compatible and properly validated to ensure the success of the system. All these components are the center of discussion throughout this book.

The approach to validation is equivalent to the validation of other pieces of equipment. The installation qualification (IQ), operational qualification (OQ), and performance qualification (PQ) are performed to assess the effectiveness of the isolator to maintain a suitable environment. Validation for isolators has been evolving since the early 1980s when experimental validations were performed. Currently, the validation program includes a number of protocols defining the application requirements, tests to be performed, methods to be used, limits, specifications, and discussion of results/data interpretation. Protocols should be reviewed by the project team including: manufacturing, QA, safety, documentation group or QA, regulatory, and vendors or consultants involved with the

Figure 1.10. Integrated validation approach.

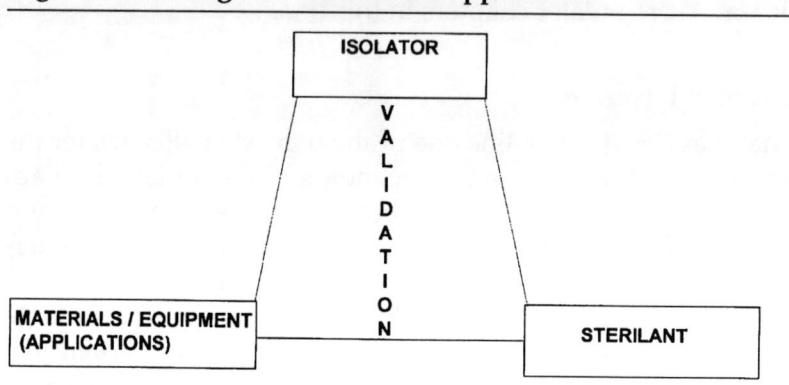

project. Protocol data should be organized for easy accessibility for audit purposes and reference.

Key validation steps include: filter integrity, leak testing, calibration of instruments, calibration of gas generators, gas distribution tests, check of chemicals used, gloves, sterilization cycle, residuals, nonviable and viable particle matter, transfer systems, bioburden testing, and media fill trials. The intensity and frequency of this testing depends on the process and the complexity of the isolator.

Sterilization

A major advantage of an isolator is that it can be sterilized to a SAL higher than that for a clean room. The sterilization cycle and other associated parameters which maintain the sterility of the system can be validated. The validation of isolators for pharmaceutical applications in Europe gained momentum in the early 1980s with experimental validations. In 1987 stable peracetic acid was made available and in 1988 further developments continued with studies of low-corrosion sterilants and improved biological indicators. Currently, the search for effective sterilants continues. VHP is popular in the U.S. and is gaining attention in Europe.

Three areas for sterilization (usually by filtration) are normally associated with isolation technology: the enclosure space, the materials entering, and the product in a production setting. It is important to remember that everything coming into the enclosure must be sterile. To ensure the sterility of the product, the equipment used for the filtration requires the same careful handling and validation as conventional clean room facilities. Isolators can be compared to fermenters, which after they are cleaned- and sterilized-in-place (CIP and SIP) are expected to maintain sterility throughout the process.

The manufacturing of aseptic products is one of the most challenging processes in pharmaceutical manufacturing. The satisfactory completion of the sterile process requires the application of a total quality system and cannot rely on results of sterility testing at the end of the process. Sterility assurance is very dependent on the manufacturing environment and the failure of one step may result in rejection of expensive product. One of the benefits of isolators is the ability to sterilize the work area and maintain its sterility when transferring materials in and out, without compromising the integrity of the interior. Sterilization is an important part of this assurance; therefore, the method chosen to sterilize the enclosure must be effective and validatable. To date formaldehyde, peracetic acid, ethylene oxide, B-propiolactone, hypochlorites and alcohol, phenolics, quaternary ammonium compounds, and VHP have been used as sterilants. Of these, the most common are peracetic acid, chlorine dioxide, and VHP. Many of the early choices such as formaldehyde and ethylene oxide were found to be incompatible with isolators for a variety of reasons.

Challenges in the sterilization process include compatibility and efficacy of the sterilant, as well as the impact of residues left after sterilization. As discussed in Richard Johnson's chapters, the approach to validation of isolators is not much different from the approach currently used for validation of equipment and facilities in the pharmaceutical industry. The main issue concerning the industry is the lack of unified understanding of what are acceptable practices and standards. As discussed by James Akers and others in this book, more guidance in this area is needed to encourage the use of isolators in the manufacturing environment.

James Rickloff and Les Edwards provide additional detail on the sterilization methodologies, and in particular, the use of VHP as a sterilizaton method. Table 1.6 compares the several methods available for sterilization of isolators, and their advantages and disadvantages.

Table 1.6. Comparison of Sterilization Methods (Courtesy of Robert Bosch GmbH)

Principle	Microbicide gas (ethylene oxide)	Spraying of liquid hydrogen peroxide	Distribution of mixture of steam plus H_2O_2	Evaporation of hydrogen peroxide and sterilization with H_2O_2 gas
General	a) well experienced b) sufficient sterilization *but* a) long aeration phase b) risk of carcinogenic traces	a) good sterilization effect b) FDA-approved *but* a) only applicable on straight surfaces b) separate fogging nozzles needed	a) sufficient sterilization on straight surfaces (in crevices condensate inhibits H_2O_2 efficiency) *but* a) large amount of H_2O_2 used, therefore high residual level b) high temp. stress on material c) machine wet	a) best sterilization effect b) no dilution of H_2O_2 by steam c) low residual level d) low thermal stress on machine e) machine remains dry f) H_2O_2 gas reaches small crevices *but* distribution must be optimized

Monitoring

Upon the establishment of validation parameters, the monitoring program should be established to help ensure the maintenance of the sterile or containment state of isolator systems. Monitoring can be performed on a continuous basis daily, weekly, monthly, or yearly depending on requirements. Routine monitoring should include, at a minimum, isolator pressure, glove integrity, HEPA filtration, transfer port integrity, sterilization reactor, chemistry of the sterilant, sterilization cycle, aeration cycle, residuals, and bioburden. Many monitoring activities can be assisted by automated recording and automated monitoring. These are viable options for the current and future users of isolators. Figure 1.11 illustrates the connection of an automated recording system to an isolator to facilitate tracking and trending of information in a computer system that has the proper security features to satisfy regulatory compliance.

Siting of Isolators

A discussion of challenges to designers and users would not be complete without mentioning the siting of isolators. To date there has been no consensus on the classification of the outside environment housing the isolator. This topic is covered well by several of the authors and its clarification is of the utmost importance for those planning the implementation of isolators in manufacturing facilities. The current view of some FDA spokespersons is to review requests for implementation of isolation technology on a case-by-case approach. This approach seems most reasonable to this author and appropriate to moving this technology forward. The ultimate standards for the siting of isolators remain to be defined. This topic is expanded by both James Akers and James Lyda.

THE FUTURE OF ISOLATION TECHNOLOGY

In this era of increasing regulatory demands and attention to cost-effectiveness, advanced aseptic processing technologies

Figure 1.11. Automated recording system. Legend: dP = differential pressure; P = gauge pressure; T = temperature; H = humidity; C = conductivity; P CTR = particle counter with 0.3 μ, 0.5 μ temperature and humidity channels. (Courtesy of R&D Scientific, Flanders, NJ)

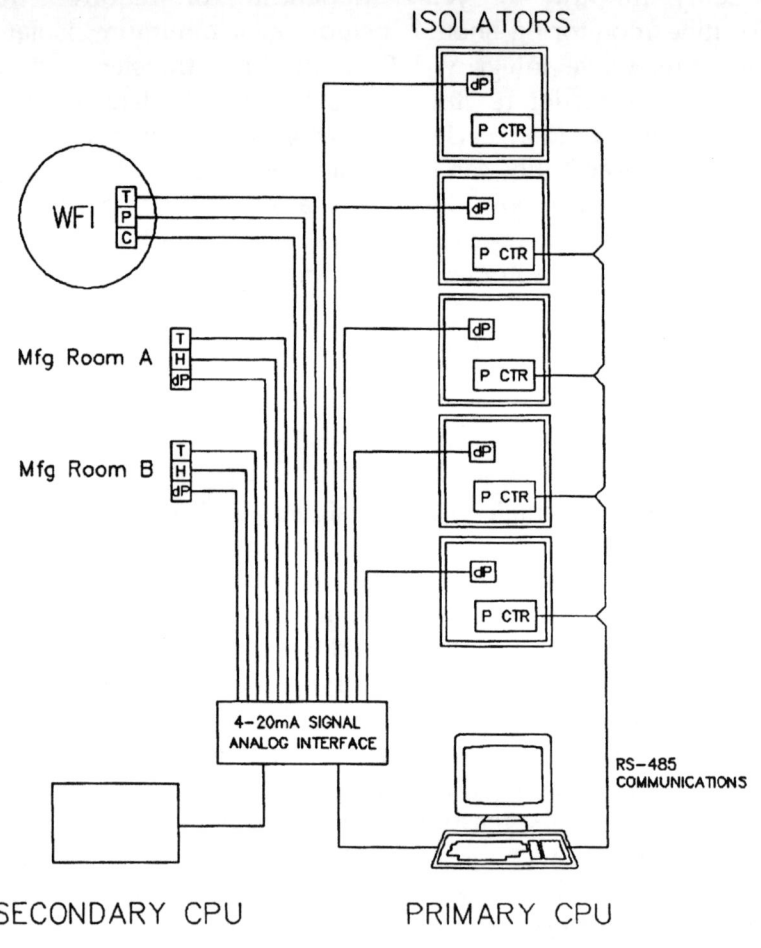

such as barrier and isolation technology, automation, robotics, and blow/fill/seal are emerging as potential solutions for pharmaceutical company challenges. Among the advanced technologies, isolation technology in particular holds many promises. As a result of their operational and economic advantages, isolators are attracting a lot of attention and their use in pharmaceuticals is expected to increase. Since the development of the DPTE, the use of isolators in pharmaceutical or other health related fields has rapidly increased. Isolators are becoming an essential element in the QC laboratory and will soon play a more important role in the production setting. They can be used at critical points during all stages of manufacturing to help maintain the integrity of the process.

The implementation of isolation technology can help improve competitiveness, cost-effectiveness, and profitability by helping to reduce operational costs, improve process control, improve operation efficiency, and reduce product waste.

Isolation technology has already impacted the quality and cost effectiveness of many pharmaceutical facilities involved in aseptic manufacturing. Now that it is possible to perform sterility testing and manufacture sterile product in a leaktight and sterile environment, isolators are destined to become an integral part of aseptic manufacturing facilities in the 1990s and beyond.

REFERENCES

Food and Drug Administration. 1987. Guideline on sterile drug products produced by aseptic processing. *Federal Register* 181–332:60360.

Food and Drug Administration. 1993. Terminal sterilization vs aseptic processing conference, October in Washington, DC.

Lee, G. M., and B. Midcalf, eds. 1994. *Isolators for Pharmaceutical Applications.* Published by the HMSO for the UK Pharmaceutical Isolators Group.

Reyniers, J. A., and P. C. Trexler. 1943. The germ-free technique and its application to rearing animals free from contamination In *Micrurgical and germ-free methods,* edited by J. A. Reyniers. Springfield, IL: Chas. C. Thomas Publishers.

Trexler, P. C., and L. I. Reynolds. Flexible film apparatus for the rearing and use of germ-free animals. *Applied Microbiology* 5:406–412.

Whyte, W. 1991. The influence of clean room design on product contamination. *J. Parenter. Sci. Technol.* 38:103–108.

Whyte, W., et al. 1982. An evaluation of the routes of bacterial contamination occurring during aseptic pharmaceutical manufacturing. *J. Parenter. Sci. Technol.* 102–107.

2

Isolator Technology: Regulatory Issues and Performance Expectations

James E. Akers
Akers Kennedy & Associates, Inc.
Kansas City, MO

Isolator technology has begun to emerge in the mid-1990s as the method of choice for aseptic processing. This emergence has been somewhat slower than many of us had hoped, but the recent interest in isolator technology manifested in virtually every quarter of the pharmaceutical industry guarantees a prominent role in sterile product manufacturing.

At the time of this book's publication there have been only limited efforts exerted toward defining standardized design, operational, and in-process testing requirements for isolator systems. This lack of standards has not been a bad thing, because experience has proved that promulgating standards is often more difficult than expected. In the past several years proposed standards for electronic particle counting in liquids, product testing using the limulus amebocyte assay, microbiological classification of clean rooms, and terminal sterilization have resulted in protracted debate on technical grounds. In recent years standards have, in many cases, arisen without a firm basis in scientific fact. Regulatory authorities have begun discussing potential requirements for the design and installation of isolator systems, but have avoided the publication of guidelines or the suggestion of hard numbers as performance or validation acceptance criteria. The conditions are now right for users, designers, and vendors, as well as regulatory agency and pharmacopeial scientists to work together to propose enlightened and technically appropriate standards for isolator systems.

The first thing any standard must consider is the definition of all the key technical terms used to describe isolator systems and their chief components. It has become clear to many of us that there is no consensus within the industry as to precisely what is meant by such terms as *barrier* or *isolator*. Without a common understanding of what isolators or barriers are and how they may be employed as clean working spaces, standards will be either excessively restrictive, or too general to be of much value.

In this book we are proposing a comprehensive glossary of terms for isolator technology. This glossary covers those areas of advanced aseptic processing technology which through some form of physical "barrier" minimize or eliminate human contact with the manufacturing environment and, therefore, reduce the likelihood of personnel borne contamination reaching the product.

A GLOSSARY OF TERMS COMMONLY USED IN DESCRIBING ADVANCED ASEPTIC PROCESSING TECHNOLOGY

Absolute Barrier—An isolator (barrier) system which completely eliminates the possibility of external contamination reaching the interior of the isolator. The term *absolute* conveys perfect air filtration and infallible physical integrity. An absolute barrier, assuming it could be sterilized to a very high sterility assurance level (SAL), would be a perfect germ-free environment. As of the publication of this book these systems do not actually exist. However, absolute barriers represent the holy grail of aseptic pharmaceutical production, and there can be little doubt that in the near future they will be a reality.

Barrier—In the context of aseptic processing systems, a barrier is a device which prevents contact between operators and the aseptic field enclosed within the barrier. These systems are used in hospital pharmacies, laboratories, and animal care facilities as well as in aseptic filling. Barriers may not be sterilized and do not have sterile transfer systems that allow passage of materials into or out of the system without a loss of sterility. Some pharmaceutical filling and bottling equipment are equipped with shrouds or covers that are in fact barriers. Some of these shrouds are equipped with HEPA-filtered air supply systems. Blow/fill/seal systems for example are equipped with barriers of this type.

Buffer Isolator—An isolator connected in series to one or more isolators. This isolator may enclose one or more processing operations, but its major function is to isolate a containment area, thereby enabling the entire system to function as a true isolator. This is accomplished by operating the buffer isolator at a positive air pressure relative to the containment barrier, thereby effectively isolating the work space. If the buffer isolator is an open isolator it must rely on the fail-safe maintenance of internal overpressure relative to the surrounding environment to maintain isolation conditions. (The buffer isolator is also called a dynamic airlock.)

Closed Isolator—An isolator that is, as much as current technology allows, a fully sealed system. The closed isolator has either a HEPA or ULPA filter on both supply and exhaust air. All passages of materials into or out of the isolator are made through special transfer doors which maintain isolation. The interior of these isolators and all contents are sterilizable to a SAL of at least 10^{-6}. Closed isolators are capable of providing both isolation of the work space from external contamination, and containment of dangerous materials within the work space.

Containment Barriers—These systems are not completely closed, but rather rely on the maintenance of a negative air pressure to the surrounding environment to provide containment. These barriers have one or more openings to the outside environment through which materials handling equipment (i.e., conveyors) pass. These systems may have sealable gates or doors which allow sterilization, but these doors are open during operation. Because these units take in air from the surrounding environment, they cannot be considered isolators. It is unlikely that systems of this type will be widely used since design alternatives exist that make isolation and containment attainable within the same unit (see Containment System).

Containment System—A containment system is designed and operated in a manner which prevents dangerous materials from being dispersed into the surrounding environment. Containment systems may be closed isolators in which both isolation and containment are possible simultaneously. Containment systems may alternatively be barrier systems which have one or more openings to the external environment for the passage of conveyor belts or other transfer devices. Containment systems may be considered isolators only if, through the use of buffer isolators or another design feature, they completely isolate the work space from the surrounding environment. Paramount is the requirement that air exchanges with the surrounding environment be accomplished only through HEPA, ULPA, or other microbial retentive filtration systems.

Doors (Air locks)—At least four different types of doors can be used with isolator systems:

1. *Rapid Transfer Door or Port*—These doors (sometimes called RTPs) enable the operator to link two isolators, an isolator and a container, or an isolator to a piece of equipment. The RTP doors consist of two flanges which can be linked together in a manner that allows the non-sterile surfaces of the flange faces to be positively locked together. A sealing gasket is compressed between the two flanges resulting in an airtight seal. Several design

variants of this system are presently available commercially. (A narrow ring typically exists at the apex of the seal that is not sterilized; this ring has been suggested by some as a potential source of contamination.)

2. *Sterilizable Rapid Transfer Ports*—Several different types of these systems have been studied. The objective of these transfer doors is to eliminate the potentially contaminated ring described in number 1.

3. *Ultraviolet Light Equipped Transfer Tunnel*—These units use ultraviolet light (UV) to kill microorganisms on the manufacturing system.

4. *Conventional Doors*—These doors, also referred to as *jam-pot* doors, have no provisions for preventing the introduction of outside air into the enclosure. Doors of this type preclude the maintenance of an enclosure at a condition of high sterility assurance. Enclosures that utilize this type of door during normal operation are not isolators. At the very best these units are barriers.

Half-suit—A flexible partial body suit that allows an operator to conduct manipulations within the isolator or barrier. These suits typically mount at approximately waist level, and the operator enters from beneath the table to which the suit is mounted. In essence, these suits comprise a portion of the isolator wall. Half-suits have their own air supply system, and incoming air is HEPA filtered.

Interface Isolator—An isolator typically attached via a bioseal or plenum to a piece of equipment such as an autoclave, lyophilizer, or dry heat oven. The interface isolator and bioseal/plenum must be sterilizable as a unit. The door and associated hardware to which the interface isolator is linked must also be sterilized to a satisfactory SAL. This must include any and all parts of the system that could be exposed to the isolated (sterile) work area during normal operations.

Isolator—Any unit that is sterilizable to a high SAL (typically 10^{-6} or less). All air that enters the isolator passes through microbial retentive filters. An isolator must never exchange air with the surrounding environment unless that air is treated by a microbial retentive filter. The surrounding environment must have no impact on the operation of the system for an enclosure to be considered a true isolator. Isolators must also prevent any direct contact between human operators and the product being manufactured or tested. Any manipulation done by operators must be conducted using gloves or partial suit assemblies.

Laminar Flow Isolator—An isolator designed to provide unidirectional airflow to the work surface. These units may be oriented either vertically or horizontally. It is important to note that the term *laminar flow,* although widely used to describe airflow in the pharmaceutical industry, is technically incorrect. In actual practice laminar airflow rarely if ever exists. It is more technically correct to call these isolators unidirectional airflow isolators.

Open Isolator—An isolator that has one or more openings to the surrounding environment such as holes for conveyor systems to pass through. These isolators must have a positive air pressurization system that prevents any unfiltered air from entering the enclosure.

Sterilization Isolator—An isolator used to sterilize production materials using a gas sterilization method. The sterilization isolator is typically part of a manufacturing system consisting of one or more other isolators. These isolators may function in either a continuous or semicontinuous manner. This isolator is similar in design and function to the transfer isolator.

Transfer Container—A container, commonly steam sterilizable, equipped with an RTP to allow sterilized goods to be transferred into an isolator. These containers are generally small enough to allow hand carrying and attachment.

Transfer Isolator—A system that can be used to transfer sterile goods from one isolator to another. The transfer is generally effected using an RTP or some variation of a port transfer system.

Turbulent Flow Isolator—An isolator with a mixing airflow rather than unidirectional or *laminar* airflow. Isolators of this design can be useful for a variety of applications including sterility testing and some pharmaceutical production activities.

It is possible to define other subsystems currently in use. However, the foregoing definitions are sufficient to allow a clear understanding of the types of barriers and isolators that can be used for various types of health care product manufacturing or microbiological testing. The distinction between the isolator and the barrier is crucial. In the author's opinion, much confusion in this field is a direct result of a failure to correctly explain an enclosure's principle of operation. This confusion can lead to interpretive difficulties on the regulatory front as well.

There have been reports that products manufactured in isolators have been found to be nonsterile, and in some cases have been responsible for patient death. Paul Hargreaves of the United Kingdom Medicines Control Agency has publicly reported the discovery of sterility failures resulting in fatalities among patients given Total Parenteral Nutrition products manufactured in isolators. According to the definitions suggested in this chapter the enclosures in which the failures occurred would not be called isolators. This is because these units are not sterilized to a high SAL, and do not completely eliminate human borne contamination from the enclosure. Furthermore, during operations these units may exchange air with the surrounding environment.

These units would be more properly termed barriers. Barriers are systems that prevent but do not completely exclude the possibility of human borne contamination entering the area of the critical zone. These units provide far less contamination exclusion capability than the closed isolators typically used for sterility testing. These units, which could more accurately be called glove boxes, are used in hospital pharmacies and have been called isolators for many years.

The regulatory concern about the use of these barriers, or glove boxes, for aseptic formulation is certainly legitimate. However, these isolators bear little functional relationship to the isolators widely used in the pharmaceutical industry for sterility testing or production. In the author's opinion, had true isolators as defined in this chapter been employed, the reported fatalities would not have occurred. Therefore, it is inappropriate to conclude from these reports that isolator technology is fraught with problems that require the imposition of severe regulatory restriction. The real problem lies with practitioners choosing the wrong tool to do a given job, rather than the performance potential of the tool. Wooden shafted golf clubs and steel or graphite shafted clubs are capable of hitting golf balls. However, a competitive golfer would certainly not choose to play with wood shafted clubs in this day and age. Similarly, glove boxes and various forms of barriers, if properly implemented, are likely to provide incremental improvements over human scale clean rooms. Proper implementation requires a careful analysis of the potential for operator interaction with the controlled environment. Sanitization and other process control (validation) issues are also of paramount importance.

Very simply put, if a system exchanges air with the surrounding environment and can only be sanitized rather than sterilized it must be considered functionally similar to a biosafety cabinet. Certainly, if the glove box or barrier system is well designed and properly installed it has the potential to reduce the likelihood of human borne contamination of the product. However, such systems, even when optimally utilized, do not have the performance potential of an isolator. Organizations proposing standards for the design and operation of various types of isolators, glove boxes, and hoods must keep these differences in mind. There are numerous functional distinctions among these systems, and lumping them all together in a performance standard without a clear recognition of their differences will do harm both to the industry and to the end users of our products.

ISOLATION TECHNOLOGY: KEY REGULATORY ISSUES

Key regulatory issues in the use of isolator systems have been discussed at virtually every technical meeting held on the subject since at least 1990. Although the emphasis has varied from meeting to meeting the key issues have generally included the following list:

1. Sterility Assurance Issues—Target performance criteria.
2. The potential for isolators to be considered equivalent to terminal sterilization.
3. Requirements for the environment in which isolators are operated.
4. The use of isolators for containment of toxic or allergenic products.
5. Environmental monitoring and control within isolators.

In spite of numerous public discussions and commentary from the regulatory agencies, most of these questions are no closer to resolution than they were five years ago. The remainder of this chapter will be devoted to a critical evaluation of the issues surrounding each of these five issues.

Sterility Assurance

The emergence of so called advanced aseptic processing technology along with the controversy surrounding the FDA's initiative on terminal sterilization has resulted in numerous discussions on sterility assurance during the first half of the 1990s. The content of these discussions has led some industry observers, including this author, to question the level of understanding that exists within our industry on the subject of sterility assurance.

A great deal of dogma has developed surrounding the concept of sterility in the pharmaceutical industry. Unfortunately, there is little or no technical data to support much of the dogma that is currently accepted by a large segment of the industry. Among the widely held notions are the following:

Sterility Assurance Assumption

The sterility assurance of an aseptic process (in conventional human scale clean rooms) can be assumed to be 10^{-3}. No data in the literature support this widely held assumption. There is no doubt that 10^{-3} came to be accepted as the performance criterion for media fill testing. However, it is not clear how this value was selected. Certainly, the selection of the 10^{-3} acceptance criterion was not based upon a scientific evaluation aimed at establishing the process capability of aseptic processes.

It is reasonable to ask how the 10^{-3} value could have become cast in stone as the acceptance criterion for media fill tests without an established basis in empirical data. Clearly there is not now, and there never has been a standard aseptic process. The 10^{-3} value was not, in my opinion, intended to be a statement of process capability, but rather a minimum acceptable level of performance. In other words, the 10^{-3} value does not represent the performance one could expect of an optimum aseptic process, nor does it reflect an average level of performance. Rather 10^{-3} is the poorest performance allowable in the validation of the aseptic process using media fill tests.

Recently, some organizations have published statistical tables indicating how many contaminated units could be observed in media fill tests of a given sample size in order to conform to the magical 10^{-3} value with a 95 percent confidence level. These tables assume that the appearance of contaminants in a media fill test is a random event that follows a Poisson distribution model. A discussion of sampling theory is beyond the scope of this chapter, but there are no data to support the notion that either media fill contamination or contaminations in actual production are random events. Quite to the contrary, it is likely that contamination is linked to human behavior in the human scale clean room and is nonrandom.

Nonrandom means that the chance of contamination is increased by certain routine and repetitive activities that occur during normal production operations. These activities are often termed *line interventions.* These interventions can include weight checks, parts hopper charging, and fallen container retrieval, as well as equipment adjustment and repairs. Many firms procedurally define these interventions as major or minor. Regulatory agencies around the world have recognized that controlling human borne contamination is the key issue in achieving high levels of sterility assurance in aseptic production. Increasingly, firms are required to characterize and control interventions, and to properly simulate these interventions during media fill testing.

Thus, contamination of a product in the human scale clean room is no longer perceived as solely the result of contamination by airborne microflora existing at some environmental background level. Experience has shown that contamination is far more likely to occur during times when people must work within the critical zone as defined by the *FDA Guideline on Sterile Drug Products Produced by Aseptic Processing* (1987). The fact that contamination in the human scale clean room is not a purely random event is actually good news, because it means that through analysis of the production operation it is possible to take countermeasures to reduce the frequency and impact of line interventions. However, we must reevaluate some of the statistical assumptions that have been applied since at least the early 1980s to the media fill test.

Publications by the Parenteral Society and the draft aseptic processing standard written by the International Organization for Standardization (ISO) technical committee 198, Working Group 9 suggest that in a sample of nearly 17,000, as many as 9 contaminants could be observed and still meet the 10^{-3} acceptance criterion with a 95 percent confidence level. Nine contaminants in 17,000 should not be considered even minimally acceptable performance in the mid-1990s. This would mean that for production lots of 50,000 units we could expect upwards of 27 contaminants—assuming the same rate of contamination was maintained. It is impossible to think that such a lot of product could be considered a sterile material. Actually, the only sterile lot is one that contains no nonsterile units.

The 10^{-3} standard has actually done great harm to our understanding of the concept of sterility, simply because a probability of a nonsterile unit of 10^{-3} or a contamination rate of 0.1 percent is not descriptive of a sterile product. The technical definition of sterility is absolute, and does not allow for rates or probabilities. It must be recognized that aseptic processes have never been perfect. Had an acceptance criterion more stringent than 10^{-3} been imposed upon the industry in the late 1970s, it is quite likely that many production operations would have been unable to comply. It is important to understand the history of the 10^{-3} criteria, and to recognize that this value has no special scientific meaning.

One of the perceived advantages of advanced aseptic processing technology in general and isolators in particular is their ability to improve upon the process capability of conventional aseptic processing. Already, we have a great deal of data concerning the performance potential of isolators. Reports by Kochansky and others have demonstrated that isolators provide great security against contamination even when worst case conditions are purposely created. Although experience with isolators is limited, the preponderance of data indicate that the traditional media fill acceptance criterion of a 0.1 percent contamination rate is too far below the performance capability of isolators to be of any value, even as a reference.

This raises the question as to what the acceptance criterion for isolators should be. This is a difficult question to answer, and one fraught with not only technical but also regulatory dilemmas. It would be tempting to set the acceptance criterion at zero. However, zero might only be appropriate for isolators and not for barrier or blow/fill/seal systems. Furthermore, from the legal and regulatory perspective it may not be acceptable to officially recognize performance differences among different types of aseptic processing operations. In all likelihood, performance differences have existed within the industry for years. However, the baseline 0.1 percent acceptance criterion has tended to mask any differences that might exist. Having three or four different standards for various types of aseptic processes would make enforcement difficult, and would create an interpretive nightmare.

At present the best advice to those contemplating the validation of an isolator system is to target a germ-free environment. The demonstration of a germ-free environment through a combination of sterilization, ongoing environmental control, and some form of media fill testing appears to be the best alternative at present. Only after additional experience, and a clear understanding of the various types of advanced aseptic processing systems in use, can more definitive performance evaluative tools be devised.

The Potential for Isolators to Be Considered Equivalent to Terminal Sterilization

The question as to whether isolator technology could be considered an acceptable substitute for terminal sterilization has been an important regulatory issue from the beginning. In the late 1980s the FDA launched an initiative to encourage the use of terminal sterilization for all applicable products. There were primarily two reasons for this initiative. First, the FDA had become aware that certain products that had been terminally sterilized by the originator were not being terminally sterilized by generic firms.

Second, the United States was unique among the major pharmaceutical producing countries in not requiring terminal sterilization for all applicable products. This initiative triggered a debate in the United States that has lasted to this day. During this debate the FDA interviewed industry representatives, including this author, in an effort to determine the financial and technical ramifications of the terminal sterilization initiative. Although the FDA published proposed rule changes in the *Federal Register*, this issue has still not been resolved.

Some industry scientists, engineers, and eventually equipment vendors began to suggest that some form of barrier or isolator technology might be considered equivalent to terminal sterilization. Some proponents of form or blow/fill/seal systems also held that the performance potential of these systems was sufficiently high that they might also be considered an acceptable alternative to terminal sterilization. At about the same time some FDA personnel, perhaps most notably Henry Avallone, suggested that there might be an overall greater benefit to the consumer in the encouragement of better methods for aseptic processing rather than focusing on the requirement of terminal sterilization.

As a result of this discussion, many people working to develop commercial isolator systems, as well as pharmaceutical engineers and scientists, began to suggest (or assume) that a probability of a nonsterile unit (PNSU) of 10^{-6} should be considered the acceptance criterion for isolator systems. This requirement has subsequently appeared in promotional literature for isolator-based production systems, and has also been widely referred to in numerous discussions at Parenteral Drug Association (PDA), Isolation Technology Users Groups (ITUG), and International Society for Pharmaceutical Engineering (ISPE) meetings, and no doubt the meetings of other associations as well.

Given the current state of technology, even the most advanced isolator systems cannot be considered to provide the same level of sterility assurance as terminal sterilization. First, it is important to recognize that the worst case conditions built into most terminal sterilization cycle designs and validations result in a PNSU significantly less than 10^{-6}. The 10^{-6} value is the minimum acceptance criterion for terminal sterilization. It is probable that the majority of terminal sterilization cycles provide PNSUs significantly better than 10^{-6}. Therefore, the 10^{-6} value that many have set as a goal for their isolator systems is actually one that terminal sterilization processes routinely exceed.

Since isolators must rely on filtration of the air and process streams to remove microorganisms, they are limited by the restrictiveness of their filtration systems. Organisms small enough to pass through the filter system may not be removed. Only the largest viruses would be removed to any degree at all by the standard 0.2 micrometer process filter. Similarly, the HEPA filters used in most isolator systems will not remove viruses. Terminal sterilization will kill viruses effectively, because they are significantly less resistant to heat than spore bearing bacteria.

The foregoing does not mean that all heat stable products should automatically be terminally sterilized. There are certainly instances in which the delivery system could provide such a marked advantage that manufacturing a terminal sterilizable product in an isolator could be justified. A delivery system that reduces or eliminates aseptic manipulations conducted by health care professionals in the administration of a product could markedly improve patient safety. An analysis of the total delivery pathway could suggest that a superior delivery system contributes more, in some cases, to patient safety than terminal sterilization. The potential for sterile products to be contaminated in the clinic or hospital environment has long been a concern in the pharmaceutical industry. This increased safety is much more likely to occur when such delivery systems can be produced in isolator systems.

Although in most cases isolators cannot be considered equivalent to terminal sterilization, it would be wise for the regulatory community to review processing requirements on a case-by-case basis. A dogmatic approach to requiring terminal sterilization for all heat stable chemical entities may, in some cases, actually reduce the microbiological safety of a product, when the entire delivery pathway is considered. The controlling principle should be to select the most appropriate manufacturing technology, taking all elements of the product and its likely use into account.

Nevertheless, vendors of isolator-based production equipment and those working to implement this technology within the industry should not consider equivalence to terminal sterilization the ultimate goal. The majority of sterile products are manufactured aseptically. It is likely that the percentage of products manufactured aseptically will continue to increase as more biotechnology products are approved. The likely increase in integrated delivery systems and home administration kits will tip the balance even further in the direction of aseptic processing. The promise of isolator technology to improve the sterility assurance of aseptically filled products is sufficient reason alone to accelerate implementation of this technology.

Environmental Requirements for the Rooms in Which Isolators Are Located

There has probably been more discussion about the environment outside the isolator than inside the isolator at industry meetings. This debate has focused on particulate air quality and classification of the room surrounding an isolator. Regulatory agency employees from both the United States and Europe have made pronouncements about the required air quality of the surrounding environment. The regulatory guidance provided thus far has been inconsistent, and has not been substantiated with any data. This intuitive or arbitrary approach to regulatory guidance has been characteristic of the general subject of clean room air quality for many years.

As this is being written, the author is not aware of any report of airborne contamination being detected within any system that meets the definition of an isolator as suggested in this chapter. Rigorous tests have been conducted and reported by some users or designers, and even in extreme challenges, breaches of the germ-free environment have not been observed. Many sterility testing isolator systems have been located in standard laboratory space, which is controlled but not classified in terms of particulate contamination. These systems have proven exceedingly reliable in terms of providing a germ-free environment. The few problems that have been reported center around leaks in gloves or half-suits.

Firm regulatory requirements for the classification of the surrounding room should not be issued. The focus should be on the quality of the environment inside the isolator and how it is to be maintained. The technical reasons for this assertion are:

1. There is no evidence that the control of microbiological quality in the surrounding room is required. The possibility of microbial contamination entering the isolator via an airborne route has proven to be exceedingly low. There have been no verified reports of entrainment of microbial contamination through pinhole leaks or required openings. The most likely entry point for microbial contamination is through direct mechanical transfer. Personnel working through gloves are the most likely source. This direct transfer of microorganisms can only be prevented by effective mechanical countermeasures. The particulate air quality of the surrounding room would have little or no positive effect in preventing the introduction of microorganisms via this route.

2. There is no need for the surrounding room to serve as a prefilter for the isolator. If the security of double air filtration is desired this can be incorporated into the isolator design. Isolators of both turbulent and unidirectional airflow design have proven exemplary in the control of particulate contamination. The background particulate counts have been at or near zero in both the flexible wall and rigid wall isolators with which the author and his colleagues have worked.

3. The room surrounding an isolator is likely to contain personnel. The goal in isolator technology is to create a germ-free environment within the enclosure. Therefore, even if the isolator were located in a Class 100 room and the people in that room gowned to full aseptic clean room standards, the environment outside the isolator would not be germ free. This environment will obviously be of lower quality than that inside the isolator.

The disparity between the quality of air even in a very good Class 100 room and the interior of an isolator is greater than that between the Class 100 critical zone and the surrounding area in the conventional clean room. Thus, unless an isolator was surrounded by another isolator, any exchange of air with the surrounding room is undesirable. Therefore, the focus must be on the prevention of contamination from entering the isolator, rather than the environment in the surrounding room.

Logic would dictate that should outside air enter an isolator, regardless of the classification of the surrounding room, resterilization should be done if a germ-free environment is the performance objective. Over the next few years not all advanced aseptic processing will be done in isolators. Since barriers will exchange air with the surrounding environment to some degree, decontamination of these systems will follow a procedure similar to the current practice for human scale clean rooms.

There is no reason to require isolator systems to be surrounded by an environment classified to a particulate air standard. Such requirements would add significant cost and ongoing operating expenses without providing the slightest increase in air quality within the isolator. It is even possible that firms might argue that since they have Class 100 air outside the isolator, entrainment of air is an issue that can be ignored. This would only be true if the firm's operational goal was something other than a germ-free environment. Clearly, to those targeting the highest possible assurance of sterility in aseptic processing, the entry of air from a room containing personnel is undesirable even if the room is technically Class 100.

The debate about the particle quality of the air *outside* the isolator has, in the author's opinion, been of relatively little importance. It should be replaced with a discussion of what design and control systems should be in place to ensure that a continuously germ-free environment exists *inside* the isolator. Provided that the proper quality of air *inside* the isolator is supplied and controlled, the quality of the environment *outside* the isolator will be inconsequential.

The Use of Isolators for Containment of Toxic or Allergenic Products

The pharmaceutical industry has been quick to recognize the advantages isolators can provide in the handling of toxic or allergenic materials. Facilities are already in place for the manufacture of both bulk sterile pharmaceuticals and final dosage forms. Handling of cytotoxic compounds or cephalosporin antibiotics to name two examples can be done safely in isolators. Containment isolator systems have the potential to restrict dissemination of these materials, particularly when handled as powders, far more effectively than is possible with conventional clean rooms as dust control systems.

A key issue in the design and operation of these units is the maintenance of both isolation and containment simultaneously. Providing either isolation (germ-free environment) or containment alone is technically challenging; doing both simultaneously is even more difficult. Containment and prevention of contamination are, by their very natures, contradictory. Conventional design of containment areas has been to maintain a negative air pressure at the critical control points relative to the surrounding areas. This can be done in continuous production isolator systems only if buffer isolators (active or dynamic airlocks) are provided so that entry and exit points of components and finished products are protected. These airlocks must be positive to both the barrier in which the powder is being handled and the external environment.

A regulatory matter concerning the use of isolators for containment that will be important to potential isolator users is multiple product manufacturing and flexibility of plant utilization. For example, it should be possible in a well-engineered containment/isolation system to safely fill penicillins or cephalosporins in a facility that is not expressly dedicated to those products. The same should also be true of cytotoxic products, hormones, or other highly toxic or allergenic products. The current requirement of essentially dedicated facilities for some types of products can impose significant cost penalties on the industry. It should be possible with the evolution of better containment capabilities using combinations of automation, barriers, and isolators to achieve higher levels of control than is currently possible in human scale facilities.

The FDA and other regulatory authorities should be prepared to view such technological advancements with an open mind. If firms can produce technical data proving that safe, controlled handling of toxic and allergenic materials has been achieved, regulatory authorities should be prepared to relax the facilities utilization restrictions that are currently imposed. In some countries, this will require changes to current drug regulations. This issue should be considered in the discussions that are now beginning on the harmonization of international GMPs. It would not be appropriate to introduce harmonized regulations in the late 1990s that are based upon facilities, equipment, control, and validation concepts that date from the 1960s.

Environmental Monitoring and Control Within Isolators

Since the late 1970s there has been a large increase in the microbiological or *viable* environmental monitoring requirements for aseptic processing operations. In addition, the industry has seen an ever increasing emphasis on viable environmental monitoring of nonsterile production operations, and closed systems such as bulk pharmaceutical chemical purification and fermentation of biological products. There seems to be a general view among many within the world's regulatory community, both reviewing scientists and inspectors, that it is impossible to do too much environmental monitoring.

Particularly in advanced aseptic processing operations that only restrict but do not eliminate the presence of human operators in the aseptic environment, the role of environmental monitoring must be critically reexamined. There are numerous instances where human interventions for monitoring exceed those for component additions or mechanical adjustments. This creates the unfortunate situation in which the monitors could themselves be the most probable cause of a nonsterile unit. It is unreasonable to assume that only line interventions conducted by production operators are likely to adversely affect product sterility. In many cases, the entry of environmental control personnel into the critical zone imposes an equivalent threat to sterility assurance.

The use of newer technologies and a greater reliance on automation requires a reexamination of the industry's environmental monitoring and control philosophy. Logic would dictate that, as equipment and facilities evolve so that less human intervention is required, environmental monitoring should decrease, not increase. Future regulatory guidance must take these newer technologies into account, or we will again run the risk of applying 1970s thinking, operation, and regulation to 21st century industry. Clearly, many of you reading this book are indeed planning facilities that will come on line in the 21st century.

In considering the environmental monitoring of isolator systems, it is even more important that the industry move away from human scale clean room concepts. It has been said that moving to new technology requires a paradigm shift. On the subject of environmental monitoring it could be said that two paradigm shifts are required, because the direction of the regulatory and standard setting organizations has arguably been countercurrent to the evolution of technology. The industry is currently increasing the level of viable monitoring for production systems that actually should require less monitoring than those of a decade past.

Isolator systems should require less environmental monitoring than any other type of aseptic processing technology. Of all the technologies currently available for aseptic manufacturing, only isolators completely eliminate personnel from the critical production zone. Based upon nearly a decade of isolator use for sterility testing and other operations, it is well known that airborne microbial contamination is essentially undetectable using conventional testing methods. The value of sampling systems that are limited to only a few cubic meters of air volume is limited. Even in conventional clean rooms upwards of 95 percent of all quantitative air samples from critical zones are free of contamination. In isolators this will approach 100 percent. In fact, unless all loading, unloading, handling, and incubation of samples is done within isolators, quantitative air sampling will be prone to giving false positive results. Some people suggest that as the probability of detecting viable counts diminishes more testing should be done. The obverse is actually true; when data indicate that the establishment and maintenance of a state of control has occurred, less testing should be needed.

As mentioned earlier in this chapter, the greatest likelihood of contamination occurring in an isolator has been through human borne contamination entering through faults in the gloves. Until more durable and puncture resistant gloves that completely eliminate this problem can be used, testing of the gloves is required. The usefulness of contact plates or swabs within an isolator is debatable. The habit of taking surface samples on walls and floors in a modern human scale clean room is well established, but is overdone and in reality provides very little useful environmental data. Surface sampling of the walls, floors, and ceilings of isolators should not be done simply because it has been done in human scale clean rooms. This is a good example of a situation in which a paradigm shift (or two) is required. The use of long exposure liquid media collection bottles in isolators may be of some interest, because very long exposures of six or eight hours are possible. It is doubtful, however, that more than one or two such bottles in even a very large isolator would be required.

The following monitoring steps are the most logical considering the way contamination could enter an isolator:

1. *Nonviable particulate monitoring.* It is possible to do 100 percent real time particle counting using remote probes strategically located in the isolator system. These probes can be oriented so that they will indicate any change in the filtration effectiveness of the air filtration system(s). Optimally, such probes could be located at the output of any air filter. Some workers have suggested that there could be some value in monitoring the return air. However, it would be impossible to distinguish between process generated particulates and particulate matter present due to a leak in the air supply system or a filter. It is not possible at present to scan the entire face of a filter during normal operation, but a single particle probe located so as to detect any change in filter effectiveness will prove a key environmental control tool, and is likely to be the most useful type of environmental monitoring.

2. *Monitoring of gloves and/or half-suits.* The introduction of microbial contamination mechanically through leaks in

soft parts will be the most useful microbiological monitoring tool. In terms of controlling the environment, it is important to realize that, since soft materials are subject to tear or puncture, care must be taken in working within these devices. It is wise to continue to adhere to good aseptic technique when working through either gloves or half-suits within isolators.

3. *Functional effectiveness of RTPs.* This is an issue that has been the subject of much discussion, and is impossible to cover in detail in a general chapter such as this. It suffices to say that users of RTP systems must be prepared to demonstrate their effectiveness. Occasional monitoring of the exposed gasket or seal region may be required in some installations. This should be reviewed on a case-by-case basis, because although the introduction of contamination through RTPs is theoretically possible, there are currently no reports of contamination resulting from the use of RTPs. In fact, there are data indicating that they work well. The industry would be well advised to take a logical scientific approach to determining the significance of any perceived problems with RTPs.

4. *Detection of air exchange with the external environment.* The use of air velocity monitors at so called "mouse holes" may be useful. These monitors may be able to alert the user to any change in airflow patterns through an opening. This can be supplemented with careful monitoring of the control of the overpressurization of an isolator, or the pressure control relationships between a chain of isolators and the outside environment. Particle monitoring probes could also be located at or in the vicinity of openings to detect any change in operation. Obviously, locations near openings to the outside are good candidates for the use of long exposure microbial sampling methods.

Some or all of the elements suggested in items one through four above should result in a suitable environmental monitoring program. These measures, in conjunction with good design verification and process control testing, can be expected to result in reliable and rugged aseptic processing environments. These monitoring activities will provide much better information about the environment than the conventional procedures now performed in human scale clean rooms and should do so at the cost of much less labor.

SUMMARY

Pharmaceutical scientists and technicians, particularly those involved in the manufacture of clean, sterile, or toxic products, must live and work in a highly regulated environment. This fact is well understood and accepted by most practitioners and their employers. However, there has been a disturbing trend, particularly in the field of aseptic processing, to increase monitoring and control activities with very little consideration given to the value of the data collected. Environmental monitoring activities are a good example of over regulation, and overreaction among firms in an effort to meet regulatory expectation. Further compounding this problem has been the tendency among standard setting groups to treat environmental monitoring as though it were a quantitative analytical assay, rather than the qualitative survey that it actually is.

Other issues discussed among these regulatory topics including such often discussed issues as the classification of the surrounding room, sterility assurance levels, and the entire debate about terminal sterilization must be treated in a scientific manner. Suggestion of, or worse, implementation of, performance requirements in guidelines or standards without consideration of scientific principles must not occur. Unfortunately, many of the suggestions made by the regulatory community thus far appear to be reactions based upon perceived problems, rather than actual problems. In some cases, the thinking expressed betrays too much carryover from the old human scale clean room paradigm.

Policy makers and regulatory inspectors have a disturbing tendency to make rules from the podium or in exit interviews. Many knowledgeable people in our industry implement these rules out of fear that the approval of a process change or product may be jeopardized by failing to adhere to a new unwritten rule. This type of imposition of regulation avoids due process, and does not allow for scientific debate on the merits of the individual inspector or policy maker's view. The word *individual* was chosen carefully because, in many cases, the entire compliance pattern for a given issue can be changed by one activist regulator or inspector.

The respected early 19th century philosopher Johann Wolfgang von Goethe suggested that ignorance acted while knowledge simply reflected and considered. The wisdom in Goethe's view can be seen in the fact that most first attempts at writing a regulation or standard are not successful. This could be the result of acting out of ignorance in an effort to fill a perceived void. If the users and the regulatory community followed Goethe's advice and waited until knowledge was sufficient to allow a sound scientific standard, the industry would be better served. If those being regulated would realize that, in some cases, it is better to resist the suggestions of a single inspector or reviewer than to implement a suggested policy they do not believe has technical merit, the industry would also be better served. If both of these things happened, regulation by podium talk and 483 would stop. It would then be possible to arrive at sound guidelines and regulations in an organized and scientific manner, without so many detours and dead ends.

RECOMMENDED READINGS

Agalloco, J. P. In press. Opportunities and obstacles in the implementation of isolator technology.

Akers, J. E. 1993. Simplifying and improving process validation. *Journal of Parenteral Science and Technology* 47:281.

Akers, J. E. Biotechnology product validation Part 6: Isolator technology applications. *BioPharm* 7 (6):43.

Akers, J. E. 1995. Commentary on the Regulation of isolator technology. *PDA Letter* (June).

FDA. 1993. *Guide to the inspections of microbiological pharmaceutical quality control laboratories.* Rockville, MD: The Division of Field Investigations, Office of Regional Operations,

Office of Regulatory Affairs, Food and Drug Administration.

Griego, V. Validation of vapor phase hydrogen peroxide sterilization. *Proceedings of the PDA/PMA Symposium on Sterilization in the 1990's.*

Haas, P. J., I. J. Pflug, and J. Lysfjord. 1993. Validation concerns for parenteral filling lines incorporating barrier isolation techniques and CIP/SIP systems. Proceedings of the Second International PDA-Congress, in Basel, Switzerland.

Hargreaves, Paul. 1995a. Unpublished lecture at the PDA Asian Symposium, in November, in Tokyo, Japan.

Hargreaves, Paul. 1995b. Unpublished lecture at the PDA/ISPE Symposium, in February, in Atlanta, GA.

Klapes, N. A., and D. Vesley. 1990. Vapor-phase hydrogen peroxide as a surface decontaminant and sterilant. *Applied and Environmental Microbiology* 56 (2).

Lee, G. M., and B. Midcalf. 1994. *Isolators for pharmaceutical applications.* Published by the UK Pharmaceutical Isolator Group HMSO.

Muhvich, K. 1995. Isolators—a FDA perspective. *PDA Newsletter* (March).

Pharmacopeial Forum. <1116> Microbiological evaluation of clean rooms and other controlled environments, Vol. 42. Rockville, MD: The United States Pharmacopeial Convention, Inc.

Rickloff, J. R., and P. A. Orelski. 1989. Resistance of various microorganisms to vaporized hydrogen peroxide in a prototype tabletop sterilizer. Proceedings of the 89th Annual Meeting of the American Society for Microbiology.

Thorogood, D. 1993. Physical and biological validation of a sterile rapid transfer system. Proceedings of the Second International PDA-Congress, in Basel, Switzerland.

Wagner, C. et al. 1988. Antifungal properties of 0.1% to 3% hydrogen peroxide in neutral buffer. Proceedings of the 88th Annual Meeting of the American Society for Microbiology.

3
Regulatory Aspects of Isolation/Barrier Technology

James C. Lyda
Parenteral Drug Association
Bethesda, MD

Author's Note: This chapter represents the best information available to the author at the time of its preparation in July 1995. The regulatory environment is not static. In late June, the European Union initiated consultation on the revision to the sterile products annex to the EU GMP directive. Also in June, ISO/TC 198 issued the third committee draft of *Aseptic processing of health care products* for a three-month ballot. Both documents contain guidance for isolation systems. The reader should be aware that changes are occurring, and be alert for important regulatory developments that may affect the issues outlined in this chapter.

Much has been said and written about isolation technology in the last few years. While the technology holds much

Copyright 1995 by Parenteral Drug Association, Inc. Reprinted with permission of *Journal of Pharmaceutical Science and Technology*.

promise and advances continue, those in the business of manufacturing health care products—be they drug, biologic, or medical device—need to keep one eye focused on, and one ear attuned to, the regulatory authorities. For it is the regulatory authorities whom we must persuade, through scientific evidence, that changes in manufacturing technology are truly improvements that will result in increased safety and quality of health care products.

This chapter will survey the regulatory statements, positions, and commentary that are available to us today. This is not a large body of information, and no one person is privy to all of the regulators' views on this subject. However, the PDA—through its meetings, journal, and international standards work—has been fortunate to be engaged in much of the existing dialogue with both the European and U.S. regulatory authorities.

THE TECHNOLOGY TODAY

It is helpful to have some understanding of where this technology stands today. In the area of sterility testing, isolation/barrier technology is clearly the preferred technology around the world. From a novel approach 10 years ago, to the industry standard today, the use of isolators has improved the reliability of sterility tests to a very large degree.

False positives for environmental and other microbiology tests have been virtually eliminated for many companies. As a result, the difficult and anxiety-producing decision of what the manufacturer should do about false positives has been largely eliminated. This is especially beneficial in light of the strict enforcement approach the FDA has taken over the past few years. This is compounded by the "Barr Decision," which has fostered some confusion regarding the interpretation of laboratory data.

WHO ARE THE REGULATORS?

I should clarify whom we are talking about when I say regulators. In the United States I am referring to the U.S. Food and

Drug Administration (FDA). In the FDA there are two components to whom we must pay attention:

1. The field investigations force, which does inspections both in the United States and internationally

2. The marketing application review microbiologists in the FDA's headquarters

While such reviewers reside in both the Center for Drug Evaluation and Research (CDER) and the Center for Biologics Evaluation and Research (CBER), it is the CDER reviewers who are currently engaged in the isolator dialogue.

The FDA's field investigators and review microbiologists work cooperatively to conduct the total review before a manufacturing system is approved as part of a marketing application. Currently in the FDA, it is the marketing application review that is impacting on isolation system approval, since these are "new" systems in the FDA's view.

In time, as more systems are brought on-line, one could expect the FDA's field investigations force to exhibit an increasing influence on this technology. This will occur as a body of experience, particularly for postapproval maintenance, monitoring, and control of isolators is accumulated. And this will manifest itself through the familiar FDA Form 483.

In Europe we have found that the Medicines Control Agency (MCA) of the United Kingdom has the lead. The European Medicines Evaluation Agency (EMEA) is just getting organized, and has not yet gained its voice. The MCA has great influence among the European inspectorates, which is likely to continue. The role of the PIC remains influential in Europe, and the meeting in Iceland in June 1995 was dedicated to the aseptic processing of pharmaceuticals, including isolation systems.

We are unaware, today, of significant policy guidance from Japan's Ministry of Health and Welfare or "Koseisho."

THE FIRST PROBLEM—DEFINITIONS

As is frequently the case in an emerging technology, the issue of definitions arises. We know the lack of formal, agreed-upon definitions hampers progress. This is especially true when that progress is dependent on one party (the regulators) fully understanding and acting on the information supplied by another party (the health care product manufacturer).

Terms we frequently hear are isolators, barriers, containment, minienvironments, and so on. Do these all mean the same thing or not? And if not, how are they different? And what about an "absolute" barrier? How is it different from a regular barrier? And can anything really be absolute?

A term that is increasingly popular in the United States is locally controlled environment (LCE). Although it does not have the verbal snap of isolator or barrier, one can convince oneself of the relative merits of that term if one thinks about it. Yet, when I last met with a European group of manufacturers, they looked at me with a blank stare when I used the term LCE.

At the recent joint PDA/ISPE Advanced Barrier Technology Meeting in Atlanta, Georgia, January 17/18, 1995, Paul Hargreaves of the MCA gave a detailed and thoughtful presentation on design, construction, and operational weaknesses associated with isolators. To highlight his observations, he referenced several deaths associated with isolator mishaps in the United Kingdom.

Afterward, it became clear to me that much of Hargreaves' comments related to isolators used in a hospital or health care environment, not an industrial environment. When the PDA talks to the FDA about isolators, we both recognize that we are discussing usage in an industrial setting, and neither of us would think about a hospital. I advocate that we need to listen carefully to each other and understand what is being said.

Definitions—FDA

What have the regulators offered in the way of definitions? From the FDA we have very little. But that is consistent with the FDA's style of regulating. Definitions will come slow, if at all, and the industry or standards bodies will have every opportunity to establish definitions themselves. The FDA has shown a willingness to adopt industry standards and terminology when they make scientific sense.

Definitions—MCA

People who have had experience with the United Kingdom in standards-setting activities recognize the skillful and precise approach the British bring to the standards process. So what do we have from the MCA in terms of definitions?

An important document is the 1994 publication *Isolators for Pharmaceutical Applications* (Lee and Midcalf 1994). This is the revision of the 1993 *Specifications for the Design and Monitoring of Isolators* with which many of you may be familiar. This document was prepared by the U.K. health (hospital) authorities, isolator manufacturers, industrial pharmaceutical manufacturers, and the MCA.

The document provides guidance for the installation and use of isolators in the health care or hospital environment. The MCA readily states that this document can serve as a starting place for discussions with the inspectorate for industrial applications of isolators.

> Further, the document offers that it has been sufficiently detailed to form the basis of a standards document that could be adopted by the BSI, CEN, or ISO committees.

So clearly we have the kernel of a standard here, and the only document in which users, manufacturers, and regulators of isolators have agreed-upon definitions, among other things.

And what definitions do we have? An isolator is defined as

> a containment device that utilizes barrier technology for the enclosure of a controlled work space.

So while the United Kingdom prefers the word *isolator* to describe the total system, we find within the definition of isolator the words *containment device, barrier,* and *controlled work space.* Very crafty, and a total of only 15 words.

Further, isolators are divided into Type 1 and Type 2. Type 1 protects the product; Type 2 protects the product and the operators. Nowhere in the definitions do we see the word *environment* or reference to microbiological quality.

The document has a total of 28 definitions that I will not detail, with the exception of sterilization, which is

> the process applied to a specified field that inactivates viable microorganisms and thereby transforms the nonsterile field into a sterile one.

Recognizing that this definition applies only within the document, microbiologists should enjoy considering the pros and cons of this definition.

This document contains much information and demonstrates an impressive internal logic. For example, it includes classification of transfer devices based on sterilization/sanitization characteristics. This classification, in turn, determines the "background environment" in which the isolator is located.

Yet we must recognize that it is intended for hospital applications, and not industrial manufacturing. It remains to be seen how much of the information survives the regulatory and standards obstacle course. There are many in the pharmaceutical industry who are not in favor of standards, citing the risks of bureaucratic control and the stifling of technology.

However, the creation of a common understanding of what we mean by isolation will be necessary if the regulators are to become comfortable with these systems and allow the industry to use them to their full capabilities. This tends to pull us toward some type of standards activity.

WHAT HAS BEEN APPROVED?

We are aware of at least two European aseptic manufacturing facilities, with different configurations of isolation systems, that have been approved by both the MCA and the FDA. Both have received much attention and have made their technologies known as they have developed.

The first, API in France, manufactures a sterile drug that can be hazardous to the operators, and uses a modular isolation system. The second, Evans Medical in the United Kingdom, manufactures a biologic in prefilled syringes and uses a custom-made isolated filling line. Representatives of both companies made presentations at the meeting in Atlanta in January 1995. Reference to these two approved facilities offers us some general insight into current regulatory expectations.

One must recognize, however, that it is official FDA policy that each marketing application stands on its own merits. One marketing application is not compared to others when the FDA does its scientific review. Therefore, the approval of a particular system must not be interpreted as generic FDA approval for similar systems in other facilities.

For the balance of this chapter, I will summarize the relative regulatory perspectives, where they can be identified, on several key issues associated with isolation technology.

ISSUE—THE BACKGROUND ENVIRONMENT

The quality of the background environment surrounding the isolator system continues to be the source of debate. The API facility specifies Class 10,000 air quality for the general manufacturing floor in which a number of isolators, both positive and negative pressure, are located. However, this air quality was specified for reasons that the manufacturer has stated are not based on risks to the product, but that are more closely associated with operator safety.

The Evans Medical filling line operates in a controlled but unclassified environment as described by both the company and the MCA in the January 1995 barrier meeting in Atlanta (*PDA Letter* 1995a). During that same meeting Paul Hargreaves of the MCA indicated it was the "feeling" of the European inspectorates working group that isolators should be located in at least a Class 100,000 environment, dependent on the intended application (*PDA Letter* 1995a).

The FDA's CDER suggested at one point that while not strictly a cGMP requirement, it would be "prudent and acceptable" for isolators to be located in a Class 10,000 environment (FDA 1994). This observation was likely influenced by the FDA's recent review of the API facility. While the FDA has not further commented in this area, there is some sense that the FDA will continue to take a case-by-case approach and not require specific background environments.

ISSUE—MONITORING OF THE INTERNAL ISOLATOR ENVIRONMENT

Evans Medical described the quantity and frequency of environmental monitoring for microorganisms in their isolated filling line. Over 6,000 settle plates were entered into the isolator in six months, with negligible results. The value of the data from such a program, weighed against the risks posed by the scale and frequency of the intrusion into the isolator environment, is open to debate.

The MCA has stated that isolators should be monitored with the same rationale and program as one would with a traditional clean room, claiming they have (to date) not been presented with data that would change this view (*PDA Letter* 1995a). To our knowledge, the FDA has not made any similar statement.

ISSUE—ASEPTIC PROCESSING VS. TERMINAL STERILIZATION

This is largely an issue in the United States, and has served as the backdrop and catalyst for much of the ferment and development in the isolator area. In 1991 the FDA proposed that all parenteral pharmaceuticals be subject to a moist heat, terminal sterilization process unless the drug product would be adversely affected (degraded) by such a process (*Federal Register* 1991). The proposal eventually exempted all products regulated by the FDA's CBER and possibly the Center for Veterinary Medicine, and would also exempt certain dosage forms.

While the regulation remains a proposal, the FDA is expected to make some determination in the near future. In the prepared comments by the FDA's Kenneth Muhvich for the Atlanta meeting, he stated that

> the frequency of contamination for products manufactured on barrier isolator filling lines should be better than those manufactured now in Class 10,000 rooms under Class 100 conditions (*PDA Letter* 1995b).

This statement was believed by some to be an agency conclusion generated by the review of comments on the proposed regulation. In the same remarks Muhvich stated,

> Until the efficacy of barrier isolator technology is proven to be equivalent, drug products that can withstand the rigors

of high thermal input should be terminally sterilized using moist heat.

Requirements similar to the FDA's proposed regulation already exist in Europe.

ISSUE—MEDIA FILLS: VALUE AND INTERPRETATION

It is the traditional regulatory and scientific view that each media fill is a discrete event, and a function of the environment and specifics associated with the tested filling line at the time of the media fill. Thus, media fills cannot be additive for the purposes of statistical manipulation or interpretation.

While this view remains unchanged, there is a growing sense that there should be some recognition and interpretation of repeated media fills with zero contamination. Wood and others suggest this fresh view toward the interpretation of cumulative media fill data is based on the reproducible process and isolator environment, which was lacking in the traditional clean room with human operators (*PDA Letter* 1994). Lacking new interpretations of data, the industry will continue to be limited by the statistical limitations of single event media fills (i.e., generation of statistics beyond 10^{-3} requires prohibitively large media fills).

ISSUE—WEAK LINKS IN ISOLATION SYSTEMS

As the environment in the isolator is recognized as a reduced risk to exposed product, other components of the total system, including the traditional filling line and sterilizing filters, become the focus of risk assessment. Hargreaves and the MCA have cataloged a lengthy list of potential design and operational defects that can affect isolator effectiveness (*PDA Letter* 1995a).

Muhvich and the FDA recognize a smaller, yet similar list of concerns (*PDA Letter* 1995b).

ISOLATOR STANDARDS—USP

The United States Pharmacopeia (USP) plays an important role in drug regulation in the United States and much of the world. The USP is a private drug standards authority specifically recognized by U.S. law, specifically the U.S. Food, Drug, and Cosmetic Act, the enabling legislation for the FDA. USP monographs for drug standards are officially recognized by the FDA and many of the USP requirements are enforceable by the FDA. However, there is an uneasy tension between the two bodies regarding who will take the lead.

During the USP five-year meeting held in Washington, D.C., the convention debated and voted on a number of resolutions. One resolution specifically proposed that the USP

> expand the scope of standards for drugs . . . to include . . . standards that govern critical processes . . . (USP 1995, Resolution 7).

The resolution went on to describe that

> Sterilization and validation have been identified as logical areas for USP standardization. . . . Barrier-isolator technology is poised to spread into both industrial and pharmacy environments.

The resolution was hotly debated, and was one of several that the FDA, with PDA and broad industry support, recommended for rejection. The resolution was finally diluted significantly with reference to information chapters, instead of product monographs, and a focus on tests for process measurement instead of a process standard.

ASEPTIC PROCESSING STANDARD—ISO

ISO Technical Committee 198, Sterilization of health care products, continues to work on a proposed international standard for aseptic processing (ISO 1995). The working group has debated the applicability of this standard to isolator systems.

Consensus wording in the current scope of the document states,

This standard was prepared to address the validation and control of aseptic processing conducted in conventional clean rooms. However, many of the principles and programs described may also apply to aseptic processing conducted in barrier/isolation systems. Requirements and guidance relating to some barrier and isolation systems may need to be considered in the future.

CLEANROOM STANDARDS—ISO

ISO Technical Committee 209 on Cleanrooms has finally activated Working Group 7 to generate standards on "clean air devices" (ISO/IES). While work has just started, this group will focus some attention on standards for pharmaceutical isolators.

ISO/TC 209 recently absorbed much of the program of work for CEN Technical Committee 243, Cleanroom technology. This elimination of duplicate work should allow the ISO work to move ahead more quickly.

THE FDA AND EUROPEAN INTERNATIONAL STANDARDS POLICIES

The FDA recently published a draft policy on its recognition and use of international standards (*Federal Register* 1994). This policy directs FDA support to international versus national standards, and describes the criteria for FDA recognition of the standard, including FDA involvement in the standard development, transparency or openness of the process, and consistency with FDA policy and rules.

The above ISO standards work meets all of these criteria. It can be expected, then, that these standards will gain some support in the FDA when finalized.

In Europe, the ISO/CEN work-sharing agreements would suggest adoption of the ISO standards in Europe where practical. This would especially apply to ISO/TC 209, Cleanrooms and associated controlled environments, which has incorporated CEN documents already in progress.

CONCLUSIONS

Isolation/barrier technology has been the subject of explosive growth and attention in the past few years. The FDA's proposed regulation on terminal sterilization sparked much of this activity in the United States. The FDA has, in general, been in a learning-and-listening mode as the resolution of the proposed regulation continues to be deliberated. Most guidance and policy statements during this time have been conservative and consistent with guidance in the traditional cleanroom area. There is evidence that the agency is aware of the issues at stake and is attempting to avoid precipitous action that would stifle technological improvements.

The MCA has been more expansive and articulate in its position on isolation technology. While conservative in most instances, and comprehensive in its description of potential isolator design and maintenance faults, the MCA has at the same time shown an inclination and willingness to engage fully in the international dialogue. In addition, the MCA's focused input into the previously described *Isolators for Pharmaceutical Applications* and the ISO/TC 198 work on aseptic processing standards (along with the FDA) demonstrates a commitment to consensus-based, standards-oriented guidance.

The development of regulatory requirements based on scientific data is the desirable policy for both regulatory agencies at this time. Arbitrary actions can prematurely slow and even stop the development of technological improvements and advancements, such as isolator/barrier technology.

REFERENCES

FDA. 1994. *Human drug cGMP notes.* 2 (1):4.

Federal Register. 1991. Use of aseptic processing and terminal sterilization in the preparation of sterile pharmaceuticals for human and veterinary use: Proposed rule. [Docket No. 91N-0074] 56 FR 51354 (11 October).

Federal Register. 1994. International harmonization: Draft policy on standards; availability. [Docket No. 94D-0300] 59 FR 60870 (28 November).

ISO. 1995. ISO/CD 13408.2 (interim draft). Technical Committee 198. Arlington, VA: Association for Advancement of Medical Instrumentation.

ISO/IES. Technical Committee 209. Chicago: Institute for Environmental Sciences.

Lee, G. M., and B. Midcalf, eds. 1994. *Isolators for pharmaceutical applications: Practical guidelines on the design and use of isolators for the aseptic processing of pharmaceuticals.* HMSO.

PDA Letter. 1994. 30 (4):10.

PDA Letter. 1995a. 31 (2):6.

PDA Letter. 1995b. 31 (3):11.

USP. 1995. Quinquennial Meeting, Resolutions for Action by the Convention, 9–12 March, in Washington, D.C.

4

British and European Experience with Isolation Technology

Gordon J. Farquharson
Tanshire Holdings PLC
Elstead, Surrey, United Kingdom

HISTORICAL PERSPECTIVE

Isolators using various elements of barrier technology are not a new concept, but many potential new applications arise almost daily. This is particularly so in the case of aseptic processing in the pharmaceutical industry. The history of isolators can be traced back more than 35 years to the nuclear industry where they have been used principally for protecting the operators from radiation and chemical hazards associated with manipulation and storage of hazardous material. The United Kingdom Atomic Energy Authority (UKAEA) was set up in 1954 to develop the civil applications of nuclear power. By 1957, isolators were being used extensively for handling hazardous materials primarily plutonium. The main function of these isolators was to protect the operator. Laboratory glove boxes were used for research and the work carried out inside changed depending on the experimental requirements. At the Atomic Energy Research Establishment at Harwell, a Symposium was held on Glove Box Design and Operation in February 1957. It was one of the earliest examples of an attempt to develop a common approach and standards.

More recently, flexible and rigid isolator devices have been designed for many other applications. Standards and guidelines for specific applications have been developed to recognise particular requirements. A good example is the microbiological safety cabinet for containment of biologically active materials. A range of well established standards exist for this type of equipment. In more recent years, applications have developed to protect and contain highly potent drug active substances, and within the microelectronics world for the purposes of avoiding particulate contamination of semiconductor devices. In the former instance, the worker is protected. In the latter case, the product is protected. These different objectives result in different strategies and significantly different technical solutions.

As the varied industrial and research applications develop, the specific needs of diverse solutions and arrangements of systems are continually growing. However, all the applications have a common thread of objectives. These can be summarised as the desire to achieve a secure micro-environment; protect products, people, and/or the environment; and minimise enclosed volumes demanding effective cleaning and disinfection, or other critical decontamination. The achievement of an effective isolator application requires a similar duty of care and approach as would be demanded in producing a critically controlled environment on a human scale such as a traditional cleanroom.

MARKET STIMULUS TO USE ISOLATORS

There are many stimuli for each particular application that may lead to the choice of isolators as the sole technique, or in combination with other methods to provide the appropriate environment within which to carry out a process or manipulation. The fundamental requirements are protecting people and conversely protecting the product. Of course, there are some applications, particularly related to parenteral cytotoxic products, whereby a combination of operator and product protection is required simultaneously. In addition, matters associated with energy conservation, improved quality assurance (particularly for sterility and cross contamination control), costs, and time to complete the implementation of a new facility will be important. It is in these specific areas that significant advantage can be gained from the appropriate deployment of barrier technology.

In Europe there are numerous examples of isolators, most commonly flexible film types, used for end product sterility testing. Such devices have been chosen principally to improve the assurance of an effective test for sterility and also to provide the testing resource at lower capital and revenue cost. As experience and confidence has grown, both these aims are now generally achieved without significant increases in initial and revalidation efforts compared to the traditional cleanroom systems. Ironically, some of the traditional arguments against the validity of the sterility testing have been removed by the use of isolators. For industrial production scale manufacturing of potent compounds, formulation, filling, and clean or aseptic assembly, individual devices or connected networks of isolators are now more common. In the cases of aseptic filling of pharmaceuticals, it is common for the total facility and process equipment capital expenditure for an isolator application to be 70 to 90 percent of that for a traditional clean room system. However, the greatest advantages are derived from improved sterility assurance levels and reduced costs. Running cost reductions of 40 to 50 percent can sometimes be achieved when considering energy, environmental monitoring, cleaning and disinfection, garment management, personnel flexibility, personnel training, equipment utilisation, and similar operational cost issues.

TYPICAL APPLICATIONS

A broad review of typical applications of isolation technology serve to show the large range of isolator devices or systems that have been deployed for specific applications. This further emphasises and amplifies some of the key objectives identified above.

Radioactive Hazard Containment Cabinets

Some of the earliest applications of isolators were for dealing with the chemical and radiological hazard associated with the nuclear industry. The devices developed to satisfy these industrial needs were containment only devices targeted at operator protection and the avoidance of discharges of contamination to the atmosphere.

Radioactive containment glove boxes have been in evidence since the early fifties for principally protecting people. Within the nuclear industry these devices were progressively developed into complex networks of isolators to house complete chemical processes. Such applications have been evolved, designed, implemented and managed within the environment of the various nuclear industry inspectorates. In certain areas the pharmaceutical industry can use some of the standards developed in the nuclear industry provided care is taken to be highly selective and to avoid over-engineering.

Microbiological Safety Cabinets

Microbiological hazard containment, particularly of category 3 and 4 pathogens, saw early use of simple glove boxes. Once again operator protection and avoidance of discharge to atmosphere were the primary objective. A review of the history of development of these devices shows a progressive evolution from simple individual glove boxes to complete networks in which organisms can be handled, as well as increasingly sophisticated entry and exit systems via autoclaves and other sterilisation and disinfection devices.

The author remembers the early days of biotechnology applications in the 1970s, when complex networks of isolators were developed for containing fermentation, as well as downstream processing. Ethylene oxide was used as the method of sterilisation and decontamination.

Laboratory Flexible Film Isolators

Laboratory users have required for many years, and continue to need effective containment systems for specific pathogen free (SPF) and infected animal work. Simple flexible film isolators are used for such applications very effectively. These systems have demonstrated an ability to achieve consistent performance when placed in controlled and uncontrolled rooms. Ultimate decontamination of the isolator envelope can be by simple incineration.

Sterility Testing Isolators

For many years the isolator has been a valuable tool for providing highly secure environments for the critical aseptic manipulation associated with end product sterility testing. For these applications both flexible film (Figure 4.1) and rigid wall devices have been utilised successfully when located within classified or unclassified laboratory environments. For well validated applications, the effectiveness of

Figure 4.1. Sterility testing in a flexible film isolator.

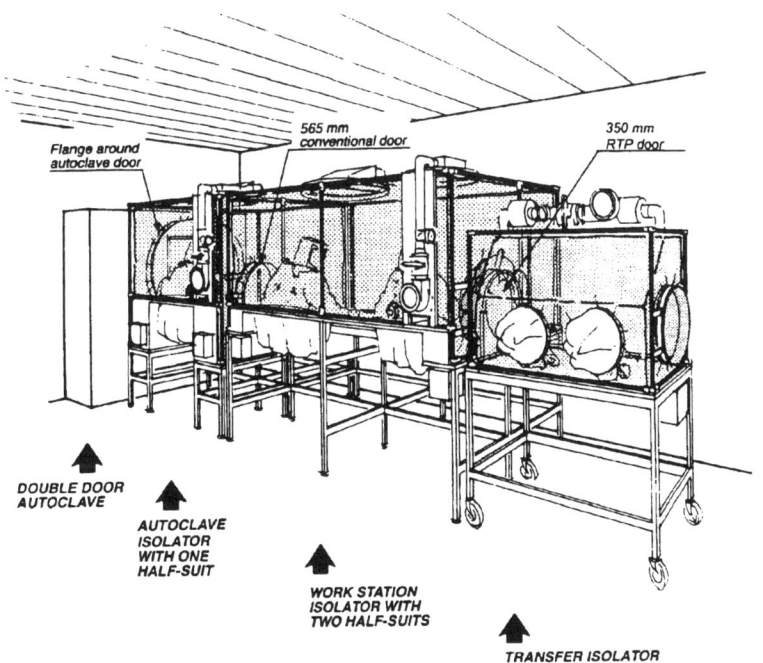

isolator technology for these processes (operating in conjunction with sanitisation techniques such as vapor-phase hydrogen peroxide (VHP), and transfer systems such as interlocking transfer ports) provide a high degree of confidence that high quality, repeatable aseptic processing environments can be achieved.

Potent Compound Dispensing Isolators

As pharmaceutical products contain more and more potent actives, and as health and safety demands gain in stature, isolators have been developed in many configurations for the safe weighing and sub-division of highly active compounds. In the most sophisticated applications, such sub-divisions are carried out under clean or aseptic processing conditions. This type of application is a good example of where both the operator and the product must be protected.

Powder Handling System Isolators

A natural extension of the handling of potent compounds is the use of isolators for transferring powders (Figure 4.2).

Figure 4.2. Powder handling in a rigid isolator.

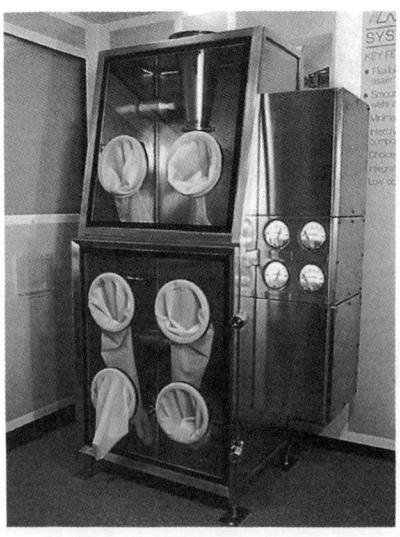

Applications in this area have two objectives. The first is protecting the operator and environment, and the second is controlling a clean or aseptic environment around the mouth of a process vessel or reactor. This type of application will normally be limited to handling lots of material of up to 50 kilogrammes.

Small Scale Clean or Aseptic Processing Isolators

Many rigid and flexible film isolators have been used for manufacturing clinical trials materials (Figure 4.3–4.5). These systems have been based on the types of isolator used in sterility testing. Advantages in this type of application are because processes often are unique and are not carried out on a continuous basis. In such situations, the security provided by isolators can reduce the opportunity of product contamination, and reduce the need to continuously maintain expensive spaces.

Large Scale Clean or Aseptic Processing in Isolator Networks

Scale up applications have led to a significant number of industrial aseptic processing systems for formulation and filling being developed and used. These have employed both rigid and flexible wall systems, and have been configured as fixed networks or with mobile transfers between fixed processing cellular isolators. Set alongside hazard containment, isolators for these applications will influence, most significantly, the attitude and approach to isolation systems engineering.

DEVELOPMENT OF STANDARDS AND MONOGRAPHS

In addition to work undertaken within organisations such as ISPE, PDA, the European parenteral societies, CEN and ISO, it is valuable to note other standards in development which can be deployed usefully into many applications of isolators. Within the United Kingdom, a hospital pharmacy guideline has been developed for the design and use of isolators. The document is called "Isolators for Pharmaceutical Applications"

Figure 4.3. Aseptic syringe filling in a network of rigid isolators.

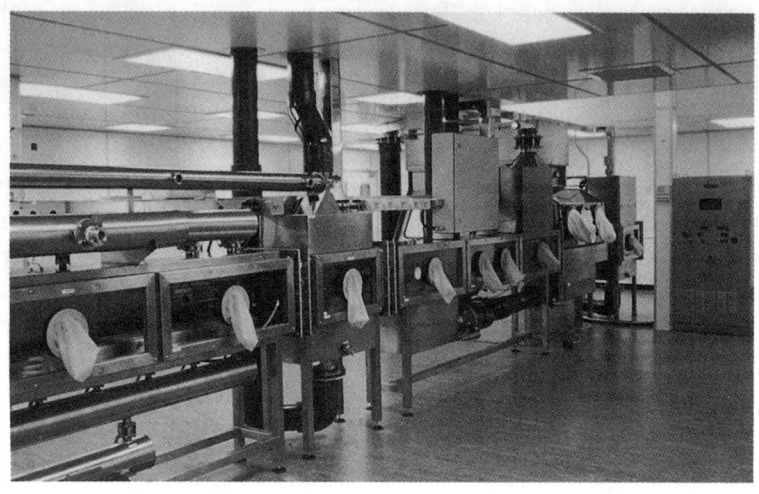

Figure 4.4. Aseptic ampoule filling in an isolator.

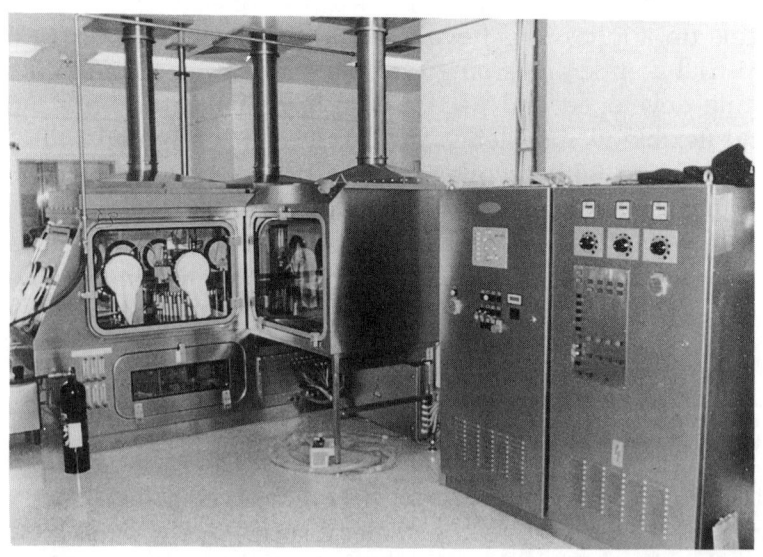

(published in the UK by HMSO with ISBN number 0 11 701829 5). This guideline focuses on applications related to total parenteral nutrition (TPN) assembly and to cytotoxic dispensing.

Figure 4.5. Small-scale aseptic filling in an inert atmosphere.

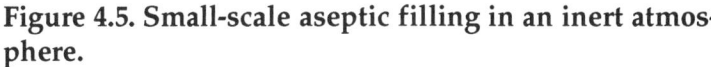

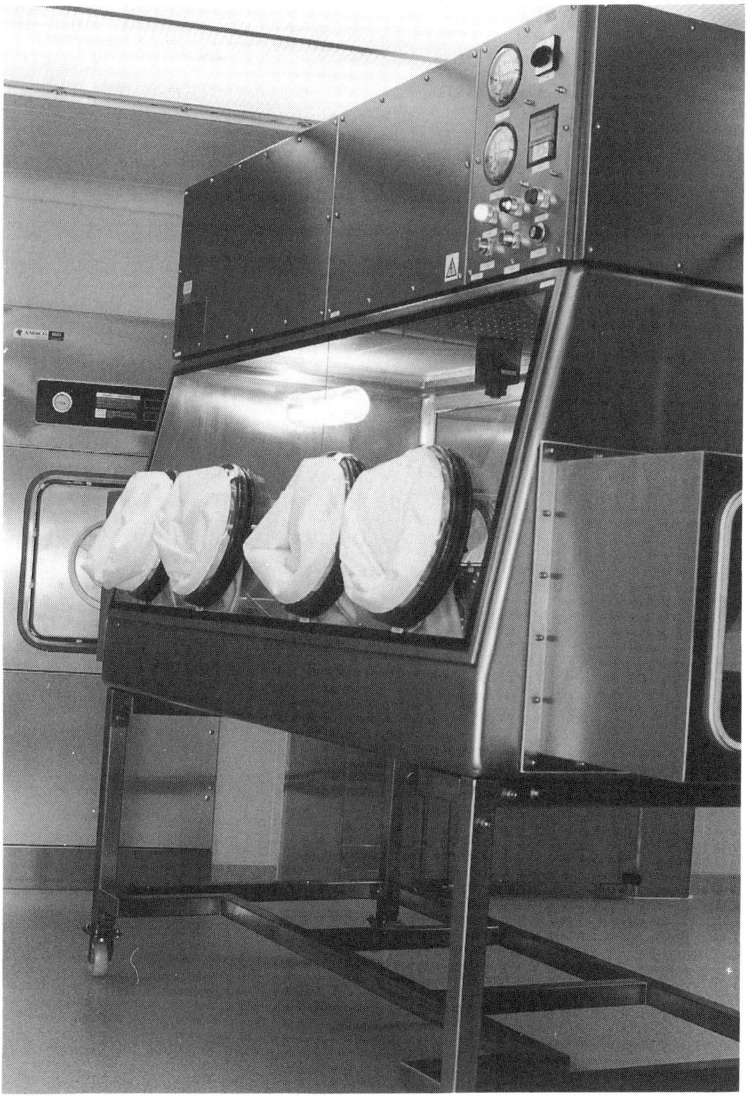

The document is a sophisticated guideline that defines the required qualities of technology used in an isolator, and sets a correlation between the appropriate surrounding environment and the integrity of the transfer mechanisms used for loading and unloading the isolator. This UK Guideline has already appeared in a mildly modified form as a draft Australian and New Zealand standard.

Microbiological safety cabinets standards, such as British Standard 5726:1992, are valuable in parts. Selected elements are relevant to isolator applications, such as those related to consideration of enclosure integrity and filtration systems. Exploring existing standards a little further, we can find standards from within the nuclear industry that, with care, can be valuable when defining aspects of pressure hold and leakage rate integrity of isolator enclosures. Such standards enable leakage rates of between 0.1 and 0.5 percent of the critical enclosure volume per hour, and a helium gas diffused leak rate of 1×10^{-2} to 1×10^{-1} cc per minute.

It is the author's opinion that national and international standards currently under development must be broad based, allowing specific industries to develop application guidance. The structure of the current ISO TC 209 work has a specific working group responsible for "Clean Air Devices". This will include isolators for pharmaceutical applications amongst many others.

In order to focus on current European practice the following structure of Standards and Guidance used is a valuable framework to be aware of.

Definitions

For clarity of understanding some essential definitions are of value. These already form part of the guidelines and monographs being developed in Europe through CEN technical committees, ISPE European technical groups, the European parenteral societies and broader contamination control organisations.

Active Isolator	An isolator employing managed air flow or air pressure as one of the elements of barrier technology used.
Barrier Technology	Specific techniques employed to provide an element of an isolator with a defined degree of containment. (*Note:* may range from absolute segregation to a percentage

	segregation of a defined challenge to the barrier)
Breach Velocity	The air flow rate through an aperture sufficient to prevent movement of airborne particles in the opposite direction to the airflow. For the purposes of this definition, the aperture should be considered as a glove port or similar size opening.
Decontamination	A process which reduces contaminating substances to a defined acceptance level.
	Sanitisation. That part of decontamination which reduces viable microorganisms to a defined acceptance level.
	Particulate Decontamination. That part of decontamination which reduces visible and sub-visible particle levels to a defined acceptance level.
	Chemical Decontamination. That part of decontamination which reduces chemical contamination to a defined acceptance level.
Docking Transfer Device	An item of isolation/barrier technology purposely designed to effect connection of one isolator or container to another without allowing external contamination to enter or internal contamination to escape.
Glove	A device that allows the arms and hands of an operator to enter the enclosed volume of an isolator whilst maintaining an effective barrier.

Half-Suit	A device that enables the head and trunk of an operator to enter the working volume of an isolator whilst maintaining an effective barrier.
Isolator	A device employing barrier technology to achieve a defined degree of segregation of an internal environment from a surrounding or adjacent external environment.
Nozzle	A fixed connection point in the envelope of an isolator for connecting pipes or ducts.
Passive Isolator	An isolator employing only physical barrier elements of barrier technology.
Sterilisation	The process applied to a specified field which inactivates viable microorganisms, thereby transforming the non-sterile field into a sterile one.
Transfer Isolator	A specific example of an active or passive isolator used to transfer materials to and from another fixed or static isolator.
Transfer Chamber	A chamber, usually with entry and exit doors, used to facilitate the transfer of materials into or out of an isolator whilst minimising the transfer of contaminants.
Transport Container	A specific example of a small passive isolator used to transport materials to and from an isolator. (*Note:* may be flexible or rigid and will be designed to interface with a docking transfer device)

Working Conditions

Passive/As Built	Isolator physically complete, but without operation of any air treatment system.
At Rest	Isolator fully functioning *without* process operational, and *without* operator interface or material transfer.
Operational	Isolator fully functioning with a defined process operation, operator interfacing and material transfer.

Other more general contamination control issues, such as air flow configuration and particulate cleanliness levels are defined in existing German, French, British and other national "cleanroom" standards. They are also fully covered in the scope of the current ISO TC 209 work items.

Specification of Requirements by European Documents

The structure and content of British Standard 5295:1989, (part 2), and the German VDI 2083 material related to the "Design and Construction of Cleanroom and Clean Air Devices" collectively provide effective methods to ensure achievement of the following:

- Project Goals
- Responsibilities of Designer/Supplier and Purchaser/User
- Process Requirements
- Internal and External Environmental Performance
- Reference to all Standards and Guidelines to be used including Regulatory Authority demands
- Definition of Hazards
- Timescale/Schedule
- Definition of Cost Boundaries

This formed an integral part of the CEN TC 243 approach, which has subsequently been evolved in ISO TC 209 within the framework of the Vienna agreement.

EUROPEAN REGULATORY APPROACH

The pharmaceutical regulatory environment within Europe operates in a more fragmented mode than in the United States. Certain European countries have differing approaches to new technologies. This writer's experience with European Regulatory Authorities has been that the more sophisticated organisations, such as the United Kingdom Medicines Control Agency, are receptive to well developed concepts and solutions, including novel and state of the art technology. Also, since there are few if any attempts by companies manufacturing sterile products in Europe to replace terminal sterilisation of parenteral products with aseptic processing inside isolators, there seems to be a positive and open desire by all parties to use the technology where appropriate.

There is now, of course, significant experience with industrial scale clean and aseptic processing in isolators in Europe. Companies such as Evans Medical, Organon, Cilag, Aquitaine, Howmedica and Baxter have all developed applications of both flexible and rigid systems. From these, very positive feedback has been received from the regulators and users. Issues such as the effects of vibration on isolator devices and the requirements of double versus single HEPA filters (for providing air filtration security similar to that achieved with traditional cleanroom technology) are frequent areas of discussion. Regulators, the UK MCA in particular, have focused on points of vulnerability of an isolator, particularly those relating to transfers in and out, manipulation techniques, and vibration. The regulators seek adaptation and deployment of tests derived from those used in traditional cleanrooms to ensure that the integrity of isolators can be demonstrated and confirmed routinely. Such tests include pressure hold and leakage rate, leak induction and a containment test developed from that used for open fronted microbiological safety cabinets. This final test is an aerosol challenge test developed to demonstrate the effectiveness of an airflow protected opening to contain a hazard. The source of the method is described in BS 5726:1992 and US NSF 49.

THE ENVIRONMENT SURROUNDING ISOLATORS

The subject of the appropriate quality for the environment surrounding an individual isolator or network of isolators, particularly those associated with the most critical demands of aseptic processing, is currently and probably will remain a major issue for debate. While some regulatory authorities have begun by making unqualified statements that isolators housing aseptic manipulations should be placed in U.S. Fed Std 209E class 10,000/M 5.5 environment, such statements have generally lacked quality in terms of risk assessment, and certainly have lacked depth in relation to consideration of air borne microbial challenge and the challenge to the manipulation and transfer. Therefore the overall judgement of what environment is appropriate must take into account a number of things and not just rely on dogma. It is first important to appreciate what might influence the quality of external environment that is actually necessary. The following considerations are the most important issues that can influence this, and are commonly used in Europe to review qualitatively the necessary relationship between the internal and external environment.

1. The Process Risk

    The susceptibility of a process to contamination would be an important consideration of risk analysis. Classically in aseptic processing, open processes are at far greater risk than closed processes. Provided that a complete evaluation of all steps of a process from the aseptic assembly of the system through to the product transfer has been taken into account, then the total activity may have low or high risk.

2. Isolator Integrity

    The higher the isolator integrity, the less opportunity there is of corrupting it; therefore, it should follow that the surrounding environment will have a lesser potential impact on the process or activity contained. Considerations of rigid compared to softwall envelopes, the quantity and quality of access panels (these always present a risk when resealing, etc.), the type and nature of joints and sealants used, the quality of fabrication, and thoroughness of fabrication tests are very important. Probably most important is the ability to routinely carry out isolator integrity tests by pressure hold or decay rate tests. The easier it is to effectively carry out such tests, the less demanding is the quality of the background environment.

3. Transfer Technique

The transfer of materials into and out of an isolator represents the most likely and most common source of loss of internal environmental integrity. The more secure the transfer system, the less demanding the external environment becomes. The simplest devices such as "jam-pot" covers or single doors present very little ability to separate the external from the internal environment during operation, and hence are unsuitable for operational transfers. In fact, in these applications, the only facet of the device's performance that provides any open cover protection is outward airflow when the door or cover is open. Improved security is achieved with a double door pass-through hatch. The performance and effectiveness of hatch devices can be progressively improved by mechanical or electromechanical interlocking of the opposing doors and by positive ventilation of the airlock space to dilute and remove contamination that may enter when the external door is open. The most secure techniques are the interlocked docking port systems (often called alpha/beta systems), and airflow protected tunnels for continuous component discharge. Whilst no generally accepted type tests or standards exist to define the performance of such devices, challenge tests which have evolved from those used for open fronted microbiological safety cabinets can be effectively used to determine a protection factor for airflow protected tunnels.

In the case of alpha/beta interlocked docking port systems, the two main manufacturers in the United Kingdom and France have developed and applied particulate and microbiological challenge tests to determine the effectiveness or protection factor achieved by the device. This can quantify the segregation achieved by such a device in simulated operation. This type of test is, in the author's opinion, likely to become a basis for performance type testing of such specialised transfer devices.

4. Internal Pressurisation

   Maintenance of a continuous internal positive pressure within an isolator greatly assists the exclusion of the external environment. The relative level of the pressurisation should also be considered to determine its ability to withstand the piston effect of rapid glove movement. It is also necessary to define whether or not the isolator air treatment system should be able to achieve a specific outflow of air in the event of partial or total glove loss. Whilst this section is focused upon positive pressure devices, the integrity and performance attributes of pressurisation apply equally to negative pressure systems. Negative pressure systems, used for clean and aseptic processing, are more likely to require a higher class of surrounding environment than that for equivalent positive pressure systems.

   The glove displacement effect in an isolator is volume related (i.e., the volume displaced by the glove compared to the volume of the isolator). As a rule of thumb, devices with a pressure difference of 15–25 pascals compared to the surrounding atmosphere are likely to be less secure due to the piston displacement effect than devices with a pressure difference of between 50–80 pascals compared to the surrounding area. When airflow protection is required to provide security in the event of glove loss or severe puncture, inflow or outflow air velocities of between 0.5 and 0.7 metres per second should be considered for negative or positive pressure systems. If extremely high velocities above these figures occur, re-entrainment of contamination due to high turbulence is a distinct possibility.

5. Sanitisation and Sterilisation Methods

There are no regulatory demands stating the required effectiveness of an aseptic processing isolator's bio-decontamination system. However, it is clear that the effectiveness and repeatability of the sanitisation method has an impact upon the quality of the surrounding environment, particularly if it is anticipated that batch changeover, for example, is carried out with an open isolator. In the event of this procedure being adopted, with an isolator being placed in a controlled but unclassified space, it is necessary first to minimise the introduction of room contamination into the open isolator by operating the on-board air system. Assuming that some minimal amount of contamination has entered the device, it is essential to use a repeatable and effective surface sanitisation or sterilisation method. Processes such as surface swabbing and aerosol spray with disinfectant are not repeatable processes of high efficacy. However, highly controlled, gaseous phase processes using agents such as formaldehyde, hydrogen peroxide and peracetic acid alone or in combination can be deployed as part of the biodecontamination philosophy. It is extremely important to recognise that most of the agents described above are toxic and in some cases corrosive and must be managed safely.

6. Regulatory Demands

It is the author's experience that since operational applications are limited, it is inappropriate to assume the regulatory authorities have the same level of confidence that has been gained with traditional cleanroom technology. It is the responsibility of the isolator user, together with the designer or supplier, to demonstrate an appropriate level of system integrity to support the selection of surrounding environments. Regulators will hope to see that the deployment of isolators brings improvements in contamination rate, other facets of product quality assurance, operator health and safety, and environmental protection. Current experience within Europe, both on the continent and in the United Kingdom, is that where effective isolator systems can be created, and the integrity continuously demonstrated as sound, the surrounding environment for aseptic processing within the isolator can be controlled but unclassified. Some knowledge of the control achieved will be required, the particulate and microbiological challenge to the isolator system being the most significant. There will also have to be clear evidence of control of access and entry of people into the operating space. The level of information and data collected and judgements made are variable from authority to authority. It is the author's opinion and experience that it is appropriate to develop a surrounding environment capable of achieving a particulate classification of Grade D/Class 100,000/M 6.5 and a microbial environment of not greater than 500 colony forming units per cubic metre. This type of condition is not difficult to achieve, and would be similar to most good quality packaging departments. More demanding surrounding conditions of Grade C/Class 10,000/M 5.5 should be anticipated where negative pressure or low technology positive pressure isolators are used.

7. Operational Issues/Revenue Costs

The final remarks above allude to the other major advantage that most of us assume can be secured by placing an effective isolator within the minimum necessary surrounding environment. This is the cost of maintaining and managing the surrounding environment in conjunction with the critical internal environment. Significant reductions in effort and associated cost can be secured related to cleaning and disinfection, and monitoring of particulate and microbiological contamination alone. By removing the need to heat and cool vast quantities of air necessary for the maintenance of cleanliness or asepsis to satisfy the occupants, significant energy savings can also be achieved. Revenue costs associated with personnel control, particularly the changing of garments, are significantly reduced by both simplified space, reduced space sub-division and associated multiple changing and by the significantly lower level and quality of garment required is significantly lower than for traditional aseptic processing in cleanrooms. Energy costs are substantially higher in Europe than the U.S., and hence are of greater importance when reviewing revenue cost advantages and payback times.

5

Developing a Barrier/Isolator Implementation Plan

Didier Meyer
la Calhène
Vélizy, France

The development of parenteral technology has caused the pharmaceutical industry to take a closer look at product safety and the need to ensure sterility. These products bypass the natural defense mechanisms and need to be completely free of microbes to eliminate the potential for patient infection. In the early days product sterility was guaranteed by autoclaving, but as early as the beginning of this century, heat-sensitive vaccines and antiserum were developed and could not be autoclaved. The number of heat-sensitive products has continued to increase, and today over 80 percent of all sterile products are produced by aseptic processing, because they cannot be terminally sterilized. Some of these products are also cytotoxic and need to be contained to protect the operators.

Existing clean room technology has served us well, but there is need for improvement. Accumulated data indicate a correlation between microbial contamination and the presence of people in the work area (Whyte 1982, 1991). Thus, the presence of nonsterile particulates and the presence of people in clean-room facilities are still concerns for aseptic manufacturers (Whyte 1984; Luna 1986; Levchuk and Lord 1989).

Several technological developments have addressed these contamination issues (Olson and Groves 1987; PDA/PMA Sterilization Conference 1990). The glove box of the 1950s focused on the "people" issue, attempting to separate people from the operation. However, its awkward ergonomics and lack of sterilization capability created concerns.

High efficiency particulate air (HEPA) laminar flow addressed air filtration and control. Through the years, laminar airflow systems have achieved sufficient filtration efficiency for Class 10 conditions (less than 10 particles of 0.5 micron per square foot) to be met. Clean room technology has continued to evolve, and better training procedures continue to ensure operator knowledge of aseptic techniques. In spite of these efforts, contamination remains an issue, and people still account for most contamination problems. Current isolators can serve the needs of companies concerned with the manufacture of sterile products and potent biohazardous materials. These improved containment units offer better ergonomics and sterilization capabilities.

This chapter addresses the major considerations for planning the implementation of isolation technology. It covers possible applications, presents options for facility design and addresses issues related to budget estimation, project time frame, scheduling, documentation, and training requirements.

DEFINING THE APPLICATION

One of the most important considerations for outlining the implementation plan, is the definition of the application and specific user's needs. Different applications may call for different design, validation and implementation approaches.

Positive Pressure Isolators

Positive pressure is used to keep contamination from entering the work space within the isolator. Positive pressure isolators can be used in the laboratory or for production applications.

Sterility Testing

One of the very first applications of isolator technology in the pharmaceutical industry was the use of isolators in the Quality Control (QC) laboratory. The goal was to improve control of sterility testing and to avoid false positives. The QC laboratory continues to be a major user of this technology. The most common system configuration in this setting includes the following:

- A workstation isolator with one or two half-suits.
- One or several transfer isolators with gloves, connected to the workstation isolator through rapid transfer ports (RTPs).
- One sterilization system, such as the VHP®1000 (Vaporized Hydrogen Peroxide sterilizer) or equivalent, that can sterilize one or more isolators.

As an option, an autoclave connected to an isolator is located between the autoclave and the workstation isolator. This allows the autoclaved products to be transferred from the autoclave to the workstation, with no requirement for sterilizing the exterior surfaces of the products or materials. The process involved is discontinuous. Once sterilized, the workstation isolator is kept sterile for the validated period of time, and all the inputs and outputs are done through the appropriate transfer isolators or specialized RTPs. This can be done without compromising the integrity of the isolator.

This design can also be used for other batch operations, such as slow speed lines or manual filling operations, research and development, scale-up, or equivalent applications.

Powder/Liquid Filling

These processes can include either batch or continuous operations. A typical example of batch filling is the processing of small lots, typically as small as 1,000–2,000 vials and/or ampoules, used in Phase III clinical trials. In the case of biotechnology, samples can be as few as 10–20.

The following equipment is usually part of this type of facility:

- One filling isolator containing the filler and product components. Some operations employ manual filling, others use slow speed automated fillers.
- One oven isolator connected to the oven in which the vials and/or ampoules are sterilized and depyrogenated.
- One autoclave isolator connected to the autoclave in which the stoppers and all the heat-stable components can be sterilized. Sterilized goods can be stored in the workstation isolator until used.
- One freeze-dryer isolator connected to the freeze-dryer in which vials or ampoules can be lyophilized, if required.
- One sterilizer that can sterilize each of the isolators.
- One mobile ancillary isolator that interconnects the network of isolators.

Continuous filling of vials and open ampoules can also be done in isolators. This set up usually calls for automatic fillers, generally having an output between 6,000 and 20,000 units per hour. The filler isolator with gloves and/or half-suits, are often made of rigid construction materials such as stainless steel, Lexan®, or glass. The filling system generally includes the following in-line connections:

- One washing machine for vials or ampoules
- One sterilizing tunnel
- One cooling tunnel

To properly use the filler isolator, the following ancillary equipment should be included:

- One sterilization system to sterilize the filler isolator. In the case of a non-leaktight isolator it is not possible to use a gas loop system (like the VHP®1000) due to the risk of exposing the operator to H_2O_2 vapor in excess of the operator exposure level (OEL) limit. Alternatively, a spray system can be used. Sprayed disinfectants, such as H_2O_2 and Alcide, have been successfully used for this purpose in Europe.

- One or more RTPs in various configurations for the transfer of powder or liquid, for the setting of pumps, for the distribution of stoppers, or other support activities.

Medical Device Production

Some medical devices cannot be sterilized by ethylene oxide (ETO) or gamma radiation, particularly combination products that include drugs or biologicals. These are usually batch processes that may include the following equipment:

- One workstation isolator with gloves and/or half-suits.

- Two or more transfer isolators to allow the discontinuous introduction of one or more presterilized raw materials. If isolators are connected, no RTP is needed because transfer can be made without compromising the microbial integrity of the isolator. RTPs can be added if introduction is going to be made from a nonsterile environment.

- One workstation isolator can be connected to one or several output isolators to facilitate the process flow of kit assembling.

- One sterilization system that can be used to sterilize each isolator.

Negative Pressure Isolators for Nonsterile Operations

Negative pressure isolators are used to maintain containment. They keep biohazardous or potent material from exiting the contained work space, thus protecting the environment and the operator.

Protection of Environment/Operators (Containment)

The use of isolators in fine chemicals and compounding manufacturing has been driven by business and regulatory requirements to improve operator protection levels and make the handling of potent products safer.

In fine chemicals isolators can be used to protect the environment and people, while charging or discharging reactors or weighing products and/or reagents. RTPs allow for the safe transfer of materials since, by design, the alpha and beta door mechanism allows the separation of contained volumes with no risk for the operators or the environment. If the enclosure and the RTPs are properly designed, built, and maintained, the system will be leaktight, and the safe transfer of potent materials can be carried out. Thus, the whole process can be isolated from the outside environment and from the user.

In compounding operations, isolators are used for raw material testing, weighing, and mixing. Depending on the size of the operation, the isolators may include gloves or half-suits.

The use of rigid construction materials is more appropriate for negative pressure isolators because this type of construction can better withstand the physical stress of this environment. Flexible materials can be used, but require design adjustments to the external frame and supports so that enclosures do not collapse when the system is depressurized. Flexible construction is not recommended for this application.

Product Recovery in Containment

Expensive products, drug substances, or raw materials need to be entirely recovered. The design of the isolator must permit the recovery of all production material, and equipment must be specially suited for this requirement.

Explosion-Proof Applications

Isolators may also be a solution for facilities that have explosion-proof requirements. The reduced sizes of pumps, blowers, and other electrical equipment help minimize the potential for sparks and explosion. In addition, the volume of the isolator can be filled with inert gases instead of air, for a non-oxygen environment.

THROUGHPUT REQUIREMENTS

Another important consideration for design and implementation is the definition of required throughput. Successful implementation of isolators should not have a negative impact on productivity.

Manual Operations

Sterility testing in the QC laboratory is a good example of manual operation. Typical throughput per operator is 15 sterility tests/day. These are highly manipulative operations, but are also highly contained. The whole operation can be easily installed within one or two half-suit workstation isolators.

Automated Operations (See Figure 5.1)

The design of the isolator must not compromise the throughput of the filler, which is typically 6,000–20,000 vials or ampoules per hour. For nontoxic materials, sterility can be maintained with positive pressure. In addition, HEPA–filtered air can constantly flush sterile surfaces. Applications requiring containment and sterility are more complex to design and implement.

Slow speed lines are easier to enclose and control, but still require careful design. This can be illustrated by a biotechnology production where only 5 or 10 ml of a biologic, such as erythropoietin, is filled, half-capped, and freeze-dried.

High speed lines are more complex and present many challenges when they are connected to isolators. The complexity of design and controls is made more difficult if isolators are to be used in a multiproduct facility or for handling different container formats. To ensure adequate throughput, isolators should be designed to include transfer mechanisms that allow for the rapid ingress or egress of materials. "Mouse holes" or "open air locks" (small openings for the conveyor mechanism to allow exiting of vials), and the connection of autoclaves and mobile transfer isolators are examples of transfer mechanisms used to date. Transfer of materials continues to be the biggest challenge for high speed line applications. Manufacturers and users continue to address this challenge.

CUSTOMIZING ISOLATOR DESIGN

Isolation technology is an essential element in the protection of product, environment, and operators. During all stages of

Figure 5.1. Example of a liquid filling isolator system with automated filling machine. Isolator is of the rigid type. (Photo courtesy of La Calhene)

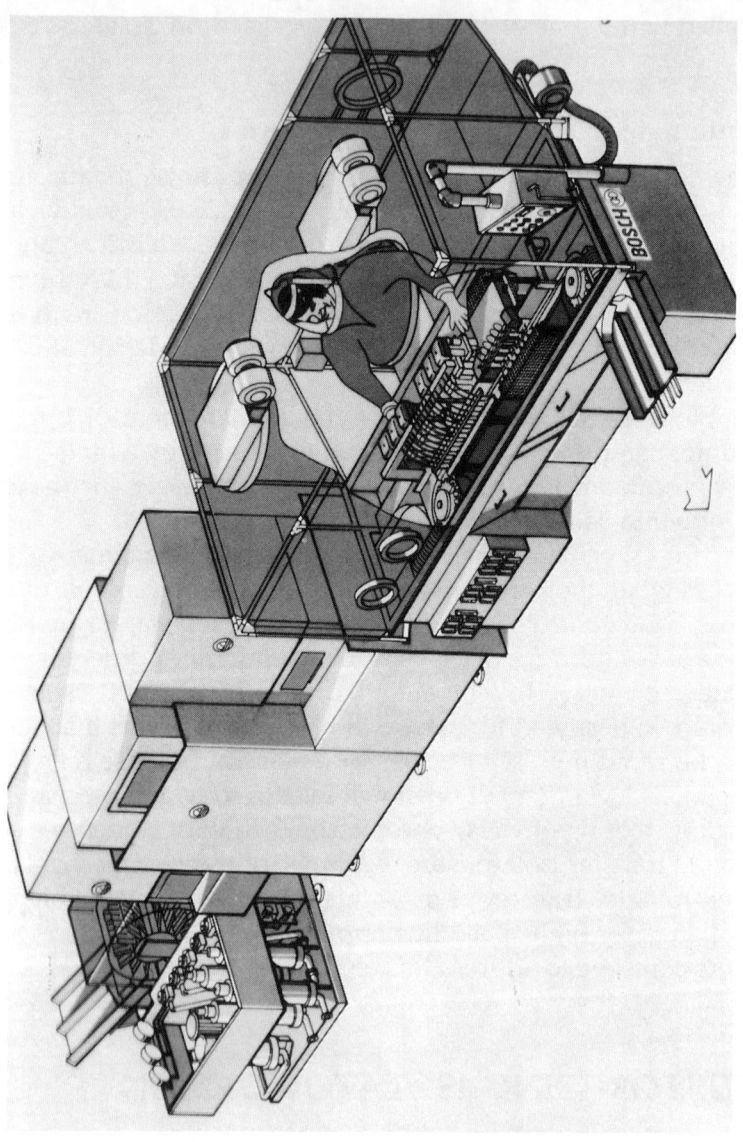

production—including mixing, filling, and/or final inspection—isolators can be effectively employed at critical points to ensure the absence of contamination. One of the benefits of isolation technology is the flexibility to customize the application (see Figure 5.2). An isolator reduces the controlled work space, limits air volume, and separates the operation from personnel and from the outside environment. This facilitates the control and monitoring of the work area.

The degree of complexity and the constraints associated with the application dictate how much flexibility and customization the user will need for the project. For example, the needs of a laboratory may be adequately served by off-the-shelf equipment that is usually less costly and more

Figure 5.2. Example of a customized isolator made of stainless steel and glass. The unit houses a high speed filling machine and has recirculating laminar airflow. (Photo courtesy of La Calhene)

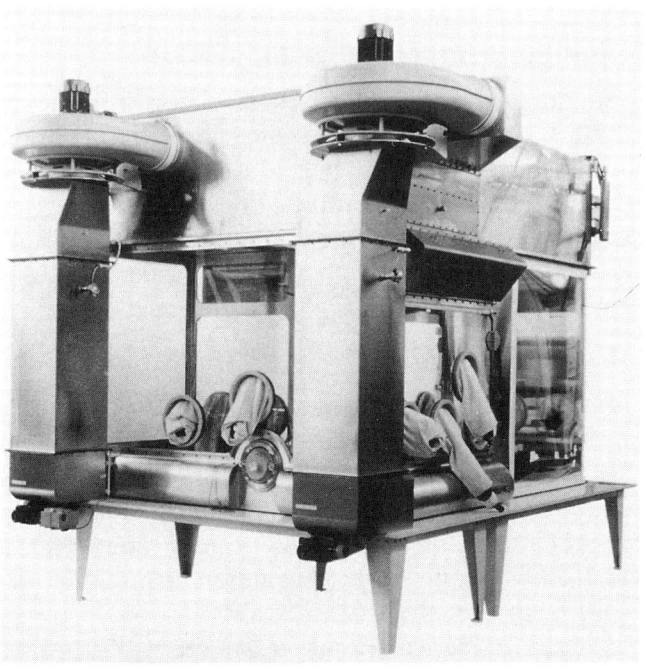

immediately available. On the other hand, a more complex production environment may call for more customization. Customized design may require minor changes to existing lines, or complete redesign of the filling equipment and enclosure.

Quality Control (QC) Laboratory—Sterility Testing Systems

Standard, off-the-shelf equipment is common in the QC laboratory. Most, if not all, QC isolators are installed in unclassified areas and use turbulent airflow. Minor customization, if needed, is often related to testing equipment. In the past users have reported difficulties with connecting test equipment and waste containers to the isolator. However, manufacturers of laboratory equipment are quickly making available new options that place mechanical parts and electronics outside the enclosure. Vendors continue to work with isolator manufacturers to ensure better compatibility of equipment with isolators.

Production Environment (See Figure 5.3)

The production environment offers more opportunities for the customization of equipment and enclosures. Here, line speed and required output should help determine how much customization is needed. For example, one must consider the different requirements for batch production versus continuous fill processes, and what kinds of changes are needed to accommodate the needs of each process.

Batch Processes (See Figure 5.4)

Slow speed lines and batch operations fit very well with the enclosing principles of isolators. In these operations one can easily go from closed system to closed system, taking full advantage of existing sophisticated transfer systems and all the benefits of controlling containment and sterility. Several European facilities have adapted isolation technology for batch processing. B. Braun Medical in Spain; Fasonut, Clintec, and KabiPharmacia in France are just a few examples of these applications. In the U.S. a small clinical production facility has been built, validated, and is currently in operation.

Figure 5.3. Isolator designs to fit different applications, including sterile toxic fill (negative pressure isolator), sterile fill (positive pressure isolator, and segregated fill of liquids, powders, and creams. (Diagram courtesy of Total Process Containment)

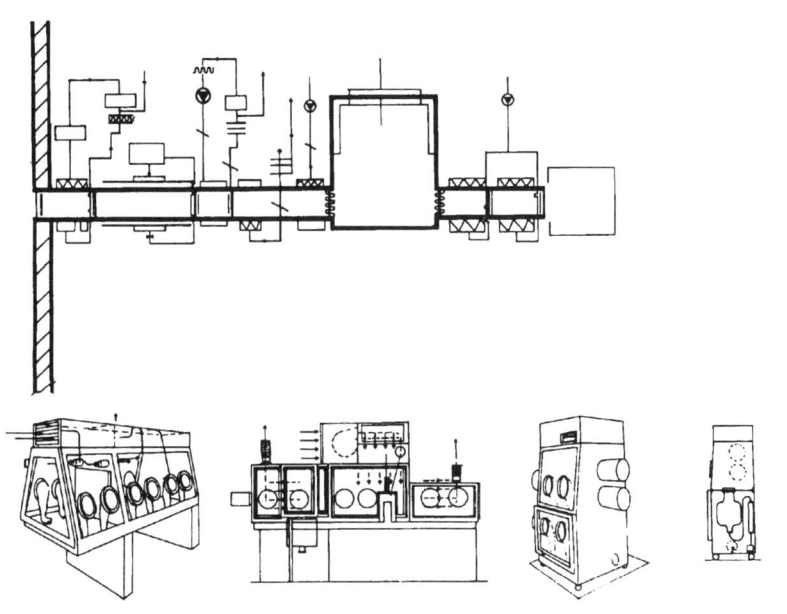

Isolators can also be used for bulk powder transfer, and weighing and compounding of potent materials. Again, several European and U.S. companies have taken advantage of this technology to improve operator and product safety. Examples include Roussel-Uclaf and Eli Lilly in France, and Eli Lilly and Bristol Meyers Squibb in the U.S.

Continuous Processes

Continuous processes offer many opportunities and challenges in the use of isolators. These systems cannot be completely sealed; thus, containment and sterility must depend on overpressure and air filtration/ventilation control. In addition, the design and monitoring of the input and output areas are critical to the maintenance of system integrity. In continuous processes the leaktightness of the whole system must be

Figure 5.4. Example of a customized isolator that can be used for batch filling processes or sterility testing. The isolator is made of glass and stainless steel, and is VHP compatible. It can also be adapted to have turbulent or laminar airflow. (Photo courtesy of Laminar Flow, Inc.)

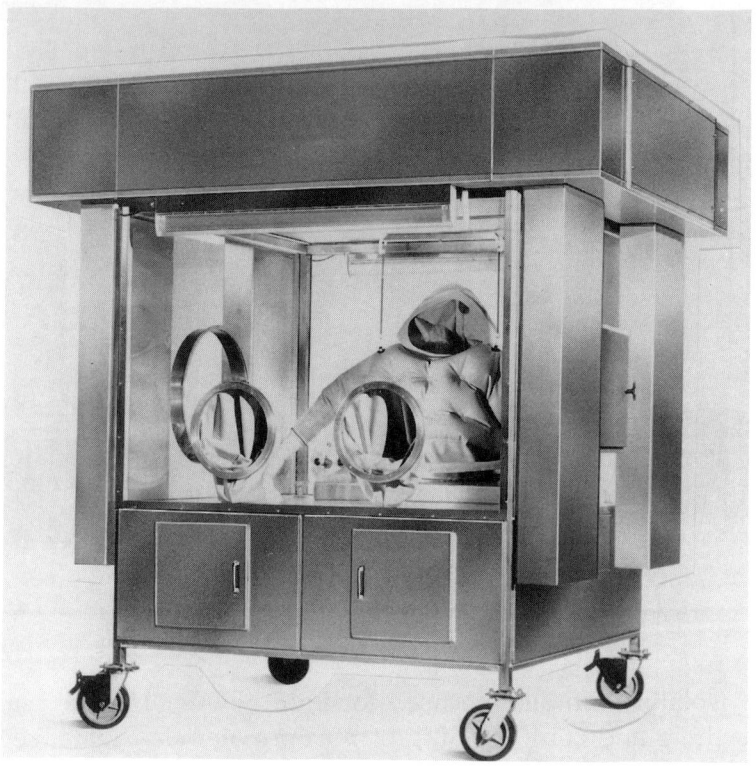

considered to ensure total system compatibility with the sterilization method.

Despite the greater complexity of these designs, many companies in Europe have implemented various applications. For example, Sandoz Pharm in France installed an open ampoule filling line in 1987 and another one in 1992. These lines contain the filling equipment connected to sterilization and cooling tunnels and to the washing apparatus. They have successfully filled more than 900 million ampoules with no contamination, in isolators housed in the equivalent of a Class 100,000 environment (Meyer and Gonzalez 1990).

Other Possible Applications

Isolators are particularly useful for applications requiring an anaerobic or other specialized atmosphere. For example, products that require low oxygen environments can easily be manufactured in an isolator. The design would require modification to allow for introduction of the desired gas and could also include modifications in the atmosphere exchange pattern.

ENGINEERING CONSIDERATIONS

Isolators can be installed in existing facilities or in newly designed and built areas. Specifications for the design of isolators should not be restrictive but should conform to some existing basic industry and regulatory expectations. Facilities must meet certain isolator installation requirements. Thus, they must be built or may need to be modified to ensure that rooms, electrical outlets, and compressed air and exhaust systems are adequate. One of the benefits of using isolation technology is the ease of moving isolators from one area to another to adapt to changes in business and facility needs (see Figure 5.5).

Existing Facilities

Existing facilities may or may not require extensive modifications to incorporate isolators. For example, sterility testing isolators can be installed in existing laboratory areas with minor or no modifications. The addition of outside exhaust to accommodate sterilization requirements may be all that is required to adapt a laboratory to isolators. On the other hand, production facilities may require more modifications to the room, equipment, utilities, and the isolator itself. The following basic design parameters should be considered:

- The siting of the isolator(s) should meet regulatory requirements. Users should be aware of conflicting information regarding regulatory expectations. Worldwide regulatory agencies should be contacted to ensure compliance.
- Temperature and humidity should be controlled, particularly if these systems use a vaporized sterilizing

Figure 5.5. Features of the installation of a system used for sterile filling. Schematic of integration of washing machine, the depyrogenation/sterilization tunnel, the autoclave, the pressure regulation unit, the isolator and filling machine, and the DPTE ports. (Diagram courtesy of La Calhene)

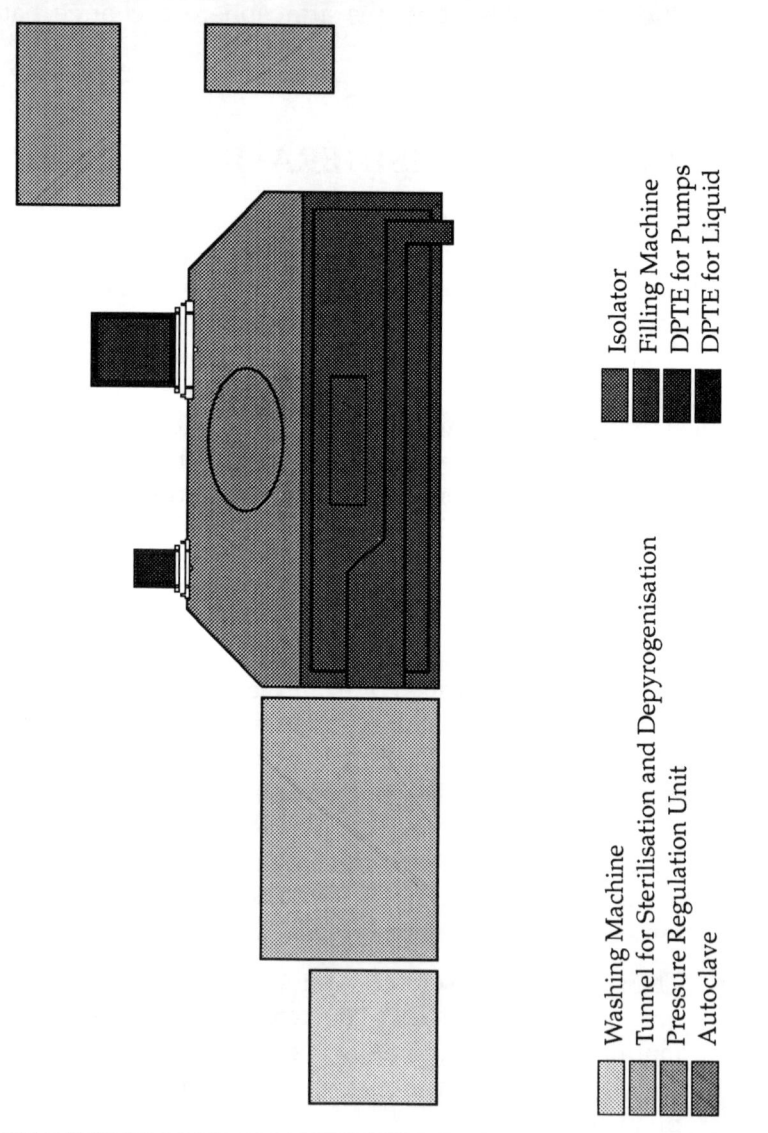

agent. Temperature control must take into account that both the washing machine and sterilizing tunnel are to be located in the same room as the isolator.

- The ventilation-filtration systems must serve only one isolator, and must include independent inlet and exhaust air systems. Air input can be unidirectional or turbulent flow.

- An ample number of electrical outlets should be strategically and conveniently located. To avoid hazards, electrical services can stem from the ceiling using twist connections. Ensure compatibility of outlet specifications with equipment requirements.

- Other utilities, such as compressed air and exhaust piping, should also match process requirements and specifications.

Production settings require that the following additional items be considered:

- Simplified gowning rooms can be used if Class 10,000 is not a requirement for the installation of isolators. This can reduce operation cost and save operator time.

- Floor drains should be considered if a clean-in-place (CIP) system will be used.

- The choice of transfer mechanisms is critical. Interlocked devices provide better security and are recommended. The size of the device should be sufficient to allow for the transfer of all equipment and materials. If the transfer device has its own air supply, it should be HEPA filtered. Openings such as "mouse holes" must be designed to ensure integrity of the process and maintenance of sterility.

- All internal areas and surfaces should be easily accessible to operators for routine work and cleaning.

- Construction materials should be resistant to corrosion and should withstand cleaning, disinfecting, and/or sterilization with gases.

- Pressure differentials should be such that if the sterile area is opened, contamination cannot pass into the controlled work area.

Newly Designed and Built Facilities

State-of-the-art design can be applied to the filler as well as the isolator. This presents an ideal opportunity to maximize the benefits of isolation technology. Some basic considerations include the following:

- Maintain or improve the original output of processing equipment.
- Build machines that are sterilant resistant.
- Include reliable transfer systems for liquid, stoppers, and other commodities.
- Include physical barriers between mechanical parts and isolators.
- Use a reproducible sterilization system and means to quantify sterilant.
- Include an automated monitoring/recording system to monitor critical parameters.

EQUIPMENT CONSIDERATIONS

Modifying Existing Equipment to Accept an Isolator

Retrofitting conventional equipment to an isolator environment requires special care. For example, when adapting filling machines to an isolator, it is necessary to ensure that the working bench of the filler fits leaktight. Whenever possible, the bench should be isolated from the mechanical parts, which are generally located beneath the working bench. Special care must be paid to the rotating parts. All materials of construction need to be compatible with the sterilant.

- The movements of operators should be studied, if possible, around a scale 1:1 mock-up.
- The safety of the operators versus moving parts and devices must be considered. For example, can a glove become caught in a moving belt?

- Ventilation-filtration has to be designed to meet laminar airflow (LAF) or engineered turbulent flow (ETF) specifications.
- Input of the sterile empty ampoules or vials must be done through a leaktight lock, such as a sterilizing tunnel connected to the isolator, to ensure maintenance of container sterility throughout the operation.
- The output of the filled ampoules or vials should be done through a protected air lock, such as "mouse holes" or buffered air volumes. In this case it is important to design the exiting system to maintain the integrity of the filling isolator and the sterility of the containers being processed.
- The supply of sterile stoppers for vials should be adequate for the filler.
- All necessary parts and equipment must be transferred within the filler isolator so that sterility may be maintained for at least one batch operation.
- All connections and exhaust systems for sterilization have to be predetermined to permit sterilization of the various subsystems within the isolator.

Modifications for Compatibility with Sterilization

- The inside of the isolator should be as smooth as possible, with round corners that will permit easy cleaning.
- The inlet and outlet of the VHP®1000 sterilizer, or equivalent system, must reach all parts of the isolator. If necessary, circulatory fans must be added inside the isolator to facilitate distribution of the sterilant.

In the retrofit of existing equipment or in the building of new systems, the end user, the filling equipment manufacturer, and the isolator manufacturer must cooperate to produce a workable system.

COORDINATION OF VENDOR EFFORTS

Successful implementation requires a well thought-out and thorough analysis of the application, budget restrictions, process limitations, and requirements early in the pre-engineering phase. Integration of vendor efforts is a must.

Engineers and manufacturers continue to work in partnership to ensure better compatibility of production equipment, sterilization systems, and isolators. Most filling machines currently available have not yet been adapted to isolators. A lack of experience in the area of isolation technology also presents challenges to many vendors used to the requirements of conventional clean rooms. To compensate for lack of experience, 1:1 scale mock-ups, plus blank production runs or, alternatively, computer simulations are recommended to help ensure accuracy of design details. Later in the project, the proper sequence of equipment delivery and installation will dictate how fast and how compatible the whole system will be. Some key considerations for successful vendor interaction are outlined below.

Preshipment Equipment Inspections

In most cases the filling equipment and the isolators are shipped to end users from several locations. Preshipment inspections should include, at a minimum:

- Isolator checks for leaktightness, HEPA filtration system(s), ventilation performance, particulate counting levels, and overall qualification of equipment according to user specifications.
- Testing of filling equipment, with qualitative and quantitative studies in a simulated production run including the washing, sterilizing, cooling, and filling of containers.

Assembly and Debugging

Equipment from the different vendors usually arrives on-site in modular format. Vendors should help with installation qualification and should be part of the assembly team, together with other highly trained individuals. Preferably, the assembly team should include people who were part of the design team and involved in the setting of specifications.

The container washer, the sterilizing tunnel, and the filler should be installed first. They should then be checked for functionality, together with all fluid utilities. Only after complete acceptance of these pieces of equipment should the isolators be assembled and tested. Leaktight testing must show that the filling system and the isolators fit correctly. A simulated, blank production run can demonstrate that the whole system reaches preestablished performance specifications and agrees with the observations documented during preshipment inspection. In general, it is more difficult to install and work with mechanical parts when using an isolator, than when using a stand-alone processing system.

Training of operation staff must be coordinated with vendors and must be included in the installation and validation program.

Implementation Time Frames—Lead Times

The projected time frame must allow for additional engineering and potential increase in validation time. The extent of the time increase will depend on the degree of customization, the amount of isolator experience within the team, and the thoroughness of the pre-engineering planning.

Delivery of isolators for a retrofitted facility could take 3 to 6 months, depending on the application. The planning and validation phases also need to be considered to calculate a complete time frame for the project. Bear in mind that it is usually harder to retrofit and make things fit than it is to plan and build from scratch. However, there will be some time savings since the need to wait for equipment and building a new facility will be significantly reduced.

The delivery time for most suppliers of automatic filling lines is between 6 and 12 months. Barrier system fabrication also requires 2–8 months, depending on the application and the number of isolators required for a given application. This time includes designing, constructing, testing, and assembling manuals and other equipment documentation for final delivery. The amount of care given to design and early evaluations will dictate the success of the system and the accuracy of the predicted time frame.

BUDGET CONSIDERATIONS

The following is an estimate of what it might cost to construct, engineer, equip, and validate an isolation system for aseptic filling. Publications and meeting presentations have reported a significant reduction in capital and operating cost. The user should keep in mind, however, that each situation is unique, and cost will vary depending on the application, level of customization of equipment, and other special requirements for each project. In some production applications capital expenses may actually increase.

Facility Costs

The budget estimates presented in Tables 5.1 and 5.2 assume a fill rate of approximately 5000–6000 vials/hr in an isolation system validated to a sterility assurance level greater than 10^{-3}, and perhaps as high as 10^{-6}. Approximate square footage is also given to provide a reference to your own target room sizes.

Equipment Cost

Equipment cost will vary. Customization could increase the cost by more than a million dollars. Expenses could amount to about $3.5 million for production equipment, including a modified (but not customized) filling line, sterilizer, stopper washer and associated isolators. The total investment cost would be about $4.8 million ($1,285,000 + $3,500,000).

The equipment cost for conventional clean rooms may be less because no modification of filling equipment is needed, and there is no expense with the purchase of isolators. The cost could be as low as $2.8 million. Keep in mind, however, that the overall savings and the reduction in operational cost will compensate for the potential extra cost of equipping the facility. The total expense for the clean room facility is calculated to be $5.0 million dollars.

In the above illustration a company using a clean room would save $245,000 in the initial facility investment.

Operational Cost

Operational cost will vary, depending on the unique features of the facility and the type of application. However, in most cases, the cost of operating a clean room is much higher than for

Table 5.1. Initial Capital Investment for Isolation Technology Facility (Updated from Czander 1994)

Area	Sq. Ft	Cost ($)
Gowning	220	$40,000
Degowning	120	25,000
Component Prep	1,500	300,000
Staging	1,100	210,000
Corridor	500	100,000
Fill Room	600	120,000
Vial Washing Room	900	140,000
Mechanical Room	4,000	350,000
Total:	8,940	$1,285,000

Table 5.2. Initial Capital Investment for Conventional Clean Room Facility

Area	Sq. Ft	Cost ($)
Gowning	225	$95,000
Degowning	150	45,000
Component Prep	1,500	300,000
Staging	1,100	500,000
Corridor	500	250,000
Fill Room	600	350,000
Vial Washing Room	900	140,000
Mechanical Room	6,000	550,000
Total:	10,975	$2,230,000

isolators. Savings are usually associated with a decrease in labor, utility cost, gowning expenses and maintenance of air filtration/ventilation equipment. The example provided by Czander (1994) illustrates these cost savings (Table 5.3).

Table 5.3. Operational Cost Comparisons[a,b]

	Cost	
	Clean Room	Isolation Technology
Labor (A)	$90,000	$60,000
Energy (B)	190,000	20,000
TOTAL:	$280,000	$80,000

[a] Based on 50% run time, labor cost addition due to difference in clean up and change over. Three (3) operators at $50,000/yr × % annual change overtime/25 shifts.

[b] Based on 60 air changes/hr with full HEPA filter ceiling in clean rooms. In Class 100,000, consider 20 air changes/hr.

This information is limited by necessity. Cost estimates are difficult because they may be based on assumptions that do not hold for all applications. Special requirements, reduction in overall labor, product quality improvements, and reduction in process failures are hard to quantify, but are, nevertheless, additional incentives for using isolation technology.

DOCUMENTATION

Documentation is an important part of any equipment/facility installation. Implementation of isolation systems requires the same care and attention that applies to the construction and implementation of other production facilities. In addition to the documents associated with the equipment (the same approach used for clean rooms applies here), the following documents should be available:

- A detailed description and drawings for the isolators and their connections to processing equipment.
- An explanation of the transfer systems and changes of the various spare parts.

- A list of the likely problems and potential solutions.
- SOPs that include, but are not limited to
  - Operation and maintenance of isolator(s)
  - Cleaning and sterilization procedures
  - Leak-testing procedures
  - Equipment/calibration schedule
  - Preventive maintenance and scheduling
  - Preparation and maintenance of biological indicators
  - Environmental monitoring
  - Sterility testing in isolators (if applicable)
  - Filling in isolators (if applicable)
  - Other process procedures adapted to isolators
  - Validation documents, including protocols

Quality Assurance should work with the manufacturer of the filling equipment and isolators to obtain operation and maintenance manuals for the equipment. Spare parts lists should also be supplied at the time of installation.

OPERATOR TRAINING

When an isolation system is to be implemented for the very first time, the operators should be involved from the beginning of the project, as much as possible. They will more readily acquire the necessary understanding and respect for the technology if they participate in all steps of the implementation program.

The manufacturer's audiovisual presentation and other training programs should include as many employees as possible. The presenter should emphasize the advantages of isolators regarding product quality and the operator comfort and freedom during the operation, compared to the constraints of gowning in the clean room. Operators must be instructed in various details of the systems. The final training should include step-by-step instruction according to in-house SOPs. Operators should also participate in sterility testing and/or media fill runs.

MONITORING

The main recording during production and off-hours is of the pressure in the isolator and the connected equipment. Each "open-lock chamber" for input and output must have an ongoing record of pressure or air flow speed. Particulate counting can also be monitored and recorded. These data provide an ongoing record of the status of the HEPA filters. The positive pressure within the barrier, relative to the room particulate counting in the final container, can also be a good indicator of filling line cleanliness. Automated recording instruments are available to assist with continuous monitoring of the isolation facility.

Microbiological monitoring of the air, surfaces, and gloves, and sterility testing on final products must be done as a matter of routine to ensure the ongoing efficacy of the isolation systems and sterilization process.

REGULATORY COMPLIANCE

The barrier system requires regulatory approval. Ideally, system design should be discussed with the appropriate regulatory authorities as early as possible to define the appropriate siting for the isolator. Other considerations include the following:

- The decontamination/sterilization system should be appropriate for the application and should be properly validated to satisfy the regulatory requirements.
- The system should be leaktight during the sterilization process, primarily if using a vaporized gas that may present safety problems for the operator.
- Upstream and downstream "open lock chambers" are monitored and can be closed.

- Operators must apply general safety rules.
- Install a monitoring system that constantly demonstrates that conditions are maintained and validated requirements exist throughout production.

CONCLUSION

Current industrial and regulatory needs dictate improved controls for contamination and containment. This chapter summarizes the decision-making process required to justify isolation technology. In the sterility testing application, the benefits are immediate, and experience easily supports the choice for isolators. In applications in the production environment, a more intense evaluation of the pros and cons of these containment systems is necessary. Isolation technology answers the regulatory requirements by addressing the following challenges:

- Reducing the size of the critical work area, facilitating its control
- Monitoring of the smaller encapsulated air volume
- Protecting the environment and the people

Isolation technology offers more flexibility for operators because of the less restrictive gowning requirements, capability for sterilization of the enclosed work area, and the potential for a lower operating cost. Isolation technology seems to be one of the best available solutions to answer the current challenges of aseptic processing. It may have been the best innovation in pharmaceutical processing during the last 30 years and may be the ideal solution for maintenance of containment and sterility in pharmaceuticals in the years to come.

REFERENCES

Czander, W., et al. 1994. New applications of containment technology in aseptic pharmaceutical operations. *Pharmaceutical Technology* 2:58–62.

Levchuk, J. W., and A. J. Lord. 1989. Personnel issues in aseptic processing. *BioPharm* 9:34–40.

Luna, C. J. 1986. Introducing people into the clean room. *Pharmaceutical Engineering* 6 (1):15–19.

Meyer, D., and J. P. Gonzalez. 1990. Advanced aseptic processing: Barrier system technology as applied to production filling lines. PDA/PMA Conference on Sterilization in the 1990s. Washington, DC.

Olson, W. P., and M. J. Groves, eds. *Aseptic pharmaceutical manufacturing: Technology for the 1990s.* Buffalo Grove, IL: Interpharm Press, Inc.

PDA/PMA 1990. *Sterilization in the 1990s.* Proceedings of the PDA/PMA conference, 26–29 August, in Washington, DC.

Whyte, W. 1984. The influence of clean room design on product contamination. *Journal of Parenteral Science and Technology* 38:103–108.

Whyte, W., ed. 1991. *Cleanroom design.* United Kingdom: John Wiley & Sons.

Whyte, W., et al. 1982. An evaluation of the routes of bacterial contamination occurring during aseptic pharmaceutical manufacturing. *Journal of Parenteral Science and Technology* 36:102–107.

Section II
Technology Implementation

6

Engineering and Project Management Issues for a Hydrogen Peroxide Sterilized Filling System

Leslie M. Edwards
James R. Rickloff
Advanced Barrier Concepts
Cary, NC

This chapter describes a typical project for the sterilization of a vial filling line using hydrogen peroxide gas. Along with project principles and concerns for managing new technology related projects, the question of whether to retrofit existing equipment or purchase a new system is addressed with a discussion of the related issues. A technical discussion follows regarding system design considerations, process control and documentation, and total sterilization cycle refinement, including strategies for accelerating enclosure preparation and hydrogen peroxide gas aeration.

COMMUNICATIONS AND PROJECT MANAGEMENT

As with any major project, proper management is critical for success. This principle is especially applicable to the implementation of new technologies, such as isolation systems and filling equipment. The typical project management model holds for the development process, with the major steps outlined in Table 6.1. Coordination of the major phases of the project differ from other projects in one major aspect, that is the education of all involved parties in the implementation of the new technologies.

Isolation technology and hydrogen peroxide gas sterilization are more than new methods for achieving results similar to previous systems. They represent a new paradigm from which many simple tasks require significant design efforts. Conversely, some previously difficult problems are solved simply and obviously by utilizing the basic characteristics of the system.

From many perspectives such as project management, engineering design, and often most important, support from senior management, strong education regarding the capabilities and limitations of the system are critical to the project's success and the longevity of the technology within the company. Too often, new technologies are introduced as panaceas to control costs and provide efficient new methods without regard for the difficulty and time required to implement the necessary changes and realize the new technology's benefits. Realistic goal setting and a keen awareness of the inherent difficulty in teaching a new paradigm will pay great dividends to a project manager who combines the necessary tasks of education, idea promotion and sales of a concept, communication, organization and coordination into the project management model.

The successful design of the filling system, including the component supply equipment and transfer systems is dependent upon the communication, cooperation and education of the various equipment vendors. A good example of this interaction is the design of a filling machine itself. The design philosophy behind an enclosed filler is dramatically different from that of a classic clean room model. "Gray-side maintenance systems" (those which place most of the utilities and motors outside of the filler), for instance, are a great advantage in an

Table 6.1. Major Steps for Project Management with an Isolation Filling Line

Step	Description
Needs Assessment	Identify basic goals of project including: production requirements, regulatory considerations, etc.
Customer Education	Learn the basic capabilities and limitations of isolation technology. Interview vendors and discuss basic needs.
Project Definition	Develop a general specification for the system defining the basic scope of the project.
Pre-Engineering Study	Develop a detailed specification and perform a basic feasibility study on various system approaches.
Request for Proposal (RFP)	From the specification and pre-engineering study results, develop a request for proposal and send to vendors for bid.
Proposal Evaluation	Evaluate the vendor proposals based upon the RFP as well as new ideas presented.
Selection of Primary Vendor(s)	Select a primary vendor who will manage either the entire project or two to three major sections.
Project Communication Meeting and Vendor Education	Set up a meeting to define the entire scope of the project to all vendors involved, including a detailed presentation of the necessary technolo-

Continued on next page.

Continued from previous page.

gies involved in the system to foster better communication and educate all vendors. Invite senior management of the client company to review the major system features and limitations as they relate to specific project goals.

Proposal Refinement, Project Scope Definition and Vendor Responsibilities

Obtain refined proposals from each vendor detailing the scope and responsibilities of each party.

Validation Strategy and Implementation Plan

Design a validation plan or outline prior to the system design. This will become the living document that forms the foundation for the validation testing to be performed during both the system development and after installation. Investment in this key component can easily save months of start-up and validation time after installation and result in more rapid line utilization. Schedule and outline regulatory events such as pre-construction review meetings and Establishment License Applications (ELA)—required for biologics.

System Design

Participate in the individual and overall system designs.

Prototype Fabrication and/or Ergonomic Modeling

Build a working or mock prototype of the system in preparation for a critical review of the system design. Consider computerized or other ergonomic models as appropriate.

Process Pretesting and Product Effects Simulations

Using either the prototype system or a laboratory test set-up, perform testing of the system

Continued on next page.

Continued from previous page.

        for product effects, including low-level sterilant residuals, product temperature extremes (due to steam-in-place of product path, etc.) or other process parameters which could affect the product.

Design Review and Refinement
        Perform a critical review of the system design and make refinements as necessary.

Fabrication
        Build the major system components.

System Integration
        Integrate components from various vendors and perform tests on the working system.

Installation
        Install the system in its final location and prepare for testing.

IQ/OQ/PQ
        Perform an Installation Qualification / Operational Qualification / and Performance Qualification.

Validation
        Complete validation testing with actual products to be manufactured. Submit any necessary regulatory paperwork, as required.

Training
        Train operational and support personnel in system operation, maintenance, and proper standard operating procedures (SOPs).

Implementation
        Implement the new technology into the production environment.

isolation filling line because they dramatically decrease the number of moving parts within the barrier, making the system easier to sterilize and maintain. Implementing such a design requires innovation and cooperation between the filling machine manufacturer and the isolation equipment vendor.

Another key member of the project team is the sterilization system vendor. This team member has expertise in the field of sterilization, and provides critical design information to the other vendors. Also, the sterilization system vendor possesses testing resources for the design of various system components, including material selection and pre-construction testing.

Often one or more key vendors takes a leadership role in the system design and is selected as the primary customer contact. Although paying a fee to one vendor to act as the primary contractor will increase the price of the system, the overall cost may be reduced due to an increased accountability placed upon the vendor and the decreased time required by the in-house project engineering staff. This is especially true for large multiple vendor projects which require many control and mechanical interfaces. A strong reason for one vendor to be generally responsible for the project is to assure that all interfaces are completed, without the juggling of multiple vendor responsibilities and the cost impact of project scope changes for individual vendors. The role of "systems integrator" for either a primary vendor or designated project manager must, therefore, be carefully assigned to a qualified and preferably experienced person with a clear view of overall system requirements and the ability to focus upon critical details. In addition, experience and/or support from a process and equipment validation perspective will pay heavy dividends during start-up and validation of the system.

RETROFITTING EXISTING EQUIPMENT VS. PURCHASING NEW EQUIPMENT

The decision to retrofit existing filling related equipment with an isolation system versus the purchase and design of a new system can be complex. Hidden costs of line downtime and start-up (including validation and regulatory agency licensing) of both new and retrofitted systems should not be minimized. Also, the level of isolation for a system may vary widely from placing rigid plastic walls and glove ports around a filling line and using a high-level disinfectant to a fully ergonomically designed filling system with sterilization and gray-side maintenance capabilities. If the goal is simply increasing sterility confidence levels within the system and there are no major economic benefits anticipated from facilities and operational savings from a stand-alone locally controlled environment sterile filling system, then a simple barrier which restricts operator access may increase sterility confidence levels over conventional aseptic filling lines appreciably. A summary of decision criteria is included in Figure 6.1.

Redesigning a system may affect its sterilization capabilities, line speed, and flexibility of use. Down time incurred during performance of an extensive retrofit may have a large impact upon the present production schedule. These extensive costs may affect the company revenue stream and must be considered in the overall evaluation of the project cost.

From a sterilization perspective, the primary factors for selecting either option (redesigning and retrofitting versus purchase and design of a new system) are process claims, material compatibility, design of the seals and mechanisms for ease of sterilization, and the acceptable total sterilization cycle time based upon system limitations. Existing systems will generally require extensive redesign in order to realize the full benefits of a sterile barrier system, unless they already employ gray-side maintenance methods or utilize clean-in-place (CIP) or steam- or sterilize-in-place (SIP) systems.

Before embarking upon such a path, a solid understanding of the following system design considerations (summarized in Table 6.2) should be achieved to appreciate the financial and operational sacrifices or gains realized by either selection. Troubleshooting, operator orientation, development of standard operating procedures (SOPs), system start-up and validation should not be minimized for either a retrofit or a newly designed system. Validation of major claims may pay the greatest dividends in operational savings, such as unclassed or minimally monitored exterior environments.

Figure 6.1. Decision criteria—Retrofit versus new system design

Establish and Prioritize Goals:
> Increase sterility assurance level (SAL) of product produced or sterility confidence level (SCL) of process
>
> Decrease clean room related costs (gowning, monitoring, etc.)
>
> Decrease facility space and utility requirements
>
> Increase line capacity
>
> Increase line utilization (uptime, productivity)
>
> Decrease manpower requirements and/or implement automation
>
> Contain pathogenic or dangerous compounds
>
> Add new products to new or existing lines without cross-contamination

Impacts of Changes:
> Process (re)validation
>
> FDA submittals and reviews (Establishment License Amendment—ELA for biologics)
>
> Downtime of existing line for retrofit (relate to current uptime and utilization only)
>
> Facility cost and utilization for new or existing retrofitted equipment
>
> Integration of related equipment (depyrogenation tunnel, stoppering, capping)

Technical Comparison for Feasibility:
> Material suitability
>
> Ergonomic suitability to barrier retrofit
>
> Maintenance access
>
> Seal and other containment capabilities and requirements

Continued on next page.

Continued from previous page.

    Control system appropriateness

    Line configuration

    SIP and CIP design constraints

System Options:
    Conventional aseptic processing (clean rooms)

    Restricted Access Barrier (RAB) systems (partial barrier systems)

    Total Barrier System

    High-level containment system

    Sterilization vs. high-level disinfection (e.g., H_2O_2, H_2O_2+steam vs. liquid HLDs)

Table 6.2. Major System Design Factors, Key Concepts and Considerations

Factor	Key Concepts and Considerations
Material Chemical Resistance	By utilizing hydrogen peroxide gas, most materials experience favorable reactions to the sterilant, although glove materials, seals, guides and most plastics should be tested by the sterilization system vendor in order to establish compatibility and anticipated replacement frequencies.
Material Surface Characteristics and Sterilization	In general, most materials should have a smooth finish to allow for easy access of a gaseous sterilant and cleaning agent. Porous, fibrous and cell structured materials may present a challenge to a gaseous or liquid sterilant by virtue of its requirement to penetrate layered inoculated spore challenges.

Continued on next page.

Continued from previous page.

Material Aeration
> The selection of material with regard to aeration is very important to the total cycle times achieved in the system. Glove ports, half-suits and many plastics may be convenient and easily available, but they may also require extensive aeration times and extend the overall sterilization cycle by many hours. Careful material selection and testing is recommended to optimize the system design.

Gas Distribution System
> Hydrogen peroxide gas may be distributed via a recirculated air stream (as in most Class 100 laminar flow systems) or may require the installation of small recirculating fans to evenly distribute the gas throughout the enclosure.

Air Handling System
> Auxiliary air handling systems can decrease the total sterilization cycle time by shortening the initial dehumidification time of the enclosure and speed aeration through more rapid removal or decomposition of the sterilant. The limit to the aeration is also dictated by the rate and extent of outgassing by absorptive materials within the enclosure.

Enclosure Volume
> The volume of the enclosure should be minimized in order to reduce the required sterilization time, maximize equipment accessibility and reduce air handling requirements.

Equipment Access
> Access requirements to equipment within the enclosure for adjustment should be minimized in the design, but within the design limitations are methods which may enhance system aera-

Continued on next page.

Continued from previous page.

tion, particularly the selection of gloves rather than half-suits, etc.

Automation/Control Systems
Control system should be appropriate for the application with proper tracking and documentation of key parameters. Include safety interlocks and independent emergency stops. Consider integrating control into a centralized supervisory control and monitoring system.

Seal Design
Seal designs must be appropriate for the particular application with containment of potent or pathogenic compounds having the most rigorous requirements. Realistic and applicable leak rates should be established in advance of design to contain the sterilant of choice for operator safety.

SYSTEM DESIGN CONSIDERATIONS

The ideal filling machine isolator design is usually a Class 100 (or better) unidirectional (sometimes laminar) flow system. Materials should be carefully selected and the design of the isolator and filling machine optimized to permit the effective sterilization of exposed surfaces. Only the active filling components and guides are located within the isolator; all other components are external for ease of servicing, in accordance with the "gray-side maintenance" design method described earlier. The design of a filling machine (either barrier or conventional) should minimize the number of moving parts in the sterile area and locate most of the major mechanical items below the deck of the filler (or behind the back wall plate when using a vertical drive system) leaving only the critical components in the sterile area. Sealing the deck at the mechanical interfaces presents an engineering challenge, but results in much simpler system sterilization (SIP), cleaning (CIP) and validation processes.

Material Selection

The selection of appropriate construction materials may be the most important design decision. It can impact total sterilization time and system performance. There are three basic criteria for material selection: chemical resistance to the sterilant, ability to be sterilized and extent of absorptivity of the sterilant.

Chemical resistance of most materials is quite good with hydrogen peroxide gas due to its relatively low chemical concentration in the gaseous phase (generally on the order of 500 to 2,000 ppm [0.05% to 0.20%] for most applications) while its efficacy as a sterilant is excellent at these low concentration levels. Certain materials, though, are susceptible to the oxidative/corrosive action of the sterilant, even at these low levels. Commonly affected items include most latex and neoprene gloves, some nylon products and natural rubbers. Generally, gloves will require replacement after as little as 1–4 weeks (depending upon frequency and duration of sterilization) while nylon products are generally restricted to near single use. Natural rubbers are to be avoided as sealing materials due to their poor chemical resistance, although many elastomers such as Viton® and Teflon® (PTFE) have demonstrated excellent long term material compatibility.

The ability to sterilize a material is generally dependent upon its physical configuration, both on a macro and microscopic scale. Most metals, elastomers, polymers and glass are easily sterilized, but cellulosic items (such as wood and paper products) should be avoided. Cellulosic products, when inoculated, tend to adsorb the spores and capture them within their mesh structure, thereby protecting them from some gaseous surface sterilization methods. Similarly, spores may be protected by layering upon one another on very rough surfaces, not allowing sterilant penetration.

Metals which oxidize readily (such as carbon steel) or other metals which catalytically decompose hydrogen peroxide must also be avoided within the system. AMSCO has performed some D-value comparison testing on various materials such as copper, brass and stainless steel and found their performance to be generally equivalent, even though copper and brass are well known catalysts for hydrogen peroxide decomposition. For cooling coils (and other piping in the system) avoid copper. Stainless steel is considered the metal of choice for most isolator components, where passivated 304 or 316L and glass are the materials of construction most often selected. Aluminum is sometimes used as a substitute for stainless steel in the cooling coils due to their location in the system (upstream of HEPA filters) and excellent chemical resistance to hydrogen peroxide gas after a very thin oxidation layer forms on its surface.

Absorption of hydrogen peroxide gas is a concern in many materials due to its impact upon the aeration time for the cycle. When hydrogen peroxide is absorbed into a plastic or elastomeric component during sterilization, significant time is generally required for the material to "outgas" or release the hydrogen peroxide so that it can be decomposed by the catalytic converter or carried away by the exhaust air system.

Major sources of absorption in a system include plastic or elastomeric filling line components, but more important are the isolator walls, half-suits, and gloves. At this writing, further development is required for the design or discovery of suitable materials to be used for gloves and half-suits that do not absorb significant quantities of hydrogen peroxide gas. Polycarbonate (Lexan®) walls were popular at first, but even when coated with other materials, significant absorption of hydrogen peroxide gas is still evident. To optimize total cycle times, glass and stainless steel wall construction is usually selected.

One design alternative could be to minimize the use of half-suits and gloves. An advantage of the glove over the half-suit is the glove's smaller surface area and lower total absorption, although half-suits offer an excellent range of motion. An alternative to gloves and half-suits is either manually actuated or automatic robotic arms. These can be constructed primarily of metal parts, thereby decreasing gaseous absorption. They have the added benefit of eliminating a glove which is generally susceptible to tearing or pin-hole leaks and widely considered a weak link in the entire isolation system. Depending upon the complexity of the robotic mechanism, though, a sleeve or bellows may be required to cover parts not sufficiently exposed during the sterilization cycle. Although some bellows no longer benefit the system from an aeration perspective, the weak-link of the glove integrity for sterility maintenance is eliminated and a major benefit is still realized. Unfortunately, robots are not always an attractive solution from a cost and maintenance perspective. If not sufficiently covered by bellows or sleeves, packings and lubricants can be contamination sources. Also added costs of automation include hardware and software development as well as computer validation.

Gas Distribution

Uniform gas distribution within the enclosure is very important for effective and repeatable sterilization. In laminar or unidirectional flow systems, which are most often utilized in a production environment with recirculated air flow, mixing of the hydrogen peroxide gas is generally excellent. This mixing yields a uniform gas distribution within the isolator, providing consistent kill in all areas. In some turbulent flow systems, the use of small recirculating fans within the enclosure to mix the gas is sometimes recommended in order to yield the desired uniform distribution.

Another technique for providing even gas distribution is the proper placement of the sterilant inlet and outlet ports. With the recirculation of the sterilant gas from the VHP®1000 hydrogen peroxide gas generator, small enclosures can often obtain excellent gas distribution without the aid of recirculation fans. Various configurations can yield good results, although often it is not possible to exactly predict the air flow patterns within the isolator prior to construction. Therefore, it is recommended that extra inlet and outlet ports be provided to allow for port location experimentation and optimization during cycle development.

Air Handling Requirements

The general air handling requirements within the isolator are most often dictated by the product requirements, but optimization of the sterilization process can also be achieved utilizing the capabilities of environmental controls within the barrier system. In general, the air handling system of the barrier or auxiliary air handling units can expedite dehumidification and aeration phases of the VHP®1000 sterilization cycle if rapid turn-around times are required.

Dehumidification of a small barrier may be quickly achieved by the VHP®1000 unit with its 20 standard cubic feet per minute (scfm) blower system, but for larger barriers, utilization of a desiccant drying system at 150 to 300 scfm or larger can significantly decrease dehumidification time. These (or similar) drying systems are also sometimes required for the isolator system itself in order to provide product fill conditions at low humidity levels (e.g., powder filling) or controlled oxygen environments where dry nitrogen or other inert gases are utilized for oxygen displacement.

For aeration, the air handling system can improve the total sterilization cycle time. A number of methods for enhancing aeration can range from direct exhaust of low-level hydrogen peroxide gas to the outside environment to catalytic breakdown of high levels of hydrogen peroxide using recirculating blowers and auxiliary catalytic converters (Figure 6.2). There is one major limitation to this method which is very important to note: the rate of outgassing from various plastics, elastomers and polymers in the system may not be significantly impacted by the use of an auxiliary air handling system. This could result in a system design which will aerate from 2,000 ppm down to the 5–10 ppm range very quickly (Figure 6.3), without significantly decreasing the time required to reach the desired residual level (the actual goal residual level may differ and will depend upon product effect testing and other factors).

Door, Seal, and Equipment Interface Designs

By far the most challenging aspect of isolation equipment design is the door, seal, and interface designs between major system components, including transfer systems discussed in the next section. The challenge is to build a door which can easily be opened during equipment operation and closed to allow for cleaning, sterilization, and leak testing of separate system segments. The Eagle 3000 SL series sliding door steam sterilizers (AMSCO) combined with autoclave interface isolators, utilize a moving door design which operates during the VHP®1000 sterilization cycle. This method insures the maximum exposure of all the door gaskets and mechanical actuators (e.g., pulleys, cables and gears) to the VHP®1000 hydrogen peroxide gaseous sterilant. A communication cable and software

Figure 6.2. Isolation filling line drawing utilizing external catalytic converters to enhance aeration. First drawing (above) shows converter placed in the facility exhaust while the second (below) utilizes an independent air handling unit in a closed-loop configuration (no outside air exchange required).

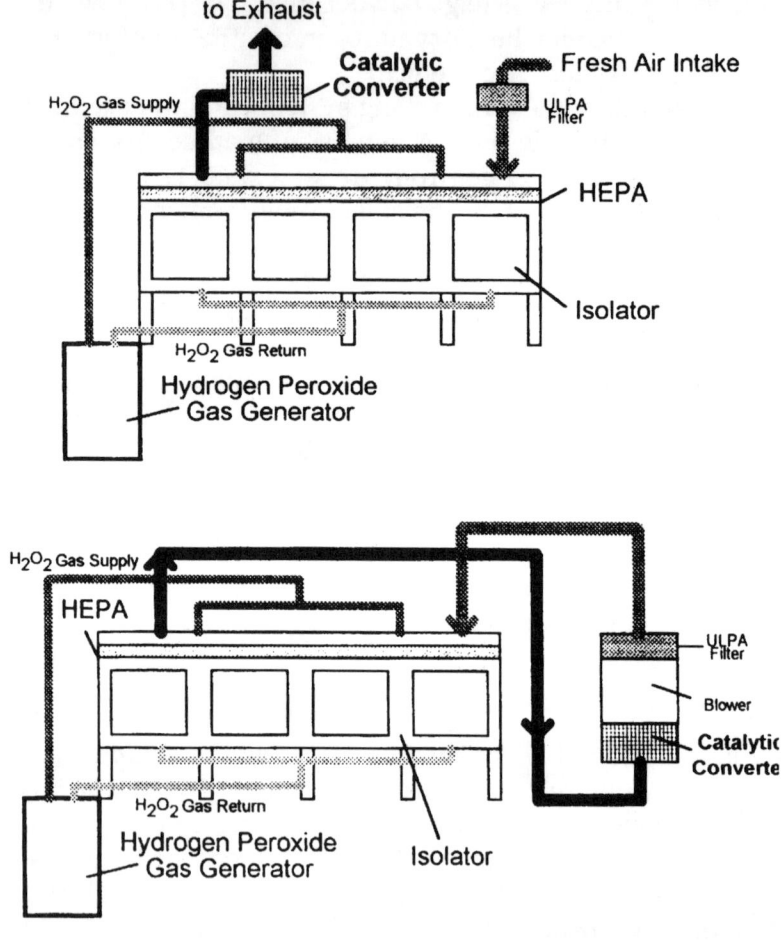

interface has been designed in this system in order to insure repeatability and detect potential errors during the cycle.

Interfaces within a filling line may be less complex than that described above, but the two main challenges remain: to

Figure 6.3. Hydrogen peroxide gas concentration in an isolator containing absorptive versus nonabsorptive materials. Concentration shown is during the aeration phase.

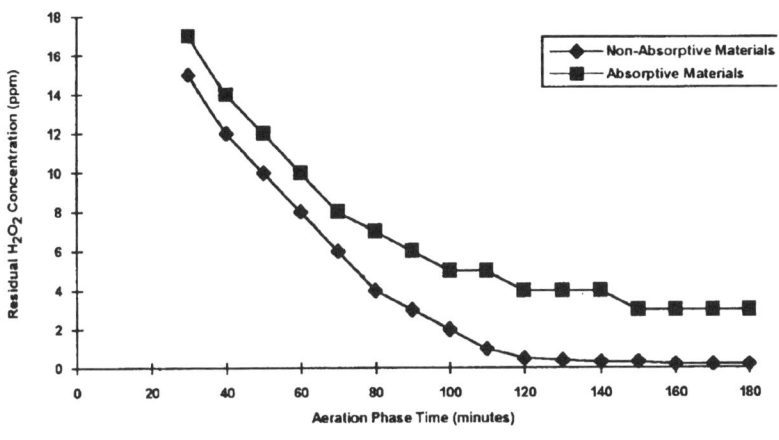

sterilize the door in the closed and sealed position to prevent the escape of hydrogen peroxide gas, and to sterilize the unexposed surfaces of the door seal. A simple (but incomplete) answer to this challenge is to sterilize all outer doors (those interfacing with uncontrolled, non-sterile environments) in the closed position and all inner doors (between areas to be sterilized in tandem) in the open position. Problems arise, though, when a sterile, enclosed area that is not intended to be hydrogen peroxide gas sterilized is connected with one that is, such as when a depyrogenation tunnel is attached to an infeed belt or accumulator table isolator (Figure 6.4). Here, if the door is left in the open position, the hydrogen peroxide gas will enter into the depyrogenation tunnel and may escape to atmosphere via the tunnel's exhaust system or inappropriately dilute the sterilant in the system. If left closed, the door seal will not be sterilized, which may lead to vial contamination because the cooling zone may not be sterilized.

One solution is to install a secondary sterilization modality for the door seal itself, in the form of a high temperature heating element within the seal. Another solution is to install a temporary outer door on the depyrogenation tunnel side and leave the standard door open with the seals exposed to hydrogen

Figure 6.4. Block diagram of a typical isolator filling system, including: (a) depryogenation tunnel, (b) tunnel outfeed (or accumulator), (c) vial infeed, (d) filling section, (e) stoppering module, (f) capping station, and (g) UV transfer system.

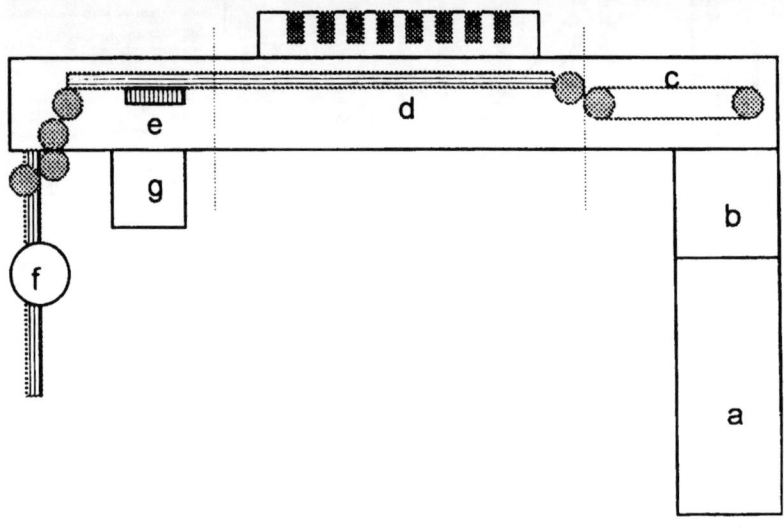

peroxide gas during the sterilization cycle. After sterilization, the standard door could be closed and the temporary outer door removed. The latter solution using a temporary outer door could also be utilized for an interface which may have interchangeable profile doors for different size vials or product containers used during a fill. The door could be removed for each sterilization, a temporary outer door installed, and any one of many profile doors could be introduced via a rapid transfer port (RTP) system and installed.

Transfer Systems

The sterile transfer of liquids, gases, mechanical parts and sterile components is a major challenge within and between isolation systems. Certain standard methods, including RTP canisters (also known as beta containers in an alpha/beta double door system) provide an excellent means for material transfer from one isolator to another and from sterile containers to isolators. The principle relies upon the integrity of a triple-lip gasket which effectively seals the two non-sterile side of two doors together and creates a single door with two sterile sides through which items may be transferred without risk of contamination. From a practical perspective, this seal is quite effective, but its effectiveness when relied upon for direct product and sterile component contact has not been proven unequivocally. A conservative approach has been adopted by many in the advanced aseptic manufacturing environment which utilizes bagged component transfers over the seals or the use of a sterile inner ring which is placed over the inner door seal to reduce the chance of microbial contamination (Figure 6.5). Other processes are being developed to provide an actual sterile seal, via dry heat after the docking process occurs and before the transfer is made.

Figure 6.5. Photograph of a dry heat sterilizable transfer port with a protective inner ring. (Photo courtesy of Central Research Laboratories, Red Wing, MN)

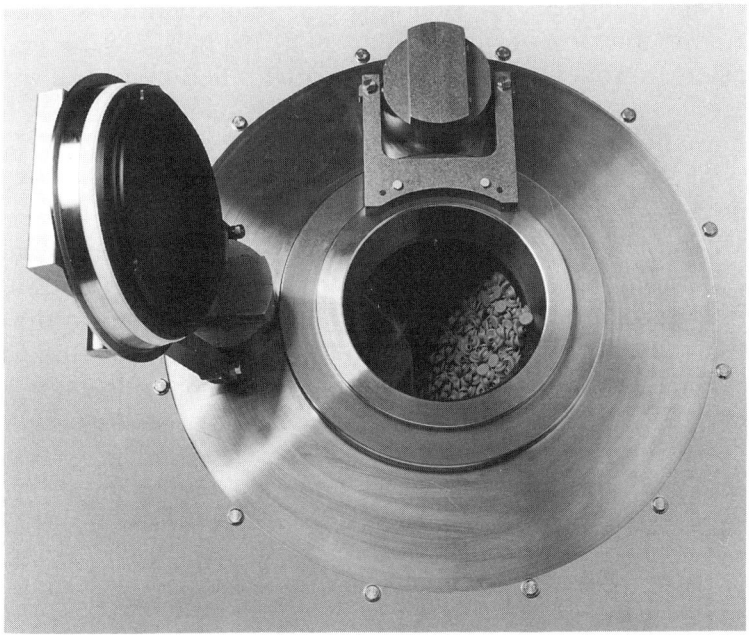

Gas and liquid transfers using the RTP system have a history of success for filling applications. The transfer of gases in and out of the barrier is a matter of providing the proper microbial filter and utilizing gas hookups and sterile tubing transferred into the barrier via the RTP. Liquid transfers can be achieved utilizing a modified RTP canister which allows for the sterilization (usually via steam autoclave or by SIP of the tubing and connections. Once the RTP canister is docked, sterile connections can easily be made in the isolation system.

Automation/Control Systems

Throughout the multiple machine system are many control systems which require various levels of integration. Certain manual operations such as docking of rapid transfer ports, tray loading and unloading, stopper handling, or other processes may be automated for ease of operator use and safety.

As a minimum, the control systems of the isolator, sterilization system, filling machine and any auxiliary air handling units should be integrated with common emergency stop buttons and interlocks for standard operating conditions. These can be in the form of simple "status OK" signals sent from one master control system or complete integration of control software. The latter is obviously a major investment, but it may be required in order to comply with the general control philosophy of the pharmaceutical company and its central production supervisory control system.

Generally, isolators are constructed with either "manual" electronic switching, a PC based computer control or common PLC based control systems. The sterilization system can either be an independent control (such as that with the AMSCO VHP®1000 control system) or integrated with the isolator (in alternative systems such as steam/hydrogen peroxide equipment). The AMSCO VHP®1000 includes a flexible input/output signal capability which can send and receive signals for triggering cycle abort conditions, valve and damper actuation, isolator pressure control, and general "status OK" signals for various cycle phases or conditions. In future generations of hydrogen peroxide sterilization products, it is anticipated that popular PLC controllers and interfaces may be included.

The filling apparatus and conveyor system is usually operated (without product or vials) during sterilization to assure that more parts are exposed to the sterilant vapors. In order to determine the necessary total exposure time requirements for the sterilant, perform a review of the filling system dynamics and predicted sterilant exposure times to insure that all critical surfaces receive the minimum required sterilant dosage to provide the desired sterility assurance level. This may require an extension of the sterilization exposure time beyond the normal requirement or system or component redesign in order to expose hidden or minimally exposed surfaces.

Control System and Parametric Documentation

The control systems of each system component must be capable of accurately and efficiently documenting the process for compliance with cGMP guidelines. Some systems allow for downloading of batch and sterilization system information onto electronic media in order to reduce paperwork.

The major items to be recorded are the critical cycle parameters during sterilization (sterilant injection rate, airflow rate, time, relative humidity, and process temperatures). During normal operation of the filling system and barrier, usually the system pressure (positive for standard applications or negative for containment fills with toxic materials) must not be held within rigid limits, except for those related to breach of containment and maintenance of sterility (the latter requiring only minimal positive pressure in most applications). In addition, the standard requirements for operation of the filling machine and other major system components should be documented.

Aeration Strategies and Considerations

The key factors for setting aeration goals are worker safety and product effect. Aeration of an enclosure to the point of an undetectable level of a sterilant such as hydrogen peroxide can be a challenging task, but may not always be a necessary goal. The Occupational Safety and Health Administration (OSHA) dictates that a safe human exposure to hydrogen peroxide must be limited to no more than 1 ppm (part per million) over an eight hour time weighted average (TWA). Because of this TWA and the general design of a barrier, human exposure is a concern, but it is generally not difficult to obtain or surpass most safety goals set for the worker.

The key point then becomes product contamination and effect. In the gaseous state, hydrogen peroxide has limited stability and readily decomposes into water and oxygen. Working against this decomposition is a new supply of hydrogen peroxide outgassing from various plastic and elastomeric components. This outgassing may extend the aeration process by several hours, emphasizing the importance of material selection in the initial system design.

The question remains, "What level of hydrogen peroxide gas can be exposed to the product without any detrimental effects?" Obviously, there is no direct answer to this question, but some general considerations may yield encouraging results. First, the level of hydrogen peroxide actually obtained during the fill can be measured with assays of various water filled vials (however, after aeration, the hydrogen peroxide level is likely to be 0.1 ppm or less). Using a xylenol orange or other spectrophotometric assay, these low-levels of hydrogen peroxide, if present, can be detected. If components are sterilized with hydrogen peroxide gas, then they can also be tested separately for residuals by an aqueous extraction technique, or can be tested as part of the previously mentioned water fill to determine the source of hydrogen peroxide infiltration.

Second, if glass vials or syringes are filled using polymer-free stainless steel filling equipment sterilized by SIP, then hydrogen peroxide will be present in the product samples in extremely low, or usually undetectable levels, because no absorption will have taken place and total aeration will have been achieved. These data can be used to determine the requirement for product effects testing.

Product effects testing should take place very early in the development of the project. Although it may seem a very early time to begin aeration studies before a system is even built, this action could be the critical point which allows a process change to be well documented and facility licensing rapidly obtained. The major reason for the product effects testing is to eliminate any doubt that residuals from the sterilization process have no detrimental effects on product stability, potency or efficacy over the long-term. Usually, a six to twelve month accelerated stability test will provide the necessary documentation and scientific evidence. Because the time required for the test is so long, one may ask how it can be achieved for a process which has yet to be developed. Simply stated, a prototype or test system may easily and inexpensively be developed which can simulate worst case conditions for the production system and allow validation off line, or at least supply a preponderance of scientific evidence to support claims made by shorter term testing on the actual production system.

CONCLUSIONS AND FUTURE TRENDS IN ISOLATOR DESIGN AND STERILIZATION

Over the next few decades, isolation technology and hydrogen peroxide gas sterilization will be widely introduced to new areas of aseptic manufacturing, research laboratories, quality control testing, and eventually health care centers where they can provide sterile environments for application of direct patient treatments or hospital pharmaceutical handling. The major advantage of isolation technology is the biological removal of the chief source of product contamination, the human. Hydrogen peroxide gas is a sterilant with excellent material compatibility, efficacy, safety, and environmental aspects. New applications for these technologies will be forthcoming through additional education about, and acceptance of, both technologies. Also, automation will play a major role in the future of advanced aseptic processing from simple interfaces and controls of sterile environments to complex product handling and transfer systems.

In addition to the continued establishment of hydrogen peroxide gas as a leading sterilant of enclosures, the other technologies mentioned such as steam/hydrogen peroxide and various liquid sterilant systems are experiencing growth. New transfer systems are presently being developed and refined using ultraviolet (UV) light pass though chambers, dry heat and steam sterilization of seals for RTP systems and integrating other sterilization modalities such as gamma irradiation of beta RTP canisters into the barrier filling systems. Many other methods are sure to be introduced and refined for easier and more rapid transfer of products to and from the sterile barrier system. More specifically, in the areas of aseptic manufacturing, refinements to the hydrogen peroxide gas sterilization process will allow for shorter exposure times and more rapid aeration of systems, either through enhanced temperature control, improved air handling systems or other means yet to be developed.

Construction materials for the isolation system present limitations to the chemical sterilization of enclosures due to their absorptive nature. In particular, glove and half-suit materials, wall construction materials, and seal development will be major areas of development. Attempts have already been made to discover appropriate coatings for plastic walls (which would allow the use of less expensive and easier to machine polycarbonate and other plastics versus glass) and many glove manufacturers are attempting to utilize puncture and tear resistant materials.

There are sure to be advancements in monitoring technologies available for hydrogen peroxide gas systems to allow tracking and documentation of sterilant gas concentrations within the enclosures, leading to an eventual parametric validation of the process, without a reliance upon extensive biological indicator validation. From a safety perspective, personnel monitoring devices such as those used for radiation safety may become available to detect and warn users of potential over exposure in addition to the automated methods presently available (although personnel are generally absent during sterilization). Improved aeration methods utilizing larger capacity generators for hydrogen peroxide gas sterilization and improved air handling systems will allow for the sterilization of much larger enclosures and more rapid total sterilization cycles for present applications.

Hydrogen peroxide gas and isolation systems will continue to provide improvements to sterile pharmaceutical processing and research applications worldwide. These advanced systems are an important step forward for the processing and delivery of safe and effective pharmaceutical products to patients as well as high quality research and development.

7

Modern Trends in Isolator Sterilization

James R. Rickloff
Leslie M. Edwards
Advanced Barrier Concepts
Cary, NC

The literature is replete with scientific evidence on the antimicrobial properties of various physical and chemical agents. This chapter will not attempt to compare the germicidal activity of these agents from the literature because of the differences in test conditions, concentrations or dosages applied, temperatures, and microorganisms used in those studies. The comments in this chapter will be directed toward the methodology involved in applying these agents to isolators and the advantages and limitations associated with each. In addition to historical data, a brief discussion of isolator sterilization processes currently under development will be provided.

The importance of choosing a disinfection or sterilization process in the early stages of custom isolator development will be touched upon during the discussion on the use of hydrogen peroxide (H_2O_2) gas. Much of the information is relevant toward other antimicrobial agents as well. Since isolators typically operate at or near ambient conditions, necessitating the use of either liquid or gaseous chemical germicides, several classical sterilization methods such as steam under pressure, ethylene oxide, and ionizing radiation will not be discussed.

TERMINOLOGY OF ANTIMICROBIAL ACTION

The terms *sterilization, disinfection, decontamination,* and *sanitization* have been defined and accepted for many years (Block 1991; Vesley and Lauer 1986). However, confusion still exists because the terms are commonly misused. Sterilization is defined as a physical or chemical process capable of destroying all microbial life, including bacterial spores. Disinfection eliminates virtually all recognized pathogens on inanimate objects, but not necessarily bacterial spores. Some disinfectants possess sporicidal properties, but only after extended contact times. Decontamination describes a process that renders an object safe to handle. Sanitization refers to a decontamination process which reduces viable contamination to a defined acceptance level. This process can range from a simple cleaning to the application of a sterilant—the choice of which depends upon the type of bioburden present and/or the intended use of the object being treated. Each of these processes can and will be applied to isolators, but one should exercise caution in making claims that specific antimicrobial processes may be unable to achieve.

ANTIMICROBIAL AGENTS USED IN ISOLATORS

Performing sterility tests, within isolators, on pharmacopeial articles purporting to be sterile has gained wide acceptance over the last decade. This is because the system isolates the primary source of contamination, the human, from the test area. A second reason is that, in an isolator, extraneous bioburden within the isolators and on the external surfaces of articles under test can be eliminated with aerosolized or vapor-phase agents, such as peracetic acid or H_2O_2.

The following sections briefly describe some of the more popular germicides used with isolators today along with those currently under development. Material compatibility, safety and environmental issues will also be discussed for some of the more commonly used germicides.

Peracetic Acid

This compound is a mixture of known percentages of acetic acid, sulfuric acid, water, and H_2O_2. The use concentration in the aqueous form is between 3.5 and 4.0 percent (w/v). The sporicidal properties of the aqueous and vapor forms of peracetic acid have been well documented although the aerosolized liquid is preferred for sterility test isolators because sporicidal levels can be attained faster (Baldry 1983; Block 1991; Portner and Hoffman 1968). The aerosol distributes itself naturally without the need for recirculation fans, is easy to use, and is relatively safe (Thorogood 1993). A typical peracetic acid spray system is depicted in Figure 7.1.

Although applied to germ free animal isolators in the United States for over 30 years, peracetic acid usage in sterility test isolators did not appear until the 1980s. Davenport (1989) provided a thorough review on the application of a peracetic acid spray for sterilizing sterility test isolators at the Upjohn Company in Kalamazoo, MI. Table 7.1 lists the sterilization cycle parameters recommended for different isolator configurations tested with 10^3 *Bacillus circulans* spores (UC 9951) per carrier. A rationale was provided for the use of the 10^3 spore titer on the carriers. The author concluded that this method could be performed under controlled conditions and was capable of producing a high degree of sterility assurance, eliminating false positive sterility test results.

Chlorine Dioxide

A sodium chlorite base with organic acid activator that can produce a sporicidal chlorine dioxide (ClO_2) solution at ambient temperature (Alcide Corp., Norwalk, CT) is commercially

Figure 7.1. Peracetic acid spray apparatus.

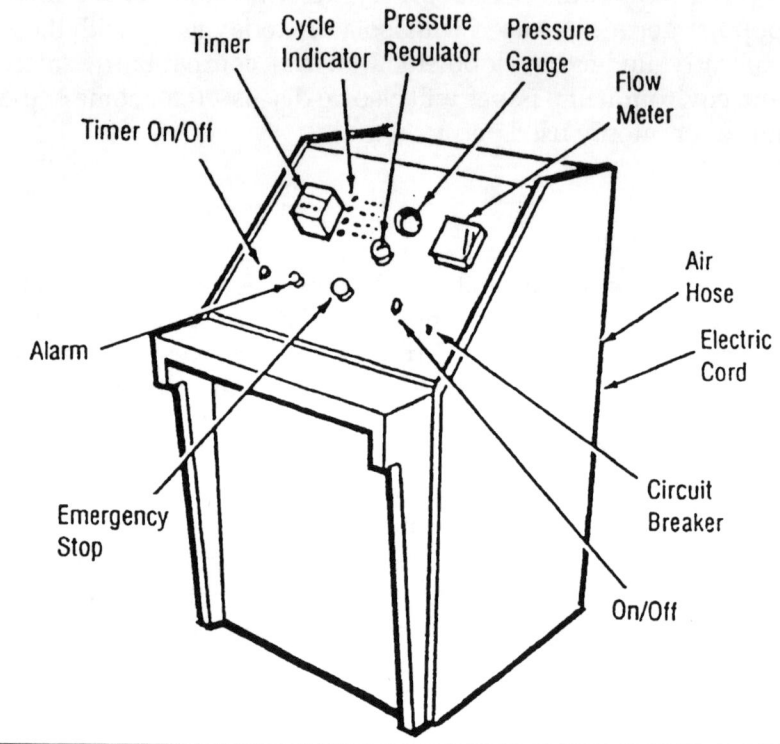

available. The solution is typically mixed and diluted to the use concentration immediately prior to use.

Chlorine dioxide has been applied with hand sprayers to flexible film isolators for the containment of germ-free animals. Production applications have involved the use of atomizers similar to the one shown in Figure 7.1. There is limited information on ClO_2 use in sterility test isolators although a Sandoz facility in France has validated on an isolated filling line that uses ClO_2 to sanitize the isolators prior to use (Gonzalez and Meyer 1990). A 15-minute spraying period (360 ml) is followed by a 3-hour exposure and 2-hour aeration. Glass carriers inoculated with 10^6 *B. subtilis* var. *niger* spores were used during the sterilization validation studies. The aeration period was shown to reduce chlorine levels (ClO_2 disassociates into chlorine) to less than 2 ppm. Information on the significance of these residue levels was not reported.

Table 7.1. Peracetic Acid Spray Cycle Parameters Used for Empty Chamber and Product Container Validation Studies at the Upjohn Company in Kalamazoo, MI (Davenport 1989)

Sterility Test Isolator Description	Volume of 4% Sterilant, ml	Phase Time, min		
		Spraying	Dwell	Aerate[a]
113 ft^3 Incubator	400	16	60	360
113 ft^3 Interface	400	16	60	360
152 ft^3 Workstation	400	16	60	360
32 ft^3 Transfer	150	10	60	360
Product in Transfer[b]	300	15	60	360

[a]outside exhaust at not less than 360 minutes
[b]peracetic acid with 0.1% Nacconal (surfactant)

Inactivation rates for ClO_2 decrease slightly when the solution is aerosolized or vaporized, but sterilization times for 10^6 *B. subtilis* spores per carrier were still within 30 minutes (Wallace et al. 1988). Jeng and Woodworth (1990) reported that ClO_2 gas sterilization times in a glove box depend on gas concentration and the level of pre-humidification. The gas was prepared by passing a 3–5 percent chlorine/air mixture through a column of sodium chlorite chips. Gas distribution throughout the glove box was accomplished with the use of a fan. Sterilization times for carriers inoculated with 10^6 *B. subtilis* var. *niger* spores (ATCC 9372) were within 30 minutes when the isolator atmosphere was pre-humidified and exposed to at least 6–7 mg ClO_2/liter at ambient temperature. Aeration times were not discussed since the glove box was used only as a research test vessel for determining kill times.

Hydrogen Peroxide

Hydrogen peroxide gas is produced by flash vaporizing a 31 percent (w/v) aqueous solution into a carrier gas (warm, dry air) which then is delivered to a sealed enclosure. The VHP®1000 Biodecontamination System (AMSCO, Apex, NC) automates this process. The VHP®1000 controls and documents all key parameters to ensure a consistent, reproducible cycle (Figure 7.2). The system can dehumidify, condition, sterilize, and aerate (typical cycle phases) enclosures with internal volumes of between 10 and 1500 ft^3. It can be interfaced electrically to auxiliary dehumidification and aeration systems if desired.

The VHP®1000 operates in a closed loop to maintain a slight positive pressure within an isolator during the cycle

Figure 7.2. Schematic of VHP®1000 Biodecontamination System.

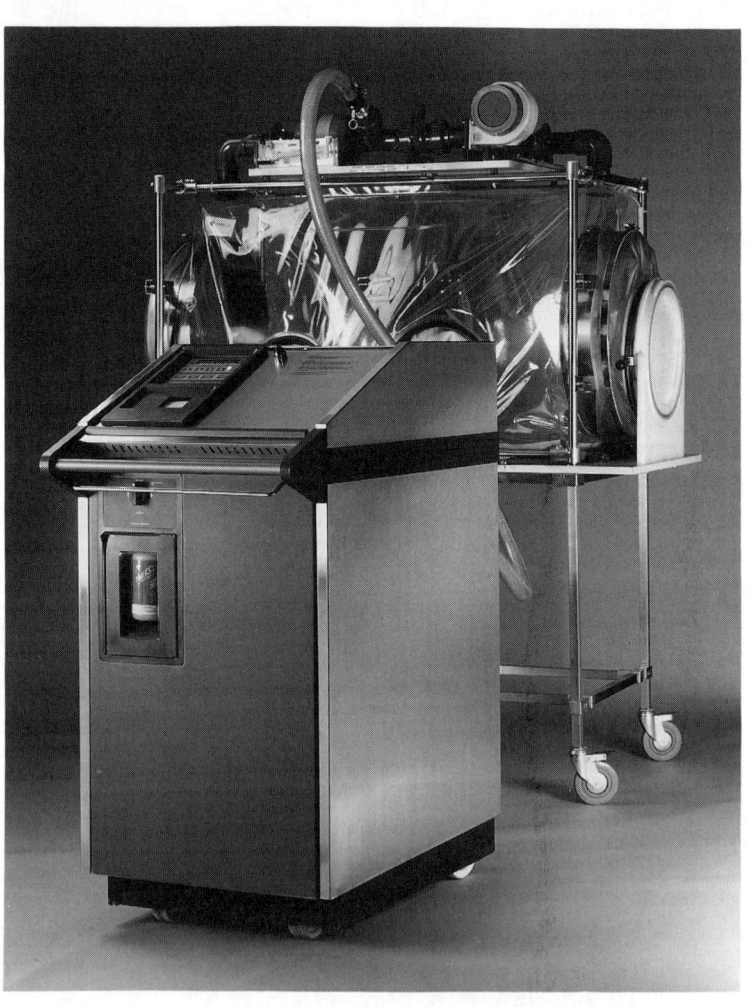

(Figure 7.3). The redundant pressure monitor provides added assurance that isolator pressure is being maintained. If the isolator has a pressure monitor capable of sending appropriate information to the VHP®1000, the redundant pressure monitor is optional. The air exiting the isolator passes through a catalyst to convert any remaining sterilant into water vapor and oxygen. An on-board desiccant system absorbs the moisture and then the warm, dry air returns to the vaporizer to deliver fresh sterilant until the sterilization countdown timer reaches zero. A Cycle Development Guide has been made available to assist the user in choosing the most appropriate cycle parameters for their particular applications (*VHP®1000 Cycle Development Guide* 1991).

Several methods have been developed to assist in the validation of isolators employing H_2O_2 gas and for their routine monitoring once validated (*VHP®1000 Validation Manual* 1991). *Bacillus stearothermophilus* spore suspensions (ATCC 12980) of known resistance to the sterilant have been available commercially for several years. These spores have been shown to be the most resistant to the sterilant (Rickloff 1988). Each lot is verified to meet a specified resistance to the gas when tested in a specially designed vessel. Users of these or any other spore suspensions should still consider performing their own studies to confirm that resistance to the sterilant meets some

Figure 7.3. Recommended VHP®1000 and pressure connections for a flexible wall sterility test isolator.

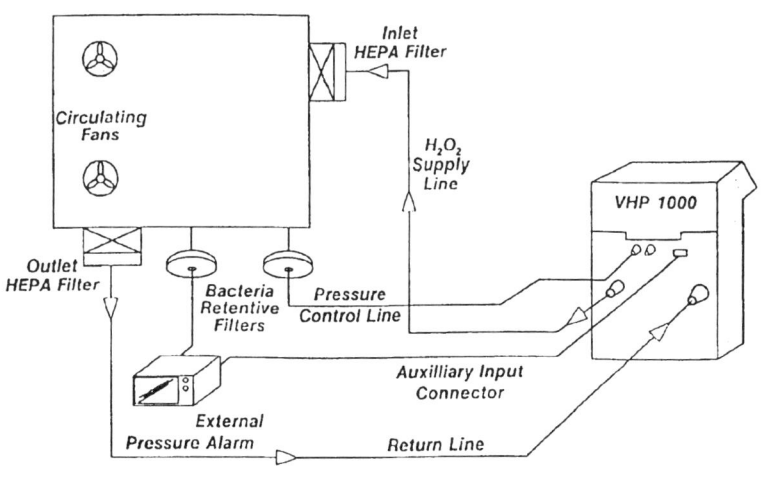

pre-established level before commencing an isolator validation. Table 7.2 lists some of the other microorganisms and viruses that have been tested for reductions in colony (or plaque) forming units when exposed to H_2O_2 gas.

A biological indicator has been developed and is available commercially for use with H_2O_2 gas. The Spordex-VHP® indicator (AMSCO, Apex, NC) is a fiberglass disc containing *B. stearothermophilus* spores in a Tyvek® package. These materials were chosen because they do not absorb the sterilant

Table 7.2. List of Microorganisms and Viruses Tested for Resistance to Hydrogen Peroxide Gas

Bacteria	*Bacterial Spores*
Brevibacterium acetylicum	*Bacillus cereus*
Escherichia coli	*Bacillus macerans*
Lactobacillus casei	*Bacillus pumilus*
Mycobacterium smegmatis	*Bacillus thuringensis*
Norcardia lactamdurans	*Bacillus stearothermophilus*
Proteus vulgaris	*Bacillus subtilis (globigii)*
Pseudomonas aeruginosa	*Clostridium sporogenes*
Pseudomonas cepacia	
Serratia marcescens	
Staphylococcus aureus	
Streptococcus faecalis	
Streptococcus faecium	
Fungal Spores, Yeasts & Molds	*Viruses*
Aspergillus niger	Adenovirus
Aspergillus terreus	Bovine Viral Diarrhea
Candida parapsilosis	Herpes simplex Type 1
Fusarium oxysporum	Influenza A2
Penicillium chrysogenum	Polio Type 1
Rhodotorula glutinis	Rhinovirus 14
Saccharomyces cervisiae	Vaccinia

(absorption could lead to lengthy sterilization times). This device currently is under consideration for inclusion into the United States Pharmacopeia Monograph on Biological Indicators as the recommended means of monitoring H_2O_2 gas sterilization processes.

Hydrogen peroxide gas distribution can be verified qualitatively within isolators with chemical indicator strips which gradually change color from light yellow to violet gray upon exposure. The rate of color change for the Chemdi-VHP® Indicator (AMSCO, Apex, NC) has been shown to be dependent upon gas concentration. Infrared spectroscopy has been used to quantitatively determine gas concentrations during sterilization although calibration techniques are still under development (Rickloff 1994). Several other means of monitoring H_2O_2 gas at sterilizing concentrations, such as guided wave technology, are also under investigation.

Recently published articles (Akers et al. 1994; Walker and Wilkins 1994) on H_2O_2 gas sterilization of exposed surfaces in sterility test and filling line isolators provide insights into the sterilant's capabilities and limitations. Table 7.3 lists typical cycle parameters that have been utilized on various flexible film sterility test isolators.

Hydrogen peroxide gas and most, if not all, of the other germicides discussed in this chapter are quite capable of sterilizing surfaces that come in direct contact with them. Complex surfaces may provide a greater challenge level to any of these germicides and this should not be overlooked during the isolator and equipment design process. Claiming complex surfaces as sterile will require the performance of direct spore inoculation studies. Sterilizing biological indicators near complex surfaces should not be considered as an adequate test challenge.

Several steps can be taken during the isolator design phase to minimize concerns over the placement of complex surfaces into isolators. Mechanical systems in critical (product exposure) areas of the isolator can be enshrouded, relocated to other less critical areas, or placed outside of the sterile environment. In addition, moveable components should be operating during the sanitization process to maximize surface contact with the germicide. Consideration should still be given toward direct spore inoculation on some critical surfaces to provide additional assurance that the germicidal process is effective.

Table 7.3. VHP®1000 Base Cycle Parameters[a] for Empty Chamber and Product Container Validation Studies

Sterility Test Isolator Description	Volume of 31% Sterilant, ml	Phase Time, min.			
		Dehumidify	Condition	Sterilize	Aerate[b]
113 ft³ Workstation	93.6	20	3	30	120
152 ft³ Workstation	144.6	20	3	40	120
180 ft³ Interface[c]	159.6	20	3	45	120
152 ft³ Workstation w/ 180 ft³ Interface[d]	236.0	30	4	60	180
24 ft³ Transfer	45.6	10	2	15	60
32 ft³ Transfer	58.6	10	2	20	60
Loaded Transfer (24 ft³)[e]	123.6	10	2	45	90

[a]Assumes minimum surface temperatures of 25°C in the half-suit and 28°C in the transfer isolators. Sterilization time set to achieve a 6-log reduction of the most resistant organism. Airflow at 20 ft³/min for all phases except for 12 ft³/min during sterilization

[b]An additional overnight outside exhaust is recommended to remove any remaining residues although product transfer to workstation isolators is possible after a 60–90 minute aeration with the VHP®1000.

[c]Assumes the isolator is connected to an Eagle® 3000SL double-sliding door sterilizer or equivalent.

[d]Sterilant delivery and removal hoses connected to each isolator. RTP or conventional door is opened between the isolators.

[e]Actual cycle times may vary considerably due to the quantity of materials and various load patterns.

Hydrogen peroxide in combination with steam at atmospheric pressure currently is under development (Despatch Industries, Minneapolis, MN) for the sterilization of custom filling lines within barriers (Pflug et al. 1993). The cycle requires the enclosure to be heated to at least 80°C prior to the introduction of the steam/H_2O_2 mixture (Figure 7.4). Temperatures stabilize near 100°C during sterilization. Test results obtained under laboratory conditions have demonstrated surface sterilization times within six minutes (Pflug 1994). Stainless steel carriers were inoculated with 10^7 spores of several different *Bacillus* species during these studies. Surface sterilization studies using steam/H_2O_2 have recently been initiated on enclosed filling line prototypes (Edwards and Porter 1995). The volume of 31 percent (w/v) H_2O_2 needed per cycle may approach 3 liters for production isolators. The introduction of warm, dry air after exposure will facilitate equipment drying and sterilant residue removal.

Wilke (1993) recently compared the application of three different forms of H_2O_2 (gas, liquid, and in combination with steam) to aseptic filling environments. The study (performed at the Robert Bosch Packaging Machinery Division, Waiblingen, Germany) indicated that each form of the oxidant was capable of rapidly inactivating bacterial spores. However, the engineering team concluded that the gas, when utilized at or near ambient temperature, offered the most advantages with the fewest limitations for isolated fillers (Table 7.4).

In the Fall of 1993, a Bosch MLF 3002 vial filler was enclosed in a flexible film, turbulent flow isolator (Figure 7.5)

Figure 7.4. Temperature-time diagram for a steam/hydrogen peroxide sterilization cycle (Walker and Wilkins 1994).

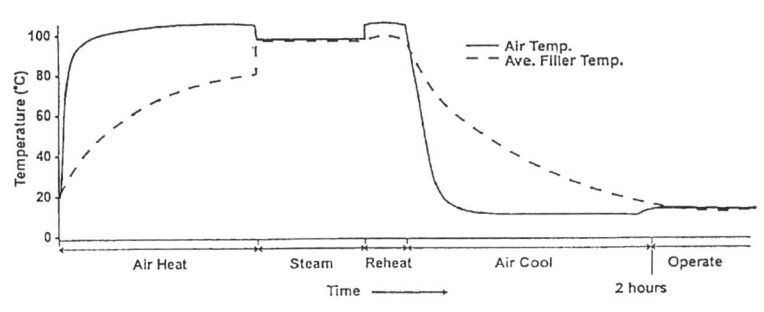

Table 7.4. Comparison of Hydrogen Peroxide Sterilization Methods (Wilke 1993)

Comparisons	Liquid Spray	Mixed With Steam	Gas
Advantages	good sterilization FDA–approved for food	good sterilization on straight surfaces packaging applications	best sterilization effect no dilution by steam low residual levels low thermal stress filler remains dry can reach small crevices
Limitations	poor penetration many fogging nozzles required	large volume of liquid high thermal stress machine wet	distribution must be optimized

Figure 7.5. Biological indicator locations in a Bosch MLF 3002 vial filler enclosed in a flexible film isolator.

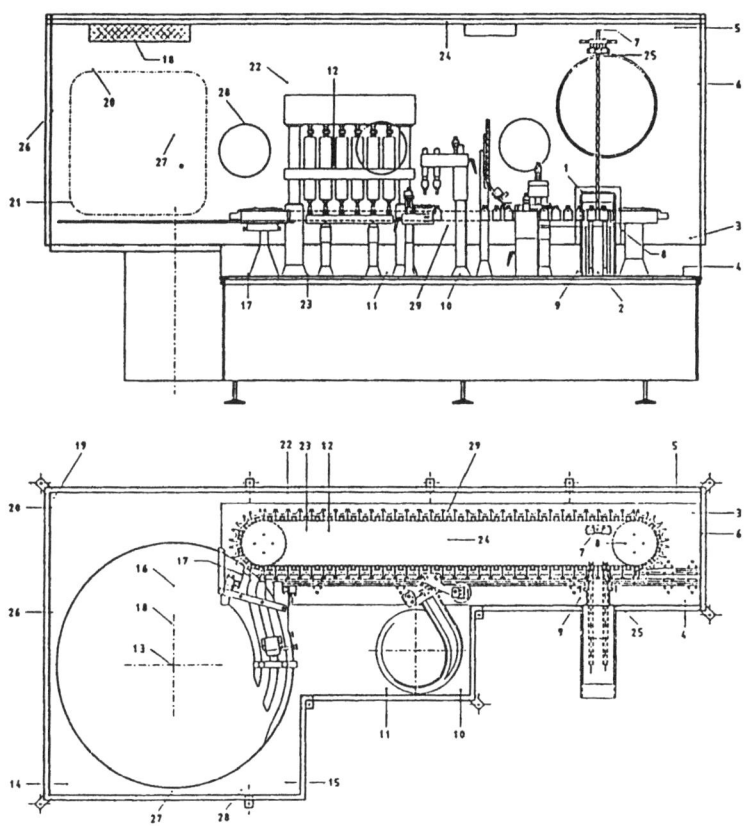

and exposed to 2.3 mg H_2O_2/liter of air for 46 minutes at 30°C (Schafer 1993). The biological test results are summarized in Table 7.5. The data clearly demonstrate the need for optimizing gas distribution within the isolator. Most positive biological indicators were eliminated by recirculating the sterilant through the isolator blower, significantly increasing the air exchange rate. Redesigning of the accumulator guide and instituting laminar flow conditions will likely eliminate areas where the gas was unable to penetrate during these preliminary studies. In addition to the biological tests, a 60 minute aeration of the isolated Bosch filler via outside exhaust reduced the H_2O_2 gas concentration to approximately 0.1 ppm

Table 7.5. Preliminary VHP®1000 Sterilization Test Results (± for Growth) Obtained in a Bosch MLF 3002 Vial Filler Enclosed in a Flexible Film Isolator

BI #	Spordex–VHP BI Location	Recirculation System Off	Recirculation System On
1	Vial Reject Tunnel	+	–
2	Vial Reject Tunnel	+	–
3	Floor at End of Reject Tunnel	+	–
4	Front Right Corner on Floor	+	–
5	Back Right Top Corner	–	–
6	Right Side Top Center	–	–
7	Top of Filling Machine Magazine	–	–
8	Right End of Conveyor	–	–
9	Floor Near Vial Reject Tunnel	–	–
10	Floor Under Stopper Bowl	+	–
11	Floor Under Stopper Bowl	+	–
12	Between Filling Heads	–	–
13	Under Accumulator Table Guide	+	+
14	Front Left Corner on Floor	+	–
15	Floor Near Front of Accumulator	+	–
16	Under Accumulator Table	+	–
17	Under Accumulator Table	+	–
18	Near Inlet HEPA Filter	–	–

Continued on next page.

Continued from previous page.

BI #	Spordex–VHP BI Location	Recirculation System Off	Recirculation System On
19	Fold of Isolator Fabric	+	–
20	Back Left Top Corner	–	–
21	Left Side on Floor	+	+
22	Back Center on Floor	–	–
23	Floor Recess Under Conveyor	–	–
24	Center Top	–	–
25	Front Right Top Corner	–	–
26	Left Side Center	–	–
27	Front Center Near Accumulator	–	–
28	Front Above Left Glove Port	–	–
29	Back Center Behind Guide Bar	–	–

in the exhaust line. Based on these and other studies, Bosch has introduced a line of vial fillers enclosed in rigid wall, laminar flow isolators.

Other Methods

A 3 percent (w/v) H_2O_2 solution in combination with 0.01 percent (w/v) peracetic acid is being spray atomized into a partially enclosed vial filling line currently in production at The Upjohn Company in Kalamazoo, MI (Davenport 1994). The mixture has been validated to obtain high-level disinfection of all internal components within the barrier and its surrounding environment. The line is enclosed within a restricted access barrier system (interim design) to eliminate operator intervention and, thus, provide a sterility confidence level approaching that of a terminally sterilized product.

The disinfectant mixture was shown to be capable of inactivating not less than 10^3 *B. subtilis* var. *niger* spores per cm^2 of stainless steel within 10 minutes under laboratory test conditions. Typical system turn-around times, to introduce and remove the disinfectant from the barrier system, were reported to be on the order of 24 hours. In addition to sub-process challenge testing, media fills, viable and nonviable particulate air sampling, and viable surface monitoring results were shown to be significantly better than industry standards previously established for conventional aseptic processing. For example, no microorganisms were recovered after sampling 15,501 ft^3 of air and 13,895 cm^2 of surface area in the restricted access barrier.

The incorporation of high intensity ultraviolet germicidal lamps into isolators has been directed primarily toward small pass-through chambers for the external sanitization of pre-sterilized supplies prior to isolator entry (Davenport and Melgaard 1995). The successful integration of this technology requires the appropriate wavelength of light (253.7 nm is optimum) for a defined period of time while minimizing shadowing effects. The Upjohn Company has validated this method on their restricted access barrier system (Davenport 1994) and were able to demonstrate a minimum 3-log reduction of *Bacillus* spores on the most difficult package surface at the lowest anticipated UV dose.

Dry heat is not an attractive option for sterilizing an entire isolator, but a dry heat process currently is under development by Central Research Laboratories (Red Wing, MN) for the sterilization of pass-through port flanges and gaskets. If successfully validated, the process will permit the sterile docking of containers eliminating concern over the transfer of sterile items over nonsterile gaskets. Preliminary results report a "dock-to-dump" cycle time of 5–10 minutes, depending upon the application (Marohl et al. 1995).

MATERIAL COMPATIBILITY

The materials of construction of an isolator or the equipment placed within them should not be compromised by the sterilization process. Many variables will dictate if the chemical germicide has an effect on a material, but the required use concentration will have the greatest impact.

Even though peracetic acid has been shown to be a reproducible means of eliminating microbial contamination in isolators, several concerns have forced the industry to seek alternative processes. The primary concerns are that the corrosive properties of peracetic acid have prohibited the placement of certain equipment within sterility test isolators. Flexible film canopies become discolored, requiring their frequent replacement at high cost. However, many facilities are still utilizing peracetic acid on a daily basis and some of the canopies are said to have lasted for several years.

Chlorine dioxide has been reported to be less corrosive than peracetic acid. Tests have shown good compatibilities with most plastics, silicone rubber, 316L stainless steel, and titanium (Rosenblatt and Knapp 1989). However, the pitting of uncoated aluminum and discoloration of polycarbonate may be a concern for some isolator applications.

Aqueous H_2O_2 capable of sterilizing surfaces at ambient temperature (100,000 ppm) has been reported to be corrosive to some materials (*Chemical Resistance Charts* 1993–1994). The major advantage of using the gaseous form of H_2O_2 is that it can sterilize surfaces at ambient temperature with concentrations in the 500–8,000 ppm range which minimizes the corrosive properties of the oxidant. Hydrogen peroxide gas is significantly less aggressive than ClO_2 or peracetic acid on aluminum or polycarbonate.

Good material compatibility results can be realized if the H_2O_2 gas concentration remains below the dew point for a particular temperature. Hydrogen peroxide has a lower vapor pressure than water, therefore, it will condense out first and very high aqueous concentrations can accumulate on material surfaces. Table 7.6 lists both the preferred and unacceptable materials of construction if H_2O_2 gas is applied to isolators. Several materials listed under the "dependent upon application" category in Table 7.6 may be compatible, but the sterilant can absorb into them. Outgassing of H_2O_2 or other chemicals can considerably lengthen aeration time of the isolator if the material is present in sufficient quantity. Materials selection for optimizing isolator sterilization cycles will be discussed in another chapter in this book.

Table 7.6. List of Isolator Construction Materials and Their Compatibility to Hydrogen Peroxide Gas

Item	Preferred Materials	Dependent Upon Their Application[a]	Materials to Be Avoided
Isolator Walls	316 Stainless Steel 304 Stainless Steel Tempered Glass	Polycarbonate Acrylic Fiberglass Polyvinyl Chloride	Cellulosics Carbon Steel
HEPA Filters	Glass Fiber Media Stainless Frames	Aluminum Frames	Paper Media Wood Frames
Gaskets/Seals	Viton®	Silicone EPDM	
Component Parts	Stainless Steel Norprene® Teflon™	CPVC Delrin® Hypalon® Polyethylene Neoprene Polypropylene Natural Rubber Kynar® Buna N Rubber Anodized Aluminum	Nylon

[a] It is recommended that the sterilization equipment vendor be provided with material lists and samples for compatibility testing under the anticipated use conditions.

SAFETY AND ENVIRONMENTAL REGULATIONS

Chemical germicides are toxic to living systems; steps must be taken to prevent unacceptable occupational exposures to them. The first safety issue that a technician will confront is the handling of the germicide itself. Peracetic acid and ClO_2 both require manual dilution to prepare their use-concentrations. The VHP®1000, on the other hand, uses a disposable cartridge containing an EPA approved sterilant, thus requiring minimal human intervention to make the connection to the sterilant delivery system.

Workplace exposure guidelines have been established for ClO_2 and H_2O_2. There is no established Threshold Limit Value (TLV) for peracetic acid by the American Conference of Governmental Industrial Hygienists (ACGIH), although acetic acid and H_2O_2 values are listed in the Material Safety Data Sheet (MSDS). The pertinent National Institute of Occupational Safety and Health (NIOSH) guidelines for peracetic acid, ClO_2, and H_2O_2 are summarized in Table 7.7. Periodic updates on various chemical hazards are provided to industry in tabular form by NIOSH (NIOSH Pocket Guide 1990). Personnel working around these environments should become thoroughly familiarized with these guidelines and then verify that all safety precautions are practiced and utilized.

Monitoring methods that can detect vapors of ClO_2 and H_2O_2 are available to determine if the work environment and/or the isolator is safe for humans. Users of peracetic acid typically sample for acetic acid vapors although H_2O_2 should be checked as well. Single-use Dräger tubes (BGI Inc., Waltham, MA) and continuous monitors (MDA Scientific, Lincolnshire, IL) work well when used within their acceptable operating ranges. Personnel should become familiar with the correct use and limitations of these devices.

Safety features should be in place when any germicide is delivered to an isolator. This applies to isolator integrity and control, and to the equipment introducing it. The VHP®1000, for example, offers an automatic pressure hold test before the cycle that will verify that an isolator is sufficiently sealed. Failure to maintain pressure within an isolator during any portion of the cycle will cause the VHP®1000 to abort.

Table 7.7. NIOSH Exposure Limits for Chemicals Commonly Used for Isolator Sterilization (*NIOSH Pocket Guide* 1990)

Chemical Name	REL[a]	STEL[b]	IDLH[c]
Acetic Acid	10 ppm (25 mg/m^3)	15 ppm (37 mg/m^3)	1000 ppm
Hydrogen Peroxide	1 ppm (1.4 mg/m^3)	No Standard	75 ppm
Chlorine Dioxide	0.1 ppm (0.3 mg/m^3)	0.3 ppm (0.9 mg/m^3)	10 ppm

[a] Recommended Exposure Limits are time-weighted averages (TWA) for up to a 10-hour workday during a 40 hour week.

[b] Short-Term Exposure Limits are a 15-minute TWA exposure that should not be exceeded at any time during the day.

[c] Immediately Dangerous to Life or Health concentrations represent the maximum concentration from which one could escape within 30 minutes without a respirator and without experiencing any escape-impairing or irreversible health effects. Values were determined only for the purpose of respirator selection.

Pressure is being put on industry to minimize or eliminate the release of various chemical agents to the outside environment. The EPA, for example, may regulate the release of formaldehyde under the Toxic Substances Control Act due to its potential carcinogenicity (Whistler and Sheldon 1989). As was mentioned earlier, H_2O_2 gas can be catalytically converted into water vapor and oxygen. The outside exhaust of low ppm levels of the sterilant, for reducing aeration times of standard or custom isolators, should have no appreciable environmental impact since the gas is diluted several fold before being emitted to the outside and decomposition into water vapor and oxygen will occur naturally over time. The environmental threat is slightly higher for peracetic acid or ClO_2 since there are currently no catalytic converters available and organic compounds are formed upon their decomposition.

All of the antimicrobial chemical agents discussed in this chapter fall under federal air emissions regulations (Clean Air Act, SARA Title III) that require permitting and annual reporting of both inventory and emissions. For example, EPA has established a reportable emission quantity for hydrogen peroxide of 1 pound in a 24-hour period; however, this requirement only applies if the chemical is used in excess of 10,000 pounds per year (Brandys 1993). Some local jurisdictions may require reporting at lower usages, therefore, one should check with local agencies for their policy on such discharges if outside exhaust of an isolator is being considered.

REFERENCES

Akers, J. E., J. P. Agalloco, and C. M. Kennedy. 1994. Experience in the design and use of barrier isolator systems for sterility testing. In *Proceedings of the 3rd PDA International Congress*. Basel, Switzerland: Parenteral Drug Association.

Baldry, M. G. C. 1983. The bacteriocidal, fungicidal, and sporicidal properties of hydrogen peroxide and peracetic acid. *Appl. Microbiol.* 54:417–423.

Block, S. S. 1991. Peroxygen compounds. In *Disinfection, sterilization, and preservation*, 4th ed., edited by S. S. Block, pp. 167–181. Philadelphia: Lea & Febiger.

Block, S. S., ed. 1991. *Disinfection, sterilization and preservation*, 4th ed. Philadelphia: Lea & Febiger.

Brandys, R. C. 1993. Regulations on worker safety and the environment. In *Sterilization Technology*, edited by R. F. Morrissey, and G. B. Phillips, pp. 491–509. New York: Van Nostrand Reinhold.

Chemical resistance charts. 1993–94. Cole-Parmer® Instrument Catalog, pp. 1463–1471. Niles, IL: Cole-Parmer Instrument Co.

Davenport, S. M. 1989. Design and use of a novel peracetic acid sterilizer for absolute barrier sterility testing chambers. *J. Parenteral Sci. Technol.* 43:158–166.

Davenport, S. M. 1994. Meeting the goals of increased sterility confidence for advanced aseptic processing—Implementation of a restricted access barrier system. In *Proceedings of the Barrier Isolation Technology Seminar*. Philadelphia: International Society for Pharmaceutical Engineering.

Davenport, S. M., and H. L. Melgaard. 1995. Ultraviolet pass-through as a transfer technology in barrier and isolator systems. In *Proceedings of the Advanced Barrier Technology Conference*. Atlanta: Parenteral Drug Association and International Society for Pharmaceutical Engineering.

Edwards, L. M., and M. E. Porter. 1995. Microbiological and physical limits testing of a locally controlled environment (LCE) prototype filling system. In *Proceedings of the Advanced Barrier Technology Conference*. Atlanta: Parenteral Drug Association and International Society for Pharmaceutical Engineering.

Gonzalez, J. P., and D. Meyer. 1990. Advanced aseptic processing: Barrier system technology as applied to production filling lines. In *Proceedings of the PDA/PMA Sterilization Conference*. Washington, DC: Parenteral Drug Association and Pharmaceutical Manufacturers Association.

Jeng, D. K., and A. G. Woodworth. 1990. Chlorine dioxide gas sterilization under square-wave conditions. *Applied and Environ. Microbiol.* 56:514–519.

Marohl, R., C. Jennrich, and R. Adams. 1995. Sterilizable transfer port (STP)—Update. In *Proceedings of the Advanced Barrier Technology Conference*. Atlanta: Parenteral Drug Association and International Society for Pharmaceutical Engineering.

NIOSH pocket guide to chemical hazards. 1990. U.S. Department of Health and Human Services. Washington, DC: U.S. Government Printing Office.

Pflug, I. J. 1994. Microbiology 101—BIT sterilization methods incorporating steam with H_2O_2. In *Proceedings of the Barrier Isolation Technology Seminar*. Philadelphia: International Society for Pharmaceutical Engineering.

Pflug, I. J., H. L. Melgaard, C. A. Meadows, J. P. Lysfjord, and P. Haas. 1993. Rigid isolation barriers for aseptic filling lines: decontamination with saturated steam at atmospheric pressure or sterilization with steam plus hydrogen peroxide. In *Proceedings of the Kilmer Memorial Conference on the Sterilization of Medical Products*. Brussels, Belgium.

Portner, D. M., and R. K. Hoffman. 1968. Sporicidal effect of peracetic acid vapor. *Appl. Microbiol.* 16:1782–1785.

Rickloff, J. R. 1988. The development of vapor phase hydrogen peroxide as a sterilization technology. In *Proceedings of the Sterilization in the 1990's Conference*, edited by J. F. Jorkasky. Washington, DC: Health Industry Manufacturers Association.

Rickloff, J. R. 1994. Hydrogen peroxide gas and its use in sterilizing barrier isolators. In *Proceedings of the Barrier Isolation Technology Seminar*. Philadelphia: International Society for Pharmaceutical Engineering.

Rosenblatt, A. A., and J. E. Knapp. 1989. Chlorine dioxide gas sterilization. In *Proceedings of the Sterilization in the 1990's Conference*, edited by J. F. Jorkasky. Washington, DC: Health Industry Manufacturers Association.

Schafer, A. 1993. New and future machinery developments. In *Proceedings of the Isolation Technology 2000 Seminar*. Durham, NC: Robert Bosch Corp.

Thorogood, D. 1993. Physical and biological validation of a sterile rapid transfer system. In *Proceedings of the 2nd PDA International Congress*. Basel, Switzerland: Parenteral Drug Association.

Vesley, D., and J. Lauer. 1986. Decontamination, sterilization, disinfection, and antisepsis in the microbiology laboratory. In *Laboratory safety: Principles and practices*, edited by B. M. Miller, pp. 182–198. Washington, DC: American Society for Microbiology.

VHP®1000 Biodecontamination System Cycle Development Guide. 1991. Part No. 129363–327. Apex, NC: AMSCO.

VHP®1000 Biodecontamination System Validation Manual. 1991. Part No. 129363–317. Apex, NC: AMSCO.

Walker, N., and J. Wilkins. 1994. Case study: Evans Medical. In *Proceedings of the Barrier Isolation Technology Seminar*.

Philadelphia: International Society for Pharmaceutical Engineering.

Wallace, J., J. Dodd, and M. Millett. 1988. Comparison of the sporicidal effect of three disinfectant solutions within an isolator transfer port. *Animal Technol.* 39:189–193.

Whistler, P. E., and B. W. Sheldon. 1989. Biocidal activity of ozone versus formaldehyde against poultry pathogens inoculated in a prototype setter. *Poultry Science* 68:1068–1073.

Wilke, B. 1993. Peroxide sterilization within an isolator. In *Proceedings of the Isolation Technology 2000 Seminar*. Durham, NC: Robert Bosch Corp.

8
Microbiological Monitoring and Control in Isolator Systems

Michael C. Carroll
The Liposome Company, Inc.
Princeton, NJ

Microbiological monitoring of the environment inside an isolator or barrier system presents a unique set of challenges to the user. Depending on the application for which the isolator system is used, there may be varying requirements for environmental monitoring. Each type of monitoring presents requirements for the introduction of equipment and materials into the isolator. The equipment may add utility requirements within the system, such as electrical power or vacuum. Use of the equipment may disrupt pre-existing conditions within the isolator. Also, every piece of equipment or material going into the system may influence the chamber sterilization parameters. The maintenance and operation of an isolator system can become a delicate balance between the amount of monitoring needed to prove—to the satisfaction of whatever regulatory agency is involved—continued sterility within the isolator system, and the amount of potential contamination introduced into the system with the monitoring equipment and materials. The approach taken to environmental monitoring within an isolator system requires a high degree of planning and foresight.

For purposes of this chapter, it is assumed that an isolator or barrier system exists which contains a process of some sort (testing system, aseptic processing or filling operation, etc.); and that the following conditions exist:

- A minimum of two (2) isolators are used: One workstation isolator, containing the process itself, and one transfer isolator that can be attached or detatched at will for the introduction of supplies for the process and removal of finished materials.

- The workstation isolator contains some fixed equipment and is equipped with any utility connections needed for operation of the equipment.

- If the transfer isolator is normally sterilized separately, validated mechanisms exist for transfer isolator attachment to or detachment from the workstation isolator without breaking the sterile environment of either isolator.

- The workstation isolator is constantly maintained at a positive pressure relative to the outside environment and any transfer isolators; the air pressure is maintained by high efficiency particulate air (HEPA)–filtered systems for both inlets and outlets.

AIR MONITORING

Sampling of the air in an isolator system presents possibly the greatest challenge of all environmental monitoring. In its simplest form, air monitoring might be performed by exhuming the venerable settling plate or the open-broth-tube method. Both methods are qualitative only; the use of plated agar media, as will be discussed later, requires qualifying testing of its ability to survive sterilization processes to enter a barrier or isolator system (*See* References). Also, since most isolators operate at fairly low relative humidity levels, settling plates will be limited in exposure time before desiccating. For the purposes of this chapter, it will be assumed that one or another of the "active" microbiological air samplers will be used, in order to provide larger volume samples and (in most cases) quantitative results.

For each type of sampler used in the pharmaceutical industry, there are several obstacles to its use in an isolator system. Table 8.1 lists the more common types of microbial air samplers, together with their modes of operation, utility requirements, etc.

Special Concerns for Isolator Systems

Airflow

For certain applications, some samplers can be ruled out. For example, in an enclosure employing unidirectional airflows, the use of a sampler which produces turbulence or disrupts the airflow is unacceptable. There will also be limits, in smaller enclosures, to the amount of air which can be pulled into a sampler without disrupting the enclosure's own air circulation and supply. High-volume sampling (e.g., Andersen-type) may be impossible.

Utilities

The sampler types described above, with the exception of the centrifugal samplers, require some utility hookups (at least vacuum; some 120V AC current as well). Each utility hookup means another entry port, if this service does not already exist in the isolator, or another tie-in, if it is present.

Access/Handling

All sampler types require the introduction of equipment and media into the isolator, and removal of at least the media at the conclusion of sampling. Samplers will also require some manipulation by operators for setting up, starting, stopping, and unloading them. Ideally, air sampling requires minimal equipment, minimal manipulation, and maximum detection near critical sites.

For manufacturing isolators, "maximum detection near critical sites" may be critical, if there is a need for continuous monitoring throughout the aseptic operations (note that

Table 8.1. Microbial air-samplers*

Sampler	Mechanism	Utilities	Advantages	Disadvantages
Slit-to-Agar (STA)	Air pulled into unit, impinged on rotating agar plate	Vacuum source, 120V AC current (Many available with built-in vacuum pump)	≥ 60' continuous sampling, minimal disruption of airflows; can sample "remotely"; sampling automatically timed	Plate changing awkward, requires much manipulation; units and media bulky (uses 15 × 150 mm agar plates)
Centrifugal Air Samplers (RCS®1. SAS®2)	Air pulled into unit by spinning impeller blades, impinged on plate or strip of agar	None (battery operated)	Rapid, easy to use, no external utilities; some use standard RODAC plates; sampling automatically timed	Battery changes difficult in-place; units won't stand sterilants and must be protected; unit can disrupt airflow (some samplers more than others); must be located near process
Liquid-Impingement Samplers	Air pulled into container, impinged on buffer; liquid later filtered and plated	Vacuum only	Continuous sampling for ≥ 1 hr; can sample "remotely"	Not quantitative; bulky; requires volumes of liquid, subsequent processing; difficult to sterilize; sampling must be timed manually

Continued on next page.

Continued from previous page.

Sampler	Mechanism	Utilities	Advantages	Disadvantages
Atrium Samplers (SMA®3)	Air pulled into metal chamber, impinged on agar plate	Vacuum only	Continuous sampling for ≥ 1 hr; all metal, no moving parts; S/S models autoclavable; uses conventional 15 × 100 mm media plates	Heavy parts; sampling must be timed manually

*Note that Andersen-type samplers are not included in this listing, as they are very bulky and difficult to introduce into an isolator system.

[1]RCS = Reuter Centrifugal Sampler: Biotest Diagnostics, Inc., Denville, NJ.

[2]SAS = SAS Air Sampler: Micro Diagnostics, Inc., Lombard, IL.

[3]SMA = Sterilizable Microbiological Atrium Sampler: Veltek Associates, Inc., Exton, PA.

current thinking tends toward a greatly reduced need for monitoring of airborne viables within a validated isolator system). For sterility-testing isolators, a "snapshot" sampling of short duration at regular intervals is almost certainly acceptable.

As a general rule, air monitoring in a processing or manufacturing operation should be performed with methods which sample over a longer period of time during the process. Most processes are performed in barrier systems rather than isolators; these are not sealed systems, but exclude the external environment with HEPA-filtered air at positive pressures. Conventional aseptic processes typically require continuous sampling throughout the duration of the process. Thus, for this type of barrier/isolator application, either the slit-to-agar (STA) or atrium samplers should be considered, and the required utilities need to be installed. For sterility-testing isolators, the centrifugal samplers may be more advantageous, since they sample higher volumes of air in relatively short periods of time (up to 400–1000 liters of air in 8–10 minutes, respectively, for the Biotest Reuter Centrifugal Sampler® (RCS® and RCS+), and disruption of airflow is usually not a concern in these isolators.

For any microbial sampler, however, the mechanisms for introduction and removal of the media must be considered very carefully. In most systems, all materials needed for an operation are prepared and sterilized in a separate sterilizer or a transfer isolator, then aseptically transferred into the workstation isolator. All the air samplers described above utilize some form of microbiological media. These media may be affected by the sterilization cycle through which they must pass. Thus, the media must be subjected to comparative growth-support testing, and special packaging may need to be obtained or developed for media transfers. Conventional agar plates (including RODAC plates) will allow penetration of, for example, gas sterilants, if they are not wrapped for protection. As with any other type of container or closure system to be used in an isolator system, the media containers and closures will need to be validated for the sterilization cycles they must undergo. Additionally, the methods of packaging the media must be very carefully controlled; if the sterilants are effectively prevented from reaching the media, there is a possibility that contaminants present on the media or plates could be introduced into the isolator system. Nearly all commonly used plastics are virtually impervious to vapor-phase hydrogen peroxide sterilization in isolators. With other isolator sterilants, it may be wise to evaluate the plastic wrappers' ability to withstand the sterilant. Many types of media are available in sterile package put-ups of various types, but these will also need to be evaluated for their ability to exclude the sterilants used in the isolators. Many of these media are commercially available in multiple-wrapped, radiation-sterilized packages. Whatever packaging is developed and validated for the media, remember that the operators must be able to unpack the media within the isolators, with minimal trouble and manipulation, using the heavy gloves provided. All of these factors must be validated, wherever possible.

For testing isolators, monitoring of nonviable airborne particulates may be required; for production isolators, it will certainly be required. For this type of measurement, the same concerns will apply: If samplers are to be used within the isolator chamber, they must have all required utilities available; they must be capable of surviving the sterilization cycles in the isolators; they must not disrupt unidirectional airflows (either with suction for pulling air samples, or with exhaust from the counter); and they must provide some means of removing the data. In the case of particle counters, it is obviously not a good idea to have a printer present in the chamber (assuming one could be gas-sterilized, paper supply and all), so provision must be made for data acquisition on an internal buffer or a diskette, or for data transmission via cable (e.g., via another entry port into the isolator system, which is not a technical problem). Particle-counter electronics and air pump motors (if included in the units), may be more susceptible to the sterilants than viable air-samplers, so the manufacturers must be contacted on this point before equipment is procured. Special packaging or protection of the units will complicate their sterilization and will increase the manipulations needed for set up and operation.

Another option for nonviable particulate counting is "remote" counting, where the actual counter is outside the isolator and air is pulled through a sampling tube. The sensitivity of particulate counting decreases sharply with each additional length of sample tubing between the sampling site and the counter. For this reason, this method is not highly desirable, unless sample volumes are high enough to overcome the loss of sensitivity. Particle counters which sample 1.0 ft^3 or more per minute are generally available; but these instruments may disrupt airflows within the chamber, and may, for smaller isolators, require "balancing" of the isolator chamber's air pressures and make-up airflows to account for the volumes of air removed in sampling. Obviously, for a 500 ft^3 isolator with 50 air-changes per hour, the volumes removed by particle-counting will be negligible.

SURFACE MONITORING

Surfaces within an isolator may be monitored by conventional sampling techniques, such as RODAC agar plates, swabs, or swipes. The only real possibility of contamination of an enclosed sterile environment is through inadvertent or accidental spillage onto surfaces, so surface monitoring should be performed at the end of any testing or manufacturing operation to maximize the chances of detecting a contaminant. The difficulties of surface sampling in an isolator environment are related, in part, to the sterilization of the environment. The gas sterilants normally used (peracetic acid or vapor-phase hydrogen peroxide) are essentially surface-active and may affect the growth-promotion qualities of the media used. If aeration and/or neutralization of the sterilant are marginal, the sterilants may leave surface residues which will negate sampling on contact. Additionally, the materials and equipment within most isolator systems are not easy to sample with RODAC plates, particularly the hardest-to-sterilize areas (half-suits, gloves, etc.). Swabs or swipes are routinely required, although these are not quantitative sampling methods and are notoriously inefficient.

Most commercially obtained RODAC plates have reasonably tight-fitting lids, particularly compared to conventional petri dish plates. However, they are not designed to be gastight. Some packaging must be obtained or developed for the RODAC plates in order to pass them through a sterilization cycle for entry into the isolator. As with the air-sampling media described above, this packaging must be done under carefully controlled circumstances to prevent contamination of the plates and the isolator system. The selection of multiple-wrapped and sterile-packaged sampling media may again be considered here, but with the same caveats as before: The media, packaging, and transfer methods must all be adequately validated for their preservation of the sensitivity and growth-support of the media, for their effectiveness at excluding contaminants from the isolator system, and for their ability to withstand the sterilant(s) used in the isolators. Also, as before, the operators must be capable of unpacking and using the materials within the isolators.

Swabs and swipes are useful for sampling those "hard-to-reach" places around half-suit and glove seals, in and around filling or testing equipment, around transfer ports, utility connections, etc. Commercially available swabs with transport medium are excellent, provided their packaging will withstand the sterilization cycles. They also have the advantage of a sealable transport tube for transferring them out of the isolator system after sampling. Alternately, swabs can be sampled and immediately inoculated into a liquid broth media within the isolator system. This eliminates another external transfer step; however, the broth tubes must be screw-top tubes and gas-tight to survive the sterilization cycles. Swipes are also useful for sampling difficult areas, but they require considerably more manipulation, particularly in inoculating them into media; this may be difficult in half-suits or gloves. Bear in mind that swipes and swabs are estimated to have perhaps as good as a 50% recovery rate, in addition to their non-quantitative nature; however, in the absence of better methods, they must be considered adequate.

PROCESS VALIDATION

An integral part of validating and maintaining any isolator system involves validation and periodic revalidation of the process(es) contained in the isolator system. Intimately involved in these validation processes is the monitoring associated with the processes.

For typical aseptic operations, whether testing or production, some form of "process simulation" is run, using microbiological growth media instead of the product or test samples. In production operations, these simulations, known as Media Fills, are the source of intense debates within the pharmaceutical industry and regulating agencies. However they are performed and interpreted, it is standard practice to perform increased monitoring and "stress" the systems during these simulations. They are thus also extremely useful for qualifying improvements in techniques, materials handling, etc., and in training and qualifying of employees. As in any operation, however, introduction of media, extra sampling materials, and process variations into the isolator system, will produce extra risks, and will require extra care in cleaning and resterilization of the systems for routine use after completion of these runs.

EXTERNAL ENVIRONMENT

Until very recently, the only published recommendation for isolators (Medicines Control Agency, U.K.) was for a minimum of a Class 10,000 environment surrounding a barrier system to be used for production. Now, a European Community Guideline has been published regarding isolators and their use in pharmacies and pharmaceutical manufacturing; this Guideline also includes recommendations for the external environment and for monitoring. Due to the nature of barrier/isolator systems, it could be argued that a manufacturing operation in such an environment could be situated in any sort of building. However, particularly when people are employed in the supplying of components to the isolated operations, it would seem wise to protect the environment external to the barrier. The "classification" of the external room environment around the barrier/isolator system can follow existing regulatory guidelines, relating the operations and personnel in these areas to the corresponding operations in support of a conventional aseptic processing operation. For example, the component preparation areas of a conventional aseptic facility are normally at least Class 100,000, frequently Class 10,000, and invariably require a fairly high degree of personnel gowning. The environment around an isolator system for aseptic processing might well be considered in the same way, with the same types of environmental maintenance and monitoring programs found in such areas. On the other hand, anterooms for a sterility testing suite are usually less stringently controlled. Since all materials passing into and out of the sterility test suite are sealed at the time of transfer, the anteroom frequently doubles as a gowning room. For the areas around a sterility-testing isolator system, only minimal environmental and personnel controls may be needed: HEPA–filtered air, at low velocities, and perhaps only hair-coverings and coats or coveralls over street-clothes for personnel.

Special concerns exist, of course, for disposal of certain types of wastes from isolator systems (e.g., sterilant wastes, cytotoxic materials, and sample or wash residues). Waste handling is also required where isolator systems are linked to autoclave, depyrogenation oven, or tunnel sterilization units. Biohazardous or biological wastes from an isolated process cannot be brought out into a totally unprotected or unrestricted area. Similarly, environmental systems must exist for sterilant venting to the atmosphere (hydrogen peroxide or H_2O_2/steam) or collection and neutralization on-site (peracetic acid, EtO). Dedicated heating, ventilation, and air conditioning (HVAC) systems and HEPA–filtered atmospheres would be recommended for such isolator rooms. Where an autoclave, tunnel, or oven is linked to an isolator or barrier system there must be a thermally protected interface, mechanisms for dissipating heat and condensate, provisions for unloading extremely hot materials into the isolator, and increased isolator airflow to maintain positive pressures. On the loading ("dirty") side of such operations, separated from the isolators by the autoclave, oven or tunnel, component cleanliness and freedom from particulates will dictate the HVAC and filtration requirements for the areas.

Human operators involved with an isolated operation are, by definition, physically removed from the protected environment by the isolator or barrier system. Operator training is critically important in ensuring that operators do not jeopardize the isolator system's integrity by improper operations and/or inadequate response to an emergency or breach of the system. However, even well-trained and experienced operators can still provide problems for the isolator system. The possibility of transferring colds or other contaminants between operators using the same half-suits clearly exists. Therefore, the insides of half-suit faceplates should be cleaned and disinfected with a mild quaternary disinfectant solution and lint-free, nonabrasive wipes between operators. The disinfectants should be wiped off thoroughly to remove residues and provide clear vision for the next operator. Alcohols, such as 70 percent isopropanol or ethanol, may also be used. They do not leave residues but may leave volatile and irritating fumes within the suits unless adequate ventilation time is given between operators. As with conventional clean-room operations, it might be a wise precaution to exclude operators with obvious skin problems or upper respiratory infections until symptoms have disappeared. The use of disposable latex gloves within the half-suit or glove-box gloves is strongly recommended, as well. However, employees with long or sharp fingernails may still present hazards to system integrity; policies and SOPs may be needed to prevent these risks.

STERILITY HOLD

Sterility Testing Isolators

The typical workstation isolator is by far the more difficult unit to validate and sterilize, due to the larger size, increased amounts of equipment, and multiple entries for routine operations. Also, the processes involved in cleaning, preparing, leak-tight testing, and sterilizing, as well as the poststerilization aeration and neutralization, can mean periods of downtime for the workstation thats last from hours to days. In an ideal situation, a workstation isolator could be gas-sterilized and then maintained nearly indefinitely sterile, with only the transfer isolator loads being sterilized for entry into the workstation. With HEPA–filtered inlet and outlet air, an isolator could effectively maintain sterility even in the event of a total power failure. The validation of a sterility hold time—a maximum time period for which, provided no breach or accidental contamination of the workstation environment has occurred, the workstation may be safely considered to be sterile—is required.

Production/Manufacturing Barriers

For production isolators or barrier set-ups, particularly aseptic filling operations, a sterility-hold period may not be possible, due to the multiple entries and the large volumes of materials introduced into and removed from the system in the course of a single operation. Barrier systems are not sealed systems, but contain mouse holes or tunnel connections for passage of components into and out of the main workstation isolator. They may have much greater positive pressures and air-volume throughput than sealed isolator systems. If multiple products are filled or processed, cleaning and sterilization between runs will be a requirement for segregation of products within the isolator environment. For operations where a sterility-hold period can be developed, the usual limiting factor is the time the operators are willing to wait, after completion of the initial sterilization validations, prior to breaking sterility, cleaning and removing all validation-related materials, and starting routine operations. In most circumstances encountered to date, the corporate impatience to begin using the system limits the sterility hold period, with validation data, to several days or a week.

Maintenance of the validated sterility-hold period can be accomplished with documentation of operations in the system and sterilization of transfer-isolator loads entering the system, and maintenance of records on pressure differentials and HEPA filtration systems. For isolator systems, document periodic leak-tight testing (which can be performed without breaking sterility on most isolators). Any breach of barrier or isolator systems and/or the validated operating procedures for the systems, will end the sterility hold period and necessitate resterilization. This would include such occurrences as leaks in the barrier/isolator or intake/outlet HEPA filters; sterilization and transfer of unvalidated or excessive loads in the transfer isolator; and spills or aerosols of potentially contaminated materials in the isolator.

Extension of the sterility hold time for an isolator system needs to be carefully planned. First, an extended period must be scheduled during a time when little or no production activity is expected (preferably no production activity, since any production activities performed in the isolator beyond the validated sterility hold time are at very high risk). Scheduled annual plant or production shutdowns might be an ideal time for such activities. Second, the workstation sterilization must be timed so that the validated sterility hold time ends at the beginning of the scheduled period of no activity. Third, a formal protocol for the validation of an extended sterility-hold time should be approved in advance, with clearly defined maintenance and monitoring activities and acceptance criteria.

Once the validated sterility hold time expires and the clock has started running on the extended time, the validation becomes merely a matter of performing and documenting whatever maintenance and monitoring activities are required by the protocol, for the duration of the desired extended sterility-hold time. It is a good idea to carry the validation out perhaps 1–2 weeks beyond the desired maximum sterility-hold time, as a cushion and for future reference. However, balance the sterility-hold time against the probable necessity to perform periodic cleaning and maintenance activities on the isolator systems. From this standpoint, a sterility-hold time beyond perhaps a few months' duration may be impractical.

CONCLUSION

The microbiological monitoring of the environment inside an isolator or barrier system does indeed face the user with a large and unique set of options and problems. There is a real balance to be maintained between environmental monitoring and potential contamination, and between monitoring and actual operational concerns. The operator of an isolator or barrier system must approach the question of environmental monitoring very carefully and very thoughtfully. Every step and decision point must be carefully documented. The potential benefits of isolator technology are so great, however, that all of this planning and troubleshooting may seem an insignificant price to pay.

REFERENCES

Buck, A., M. Carroll, and C. Wagner. 1992. Validation of isolators for sterility testing applications. Unpublished observations. (Includes demonstration of reduced growth-support capabilities in tubed and plated microbiological media in non-vapor-tight containers, after exposure to VHP sterilization.)

European Community Guideline. 1995: Isolators for pharmaceutical applications. Edited by G. Lee and B. Midcalf. UK Pharmaceutical Isolator Group.

Griego, V. 1990. Efficacy of hydrogen peroxide vapor as a sterilant. Presented at the PDA/PMA Conference: Sterilization in the 1990's, 26–29 August, in Washington, DC.

Meyer, D., and J. P. Gonzalez. 1990. Advanced aseptic procesing: Barrier system Technology as applied to production filling lines. Presented at the PDA/PMA Conference: Sterilization in the 1990's, 26–29 August, in Washington, DC.

Rickloff, J. 1988. The development of vapor-phase hydrogen peroxide as a sterilization technology. Presented at the HIMA Conference: Sterilization in the 1990's, 30 October–1 November, in Washington, DC.

Rickloff, J. 1989. Use of vapor-phase hydrogen peroxide (VPHP) for sterilization and biodecontamination applications. Presented at the PDA Annual Meeting, 30 October–1 November, in Hollywood, FL.

Wood, R. 1990. Advanced aseptic processing: Barrier technology sterility testing laboratory. Presented at the PDA/PMA Conference: Sterilization in the 1990's, 26–29 August, in Washington, DC.

9

Introduction to the Validation of Sterile Processing Using Isolation Technology

Richard M. Johnson
Alcon Laboratories
Ft. Worth, TX

The primary objective in employing isolation technology for sterile pharmaceuticals currently produced using aseptic processing is to achieve a verifiable contamination rate (aka, sterility confidence level (SCL)) higher than the current standard of 10^{-3}—if possible, equal to or better than terminal sterilization. Based upon industry and regulatory discussions in the U.S. and EC over the past few years, it is clear that achieving parity in SCL with terminal sterilization will be expected for aseptic processing, once such technology is proven.

Sterility is a concept that cannot be practically proven; the test itself is destructive. Therefore, proof of sterility requires both statistically valid sampling with destructive testing and sufficient process controls to assure that critical process parameters that have been proven to yield sterility can and will be met. Validation of sterilization processes traditionally has involved a specific process with a known, controlled, and finite number of variables that are evaluated, tested, and challenged with resistant microorganisms, in order to prove the statistical certainty of achieving an acceptable safety factor (sterility assurance level) of 10^{-6} (i.e., less than one in one million chance of a nonsterile unit). If these specific, measurable variables are repeated, it is concluded that this process will yield a sterile product.

Aseptic processing as currently practiced contains far more variables than controlled sterilization processes. For this reason, the same approach to validation of the aseptic process has been impractical; validation of aseptic processing has been inferential. Once an aseptic process is well defined to prevent potential contamination, representative trials (media fills) using growth media instead of product are performed. Media fills attempt to simulate production operations. If any of the units so processed are contaminated, they can be easily identified by visual examination. If none (or a very small number) of these media units are contaminated, a probability of contamination level is calculated. It is inferred that if the process is repeated, it will yield sterile products. The difficulty with this approach is that it is difficult (or impossible) to assure that all of the variables are the same for routine processing as for the media fill. Generally speaking, due to practical limits on the number of media units that can be processed, and a perception of a higher probability of contamination, a lower acceptance criteria of less than one contaminated unit out of 1,000 (10^{-3}) has been applied to aseptic processing. This is several orders of magnitude less safety than terminal sterilization or any validated sterilization process. As concerns about the safety of sterile medicines have grown within regulatory agencies, this dual set of standards has been called into question. The U.S. Food and Drug Administration has indicated that all sterile pharmaceuticals should be terminally sterilized, if possible, and improved SALs for nonterminally sterilizable products should be achieved.

The pharmaceutical industry has responded to this challenge. Some industry associations and companies have agreed that, where possible, sterile pharmaceuticals should be terminally sterilized. However, many pharmaceuticals are incapable of withstanding terminal sterilization. The cost of assessing the compatibility of existing pharmaceuticals to terminal sterilization, or even sublethal heat treatment, may exceed practical limits. Heat labile ingredients (including most biologically derived products) or delivery systems (such as pre-filled syringes) may make steam sterilization impractical or even impossible. Ionizing radiation (gamma, electron beam, UV, or X-rays) or other methods of terminal sterilization are unproven or incompatible with most pharmaceutical finished dosage forms. This leaves most of the present, and a majority of the future, sterile pharmaceutical preparations dependent upon enhancements to current aseptic processing to insure their freedom from microbiological contamination.

The validation of advanced aseptic processing, designed to demonstrate higher SCLs, must include the possible configurations of the processes designed to be compatible with higher SCLs. In order to assure sterile products, a process must be designed to kill any microorganisms that may be present, to exclude potential contaminants from contacting the product, or a combination of both.

Terminal sterilization starts with a premise that the product is contaminated, then applies some treatment designed to render those contaminants nonviable after the product is packaged in its final container. The integrity of the container in preventing the intrusion of live organisms under all conditions, including the sterilization process itself, must be proven for this process to be utilized. Overkill terminal sterilization cycles, as frequently used in the pharmaceutical industry, take this concept one step further, and presuppose that the contaminant in the product to be sterilized is the most resistant organism possible (i.e., a biological indicator), in numbers sufficient to demonstrate a 6 log reduction.

Isolation technology includes rendering various components sterile by applying sterilization technology, then bringing the components together in an environment that excludes outside contamination. The application of this principle forms the rationale for this technology.

What are the components that will need to be sterilized and brought together? They can be divided into three categories: primary packaging, product, and gases.

MATERIALS STERILIZATION

Primary Packaging

The primary packaging of a drug product for most sterile pharmaceuticals generally consists of a glass or plastic container and elastomeric closures. The container can be an ampule, a vial, a bottle, an IV bag, or a prefilled syringe. They can be sterilized by thermal processing, either saturated steam or dry heat. In-line dry heat sterilization (and depyrogenation) is commonly used for glass containers today, and is validated to achieve a SAL of at least 10^{-6}. This process is monitored through physical parameters such as temperature, belt speed, and air flow to insure that sterilization conditions are delivered to every unit passing through the dry heat sterilizer.

Elastomeric closures can be natural or synthetic rubber stoppers, seals, or plungers that are generally compatible with steam sterilization, but incompatible with dry heat. The difficulty in designing in-line steam sterilization systems usually results in these components being batch processed and sterilized. Various "terminal" package configurations are available. They can allow these components to be batch sterilized in an autoclave in a closed package then transported to another location for use.

Product

The pharmaceutical solution or suspension is the therapeutic material, but its thermal and radiation sensitivities are the predominant reason for eliminating terminal sterilization. Sterilization by membrane filtration is employed, and can be validated to achieve log reduction values of indicator organisms in excess of 6 (e.g., SAL of 10^{-6}). Redundant filtration as an added safety measure has become common practice. Verification of the integrity of the membrane filter post-sterilization via integrity testing is a necessary part of process monitoring.

Gases

Various gases are introduced either into the product/container or into the environment immediately surrounding the open container or components. The most ubiquitous of these is the air in the environment. It is through this air, and the airborne particles that may be present, that most microbial contamination may occur. For this reason, existing technology may use high efficiency particulate air (HEPA) filters to exclude particles, both viable and nonviable, of a size which might indicate potential contamination. HEPA filters can effectively exclude particles of ≥ 0.5 μm in size to less than 100 per ft^3. The integrity of this filter may be verified through challenge testing, and through continuous monitoring of the pressure drop across the filter.

Other service gases which may be employed, including nitrogen or compressed air, may be sterilized by filtration at the point of use (i.e., at the point of entering the sterile area). These filters can be tested for integrity in much the same way as product filters.

ISOLATION TECHNOLOGY

If we can effectively sterilize and bring each of the materials which are necessary for a sterile pharmaceutical to a common area, the question becomes: How can we sterilize such an assembly area, and how can we be sure it will remain sterile during a dynamic process such as that required for modern pharmaceutical production? Isolation technology is designed to provide the answer to this question.

Isolator Design

The isolator is a primary barrier between potential sources of contamination and the sterile environment of the filling and closing process. The primary sources of microbiological contamination in traditional clean rooms are the operators. Current aseptic processing areas and processes rely heavily upon operator training and compliance to assure process reliability. This dependency represents the most significant difficulty in process validation. The isolator, and the equipment designed to be contained within, therefore should be designed to minimize the amount of human intervention required. Automated systems for performing "operator" activities, such as checkweighing may be employed. Adjustments and maintenance locations should be designed, as much as possible, outside of the barrier (either underneath, or along one wall).

Where human intervention is unavoidable, half-suits or glove ports can provide opportunities for sterile manipulation within the isolator. To facilitate this, the machine/line configuration will become narrower, to allow access within arm's length of all areas within the chamber. The walls of the isolator will most likely be clear glass or plastic, allowing an unobstructed view of the sterile operations.

How materials enter and exit the isolator is critical to maintaining the sterile environment during dynamic production operations. Materials, such as glass vials, may enter through a sterilizing tunnel. Sterilization of the components is assured through process monitoring, and the airflow balanced to verify unidirectional flow from the isolator to the tunnel. Materials may need to enter in a "batch" process, for example one container of pre-sterilized stoppers at a time. This requires some type of connection mechanism, which might include a sterilizing antechamber or a sterile transfer system (e.g., alpha-beta mechanism) to connect the sterile isolator to a sterile container of components. How well this is designed and validated will dictate the type of environment required outside of the isolator (the higher the level of control/confidence, the lower the control requirements for the environment surrounding the isolator).

Since the isolator will be designed to minimize human intervention, the equipment inside should be designed for easy cleaning and sterilization, in place if possible.

Due to the large number of critical parameters that require continuous monitoring, a computerized control and monitoring system may be employed. Such a system requires full documentation and verification during the validation process.

RECOMMENDED READINGS

Cooper, M. S. 1992. The compendial, industry, and regulatory initiatives regarding aseptically processed sterile products. *J. Parenteral Sci & Technol.* 46 (2).

Dixon, A. M. 1991. Training clean room personnel. *J. Parenteral Sci & Technol.* 45 (6).

Federal Standard 209E. 1988, rev. 1992. *Airborne particulate cleanliness classes in cleanrooms and clean zones.* Institute of Environmental Sciences.

FDA 1978. Current good manufacturing practices for finished pharmaceuticals. *Federal Register* 43:45077 (September 29, 1978).

FDA. 1987. *Guideline on sterile drug products produced by aseptic processing.* Rockville, MD: Government Printing Office.

FDA. 1991. Use of aseptic processing and terminal sterilization in the preparation of sterile pharmaceuticals for human and veterinary use. *Federal Register* 56:51354 (October 11, 1991).

Frieben, W. R. 1993. Presentation at FDA Open Conference on Sterile Drug Manufacturing, 12 October, in Bethesda, MD.

ISO/CD 13405. 1993. Aseptic processing of health care products. ISO/TC 198 N171.

Melgaard, H. L. 1994. Barrier isolation design issues. *Pharmaceutical Engineering* 14 (6).

PDA 1980. Validation of aseptic filling of solution drug product. Technical Report No. 2. Parenteral Drug Association.

PDA. 1991. Aseptic processing and terminal sterilization. *J. Parenteral Sci & Technol.* 45 (6).

PDA. 1993. PDA Presentation at the FDA Open Conference on Sterile Drug Manufacturing, October, in Bethesda, MD.

PDA/PMA. 1990. Sterilization in the 1990's. Joint Conference sponsored by PDA and PMA, 26–29 August, in Washington, DC.

United States Pharmacopeia 23 (1995). 1994. Rockville, MD: United States Pharmacopeia Convention.

10
Guideline to the Validation of Isolation Technology

Richard M. Johnson
Alcon Laboratories
Ft. Worth, TX

The validation of an isolator system depends upon the level of isolation in the system, and the claims to be made. The basis for the sterility assurance of the system is the ability to sterilize the isolator and to maintain exclusion of external contaminants to the system. Verification of this is the aim of the validation program.

ISOLATOR INTEGRITY

Once an isolator is sterilized, the maintenance of that condition must be assured. Leak testing of the isolator may be used, and/or the maintenance of the correct positive pressure differential. We currently apply similar technology to the maintenance of sterility of materials held within an autoclave or a lyophilizer. Monitoring of the differential pressure of the air supply across the high efficiency particulate air (HEPA) filters to the isolator provides assurance of the continued integrity of the filters (after initial integrity challenge). Nonviable particulate monitoring must be done continuously in critical locations. Alarms that identify and record any breaks in the system (e.g., human intrusion) are required.

ISOLATOR STERILIZATION

Sterilization of the isolator is a primary differentiator of this technology from current aseptic processing. By sterilizing the environment in which the sterilized materials are brought together and assembled, and maintaining that state, the product can be concluded to be sterile. Sterilization of the enclosure, and the equipment contained within may be a combination of separate processes, or an integrated, single process. Machine and fluid contact parts could be sterilized separately and sterile-transferred into the sterilized enclosure, or they could be sterilized in place. Sterilization-in-place using saturated steam requires a system to capture and remove the steam from the enclosure, monitor the temperature and pressure, and prevent the build up of condensate.

The isolator itself and enclosed equipment might be sterilized by a chemical sterilization process, with or without steam to enhance the distribution and efficacy of the sterilant. In order to assure adequate contact of the sterilant to all surfaces, the system should be designed to allow free flow of the sterilant throughout the isolator. The floor of the isolator might be sloped to facilitate cleanup and elimination of residuals. The system must be designed to achieve uniform, adequate, and reproducible sterilant concentration throughout the enclosure. Factors which might affect the sterilization efficacy, such as temperature, fan speed, air flow, etc., will need continuous monitoring. If the sterilant is a hazardous material, secure and verified methods for assuring closure of the system prior to sterilization will be required, as well as methods to test residuals in the enclosure, and airborne concentrations outside of the enclosure.

ISOLATOR VALIDATION

Validation of the overall system, and its ancillary subsystems, is necessary to prove that the process will deliver sterile products. All validation activities should be performed according to predetermined protocols and acceptance criteria, and must be documented.

Installation Qualification

This activity is a documented verification that all key aspects of the installation adhere to appropriate codes and approved design intentions. Some of the key components of an installation qualification (IQ) protocol are:

Equipment/System Description

Each component or subsystem is described as to its intended function and location. Functional requirements are identified.

Equipment/System Specifications

Design and/or vendor specifications are detailed for each element of the system. Critical operational parameters are included.

Installation Verification

Drawings and documentation of the final, installed systems will serve as the basis for future change control.

Utility Connection Verification

Verification of necessary and correct utility connections insures the safety of both the equipment and operators, and documents the integration of the systems into the facility.

Maintenance Procedures

Approval of maintenance procedures, including calibration, ensure that the equipment will be kept in the same operating condition as when validated.

Instrumentation Calibration

All critical measurement instruments and devices must be adjusted and verified to be accurate within specified tolerances.

Operational Qualification

This consists of documented verification that the system or subsystems perform as intended throughout all operating ranges of the equipment. Operational qualification (OQ) consists of the following:

Process Description

Processes to include the operation of the filling/closure machine, the isolator air systems, the isolator sterilization systems, clean-in-place/steam-in-place (CIP/SIP) systems, component entry processors (e.g., glassware depyrogenation tunnels), and sterile transfer systems.

Process Variables and Limits

Variables include line speeds and capabilities, HEPA filter integrity, air flow and air balance, and time/temperature/pressure/gas concentration of sterilization.

Process Verification

Studies designed to verify the operational performance of the system at the upper and lower specified limits of each controlled process parameter, and that all controllers, monitors, alarms, and interlocks are functioning properly.

Performance Qualification

This activity identifies the critical process parameters to produce a sterile pharmaceutical product, establishes acceptable operating ranges for those parameters, and verifies that they can be controlled and monitored consistently. Studies will be performed in triplicate to assure reproducibility. Traditional aseptic filling process validation has relied upon environmental monitoring, personnel training, and media fills to demonstrate process adequacy. The principal difference in isolation technology is the concept that if each part of a system is validated to a known sterility assurance level (e.g., 10^{-6} SAL), and the integrity of the system is continuously monitored and assured, and the interfaces between parts of a system are integral, then the sum of the process can be said to be validated to that same SAL (i.e., not less than 10^{-6} SAL). Validation approaches for many of the support subsystems are well known. Some of the processes for isolation technology are unique. Validation of these processes includes:

Sterile Transfer Mechanisms

The integrity of the sterile containers can be verified as with container/closure integrity testing. These studies challenge the transfer device using biological indicators, and leak testing. Any sterilizing antechamber requires physical and/or chemical verification of sterilizing conditions, as well as microbiological challenge with appropriate indicator microorganisms. Emphasis on the juncture of the sterile/nonsterile contact parts is required to ensure that sterile connections are possible.

Isolator Integrity

Studies are performed to verify the ability of the isolator to exclude external contamination once sterilized. This is demonstrated via a controlled leak test, and continuous monitoring of differential pressure between the isolator and its environment, as well as the HEPA filter differential pressure (Δp). Maintenance of integrity must be demonstrated during the sterilization process.

Sterilization

Validation of a chemical or chemical/steam sterilization process is similar to that currently used for ethylene oxide sterilization. The studies consist of a combination of physical and chemical monitoring, and biological challenges to assure sterilization.

Depending upon the sterilization process chosen, critical parameters include temperature of the gas vaporizer, temperature within the isolator, volume of sterilant used, gas concentration throughout the isolator, time of sterilization, and time of evacuation. Use of a chemical sterilant requires verification of removal of residuals to an acceptable level.

For validation approaches dependent upon known bioburden, microbiological monitoring of the isolator prior to sterilization is performed. Current environmental monitoring methods for aseptic processing areas (e.g., active air samplers, swabs, and RODAC® plates) are used to gather the data. The resistance of these organisms to the sterilization process can then be demonstrated. This requires ongoing microbiological monitoring to assure no changes in the quantity or variety of bioburden. The minimal expected contamination, coupled with the inefficiencies of microbiological monitoring, will make this approach difficult.

If a biological indicator (BI) log reduction validation approach is used, care must be taken in the selection of the appropriate BI, and the carrier vehicle of the organism during exposure. The BI should be of proven resistance to the sterilant, and should be verified and enumerated prior to all validation trials. *Bacillus stearothermophilus* is widely used as an indicator organism for vapor-phase hydrogen peroxide. Stainless steel coupons or fiberglass discs have been used as carriers.

The selection of chemical, physical, and biological monitoring locations should be designed to assure complete coverage of both the complete isolator, and the most difficult to sterilize locations. These include geometrically distributed points throughout the isolator, selected locations such as heat sinks, and locations where gas/steam distribution may be more difficult.

Revalidation

Once specified parameters of sterilization are validated, with defined safety factors, ongoing monitoring will assure process performance without dependence upon inferential media fills or environmental monitoring. As with any validated process, an effective change control process and revalidation program must be implemented.

RECOMMENDED READINGS

Federal Standard 209E. 1988, rev. 1992. *Airborne particulate cleanliness classes in cleanrooms and clean zones.* Institute of Environmental Sciences.

FDA. 1987. *Guidelines on general principles of process validation.* Rockville, MD: Government Printing Office.

FDA. 1987. *Guideline on sterile drug products produced by aseptic processing.* Rockville, MD: Government Printing Office.

ISO/CD 13405. 1993. Aseptic processing of health care products. ISO/TC 198 N171.

Pflug, I. J. 1993. Introduction to the kinetics of bacterial destruction, treatment of bacterial destruction data, results of bacterial destruction tests in a laboratory apparatus using atmospheric steam plus hydrogen peroxide in the 2,000 to 8,000 ppm range. Presented at International Congress of Pharmaceutical Engineering, May, in Philadelphia, PA.

Regional Quality Control Sub-Committee of Regional Pharmaceutical Officers. *The design and monitoring of isolators.* Ed. 1.

Rickloff, J. R., and P. A. Orelski. 1989. Resistance of various microorganisms to vaporized hydrogen peroxide in a prototype tabletop sterilizer. Presented at Annual Meeting, American Society of Microbiology, May, in New Orleans, LA.

Rickloff, J. R. 1993. VHP Sterilization. Presented at International Congress of Pharmaceutical Engineering, May, Philadelphia, PA.

United States Pharmacopeia 23 (1995). 1994. Rockville, MD: United States Pharmacopeia Convention.

11

Points to Consider in the Use of Sterility Testing Isolators

Richard T. Wood
Pfizer Incorporated
Terre Haute, IN

End-product sterility testing is widely practiced in the pharmaceutical and medical device industries for aseptically produced products. Although sterility testing has been dropped for some terminally sterilized products, it remains an absolute requirement by law for the large number of products that are sterilized by filtration and filled aseptically. The United States Code of Federal Regulations, Part 21, Section 211.167(a)., states "for each batch of drug product purporting to be sterile and/or pyrogen-free, there shall be appropriate laboratory testing to determine conformance to such requirements. The test procedures shall be in writing and shall be followed." Examples of products tested are biologicals, small and large volume parenterals that cannot be terminally sterilized, lyophilized products, oil-base products, ointments, ophthalmics, surgical implants, and sterile medical devices.

Sterility testing of injectables was first required in Great Britain around 1925. By 1936, both the United States

Pharmacopeia and U.S. National Formulary included sterility test procedures (Olson 1987). The methodology has evolved over the years to the present tests which appear in USP XXIII. Two different tests are described in USP Chapter <71>: a direct test for insoluble products (in which product is added directly to culture media) and a membrane filtration test for soluble products. The membrane filtration test is preferred because there are fewer manipulations, it is less expensive to run (needing less culture media), and it is easier to evaluate.

STERILITY TEST LIMITATIONS

Sterility testing has serious limitations and cannot prove that a batch of product is sterile. This follows from basic considerations of sampling statistics. The probability of rejecting a batch of product depends upon the number of samples tested and the frequency with which those samples are contaminated (Harbord 1986). The probability of rejecting a lot can be calculated using the following equation.

$$\text{Probability of rejection} = 1 - (1 - p)^n$$

where p is the proportion of samples contaminated and n is the number of sample items tested.

For example, a sampling plan of 20 items taken at random across a lot where the normal batch size is 10,000 units and the contamination rate is 1 percent would be expected to have only one chance in five of detecting contamination (see Table 11.1). Although the sterility test has difficulty detecting intermittent, low-level contamination, it will detect grossly contaminated products that might result from a manufacturing process breakdown. Therefore, the test has some value as a useful adjunct to a fully validated process.

In addition to the difficulty of detecting low level contamination, the sterility test suffers from other weaknesses that can lead to both false negative and false positive results. To minimize the possibility of false negative results, the sensitivity of the method must be demonstrated for each individual product through validation of test media and sample preparation. Biological challenge studies are conducted to rule out bacteriostatic or fungistatic activity that might be caused by product interference.

Table 11.1. Probability of Lot Rejection Based on Contamination Level and Sample Size

Sample Size	% Contamination			
	0.1	1	5	10
10	0.01	0.09	0.40	0.66
20	0.02	0.18	0.65	0.89
50	0.05	0.34	0.92	0.99
100	0.09	0.63	0.99	
300	0.26	0.95		

False positive sterility test results can occur from accidental contamination while the test is being performed. Thus, even though a product is sterile, it may be rejected through poor laboratory technique. Potential sources of contamination are the person doing the test, the testing environment, the test equipment, and the outside of product containers.

USP XXIII, Chapter <71>, recommends that

> The facility for sterility testing should be such as to offer no greater a microbial challenge to the articles being tested than that of an aseptic processing production facility. The sterility testing procedure should be performed by individuals having a high level of aseptic technique proficiency. Appropriate, known-to-be-sterile, finished articles should be employed as negative controls as a check on the reliablility of the test procedure.

Despite these precautions, it is still possible to have a relatively high false positive failure rate.

Even when the test is conducted in a cleanroom environment on a laminar air flow (LAF) bench by skilled staff who are highly proficient in aseptic technique, there is always a finite possibility that a false positive test can occur. False positive rates ranging from 0.1 percent to 2 percent are not uncommon depending upon the complexity of test manipulations. A high background of false positive tests makes it very difficult if not impossible to detect true positive results.

ISOLATOR TECHNOLOGY

Isolator systems provide an ideal environment for sterility testing and are currently very popular in the pharmaceutical industry. Typically, an isolator is a free-standing, sealed enclosure constructed of impervious plastic material. It is ventilated through high efficiency particulate air (HEPA) filters to exclude contamination from the external environment. Chemical sterilizing agents such as peracetic acid, hydrogen peroxide, or chlorine dioxide can be used to eliminate microorganisms inside the enclosure, and materials enter and exit the enclosure in such a way that the sterile environment is preserved. Sterility tests are conducted by personnel working through glove ports or flexible, ventilated, half-suits attached to the enclosure to further prevent the introduction of microbial contamination (see Figure 11.1). The half-suits provide a greater range of movement inside the enclosure than glove ports.

Figure 11.1. Sterility test isolation chamber components. Clockwise from the bottom: half-suit; glove port; inlet air / HEPA filter; transfer isolator / rapid transfer port; double-door autoclave; outlet HEPA filter.

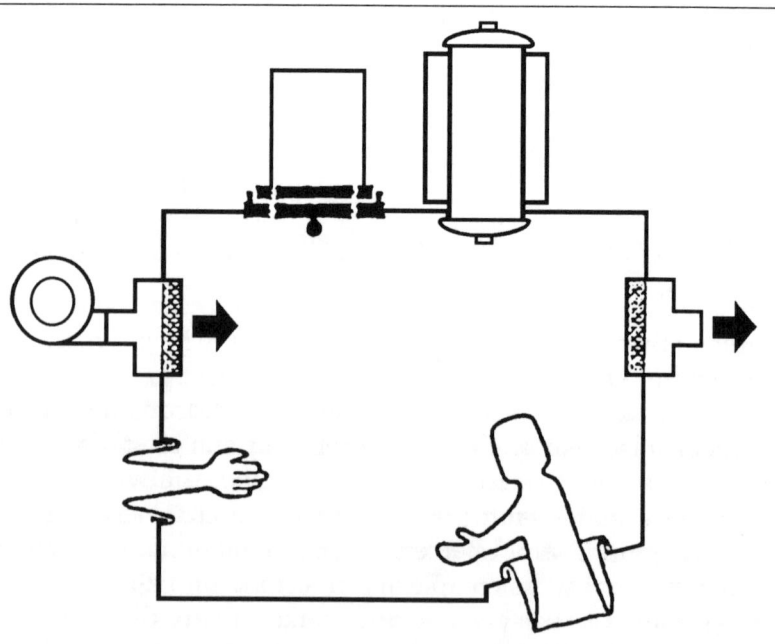

Isolator systems used for sterility testing normally consist either of a tubular steel framework supporting a flexible polyvinyl chloride (PVC) envelope, or of rigid plexiglass walls and framework on a steel base. Rigid isolators are more durable, but they are also more expensive. On the other hand, the PVC envelope, which is the most expensive part on a soft-wall isolator, must be replaced every 3–5 years.

The internal environment of a sterility test isolator must be free of microbial contamination, but Class 100, unidirectional air flow conditions are not required. Most systems have turbulent air flow which is only a disadvantage when sterilization with chemical vapor is attempted. In this case, the sterilizing atmosphere must be vigorously mixed and distributed by electric fans so that it contacts all areas inside the enclosure.

Rapid transfer ports (RTPs) are a unique feature of barrier isolator systems that distinguishes them from conventional glove boxes or biohazard hoods. An RTP can be used to connect two sterile enclosures together in a non-sterile environment and to interchange sterile materials without exposing them to contamination. After the non-sterile surfaces of the two RTP flanges are mated together to form the RTP door, the door can be safely opened and taken into one of the isolators to provide a passage way between the two sterile chambers.

Advantages of an Isolator Laboratory

There are many advantages to using an isolation chamber for sterility testing. To begin with there is a greater assurance of sterility of the testing environment. False positive test rates decrease dramatically, approaching zero. Many of the precautions required in the conventional laboratory to prevent contamination are unnecessary in a sterile isolator. For example, a supply of sterile filter funnels can be maintained in the workstation and funnels can be replaced on a single manifold as many times as is necessary to complete the workload.

The need for personnel gowning is eliminated. Sterile gowning supplies and other costs associated with gowning and maintaining a conventional clean room laboratory are eliminated. Strict aseptic technique is not required during testing. The need to run manipulation controls and to test known sterile materials on a routine basis as suggested in the USP should not be required.

Labor associated with material preparation is reduced, especially if an autoclave is interfaced with a workstation isolator. In this regard, sterile instruments and supplies do not require wrapping which saves preparation time. Sterile test equipment and culture media can be stored on shelving in the work station isolator which permits the laboratory to operate at peak efficiency. The savings in preparation and testing time mentioned above contribute to greater productivity.

The cost of constructing an isolator laboratory is much less than a conventional clean room. Isolators can be placed in practically any space that provides adequate services such as air conditioning, electricity, and a source of vacuum, compressed air, and steam. HEPA–filtered air under positive pressure is not required in the room that houses an isolator.

Disadvantages of an Isolator Laboratory

A major limitation of an isolator laboratory is lack of internal workspace. Careful planning must be exercised if many lots of product are to be tested in a single day. There is a maximum workload that the work station can handle at any one time, and with that volume it is necessary to remove empty reagent bottles and inoculated containers as each test is completed in order to maintain an open, uncluttered working environment.

Another limitation is reach. When working in an isolation chamber with two half-suits, all locations are not within reach. This requires moving from one half-suit to the other in order to reorganize supplies, samples, and empty containers, and a second person to assist with the transfer of materials between chambers.

Flexible isolator enclosures, half-suits, and gloves are also fragile and they cannot be handled roughly. Although these plastic components are easily repaired, small perforations that could compromise chamber integrity are not always apparent. There is no way to be absolutely sure at any given moment that integrity of the isolator has not been compromised. Gloves and half-suits can develop small leaks during normal operations. The leak problem can be controlled to some extent by maintaining a positive differential pressure in the enclosure at all times. In addition, microbiological environmental monitoring efforts should be directed at leak detection.

Operation and maintenance of an isolator laboratory operation are more complicated than in a conventional clean room. Detailed procedures are required for every aspect of isolator operation and maintenance. Minimally, an isolator should be recertified on a semiannual basis. At this time, the HEPA filters are tested for integrity, and the isolator is thoroughly leak tested.

The consequences of a first stage sterility test failure are more serious when the test is conducted in an isolator laboratory that is purported to provide an absolutely sterile working environment. To quote the FDA (1993),

> If an initial test failure is noted in a sample tested in such a system, it could be very difficult to justify release based on a retest, particularly if test controls are negative.

On the other hand, the May–June 1995 issue of *Pharmacopeial Forum* states

> If microbial growth is observed and confirmed (in a sterility test conducted in an isolator), the article tested fails to meet the requirements of the test for sterility. DO NOT RETEST.

The latter statement represents an extreme position. In this regard, a sterility test investigation should always be conducted for every failed test, including those conducted in an isolator. If environmental monitoring in the isolator shows contamination unrelated to the test samples, or test controls are positive, it might be possible to invalidate and repeat the first stage test.

DESIGNING AN ISOLATOR LABORATORY

Location

No special air cleanliness class is necessary for a room in which an isolator laboratory is located, but temperature and humidity must be controlled. Low humidity is especially important when vapor-phase hydrogen peroxide (VHP) is used to sterilize enclosures, and both humidity and temperature control are important for the comfort of personnel working in half-suits. It should be emphasized that personnel do not have to wear cleanroom garments to work in or around a sterility test isolator, but they should observe good hygienic practices.

The room in which an isolator is located should be large enough to permit access to all sides of the workstation, and for the movement and docking of transfer isolators and sterilization equipment, and so on. It is also advantageous to locate the test incubators in the same room.

Size

Isolators are commercially available in a range of sizes to fit almost any application. In addition, custom designs are easy to fabricate. Factors that should be considered when determining the size of an isolator workstation are the amount of internal space that will be required to handle the expected daily workload, and whether the intent is to store materials in the isolator or to take in fresh supplies each time a test is run.

A one half-suit workstation supplied by a single transfer isolator is suitable for small workloads (see Figure 11.2). This type of system takes up the least amount of space, but efficiency suffers due to material transfer and storage problems.

A two half-suit isolator containing storage shelves is much more efficient. This type of workstation can be supplied simultaneously by two transfer isolators, or one of the transfer isolators can be in service while the other is used to sterilize a load of materials, etc.

For greatest versatility and convenience it is recommended that an isolator be attached to the output side of a double-door autoclave to permit materials sterilized by moist heat to be transferred from the autoclave to the work station without having to expose them again to a nonsterile environment. Material transfer can be accomplished using a transfer isolator that can dock with both the autoclave interface and workstation isolator. The obvious advantage of this system is that sterile instruments and supplies do not require wrapping or further processing before they are taken into the workstation. This saves a significant amount of preparation and testing time, and helps to preserve the sterility assurance level in the isolator.

The ultimate sterility test system is a workstation isolator connected directly to an autoclave interface isolator on one side and a transfer isolator on the opposite side (see Figure 11.3). This arrangement permits maximum efficiency in transferring materials sterilized by moist heat or exposure to a chemical sterilant, and in handling large workloads (Wood 1990).

Material Flow

A basic premise on which isolator systems operate is that the work environment is sterile, and that all materials and test articles are sterilized (at least on their outer surface) before they

Figure 11.2. One half-suit workstation with transfer isolator attached. (Diagram courtesy of la Calhène, Inc.)

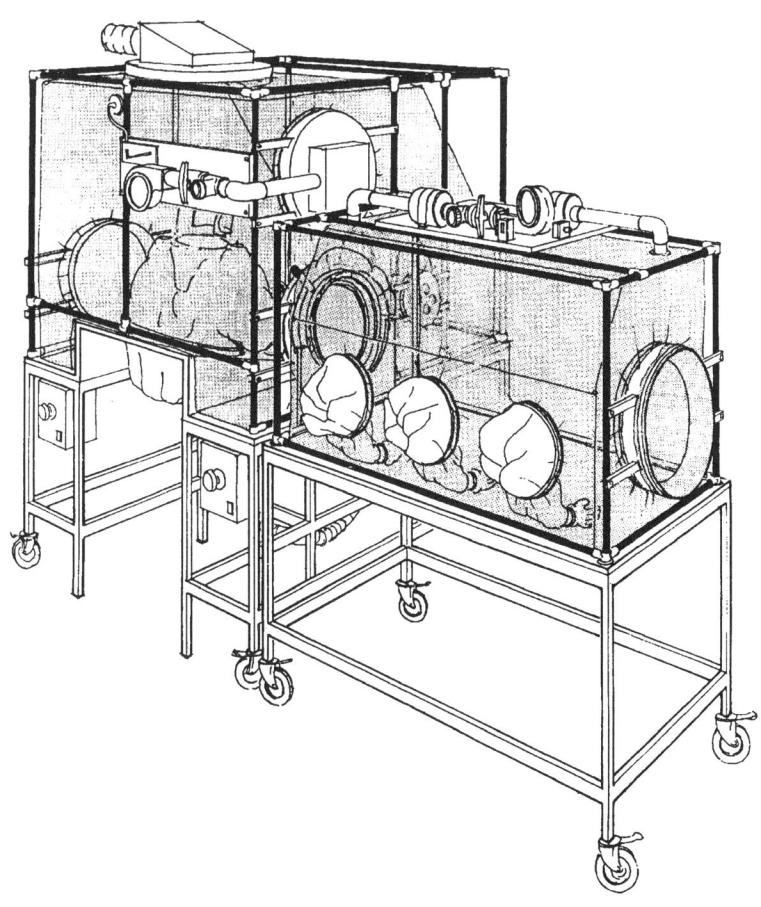

Figure 11.3. Two half-suit sterility testing isolator with autoclave interface. (Diagram courtesy of la Calhène, Inc.)

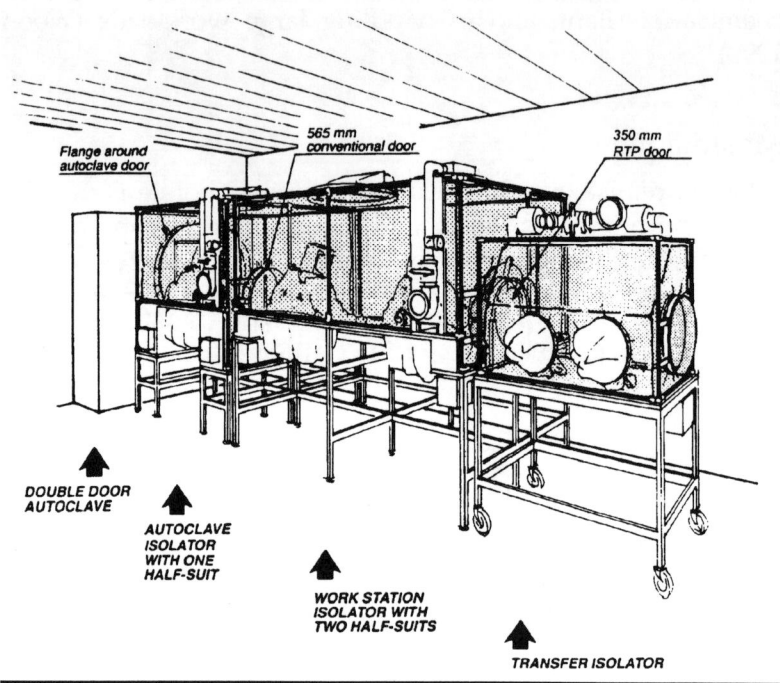

are handled in this environment (Akers 1994). Thus, although strict aseptic technique may not be required to conduct a sterility test in a barrier isolator, good technique is still important to protect the environment from test samples that could contain microorganisms.

Special problems are caused by items that have to be reintroduced into an isolator, such as direct inoculation sterility tests that require subculturing after incubating seven days. One solution is to retain the inoculated tubes in transfer isolators that are wheeled directly into the incubators.

Integrated Systems

The Steritest™ System developed by Millipore Corporation utilizes a self-contained, membrane filtration device for sterility testing. Filter handling is eliminated by enclosing the filters in sterile, disposable, plastic canisters through which liquid samples and rinse solutions are pumped. A sterile culture medium is added directly to the canisters, which are then sealed and incubated. Use of Steritest™ in an isolator will further reduce the chance of false positive results. In addition, since the canisters are sealed in the isolator, the possibility of picking up contamination in a nonsterile incubator is practically eliminated.

Until recently, the use of Steritest™ in isolators has been hampered by the difficulty involved in sanitizing the pump and electronic parts. However, an advanced unit called the Steritest™ Integral 316 II is now available that can be mounted directly in the floor of an isolator, as shown in Figure 11.4. The peristaltic pump head, controls, and accessories are the only items protruding into the workspace. These parts are made of 316L stainless steel and are unaffected by aggressive sanitizing agents. All sensitive mechanical and electronic systems are contained under the work surface in a metal cabinet, and an external footswitch operates the pump (see Figure 11.5).

Utilities

The utility requirements for an isolator laboratory will vary depending upon the complexity of the system. Ventilation and air

Figure 11.4. The Steritest™ Integral 316 II mounted in the floor of an LAF hood. (Photo courtesy of Millipore Corporation)

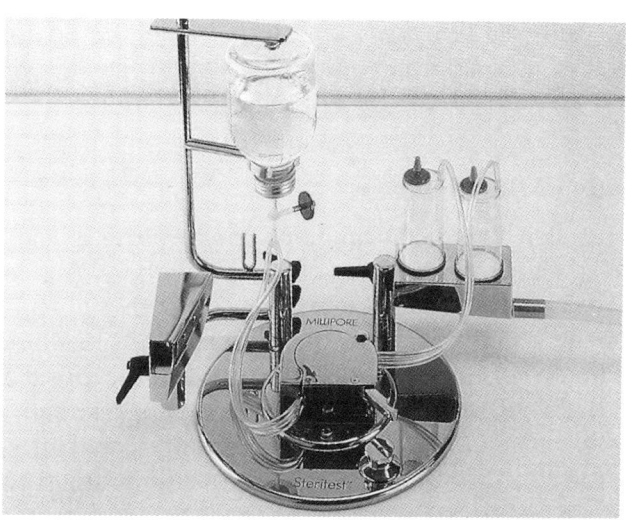

Figure 11.5. Cutaway showing method of mounting the Steritest™Integral 316 II. (Photo courtesy of Millipore Corporation)

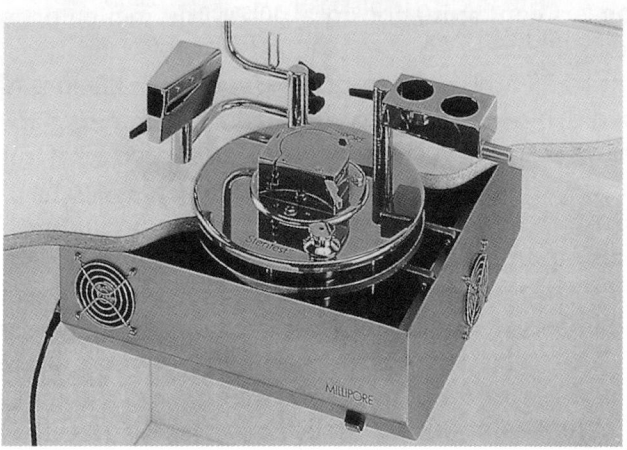

pressurization are an integral part of all isolators as mentioned previously. Sterilization gas must be exhausted to a roof vent when peracetic acid and chlorine dioxide are employed, but VHP can be handled by a self-contained, closed-loop system that requires no special venting. A vacuum source with backflow prevention is required for membrane filtration sterility tests that utilize replaceable filter cups and a vacuum manifold. Dry, oil-free compressed air is used with liquid spray and some vapor sterilization equipment. Finally, steam will be required if an autoclave is part of the isolator system.

Methods of Sterilization

Chemical sterilization at ambient temperature is the current method of choice for barrier isolation chambers. Peracetic acid (PAA) was one of the first agents used for this purpose. PAA solution at a concentration of approximately 3.5 percent is heated in a reservoir at 45–52°C to produce a vapor that is delivered to the isolator in a closed system using a stream of compressed air. The isolator is maintained at a constant pressure during the sterilization cycle by controlled venting through an exhaust system to the atmosphere outside the laboratory. PAA vapor rapidly decomposes to innocuous acetic acid and water vapor when it contacts air.

Table 11.2 shows typical PAA sterilization parameters to produce a 6- and 18-log cycle reduction of *Bacillus subtilis* spores in a transfer isolator and workstation, respectively. Additional reduction of spores occurs in the transfer isolator prior to sterilization from PAA vapor released during the wipe down of sample containers. It may be seen that the sterilization dwell time varies depending upon the volume of the isolation chamber, and that aeration times can be quite lengthy for large isolators.

During the sterilization of leak-tight systems, the sterilant vapors should be completely contained inside the enclosures and nothing should escape into the room environment. One advantage of working with PAA is that the vapor has a pungent acetic acid odor that is easily detected at very low concentrations. When this odor is present, it is a warning that there is a leak somewhere in the system. A self-contained breathing apparatus should be available in the laboratory for worker safety in the unlikely event that a major leak occurs.

Davenport (1989) described an automated system for sterilization of isolators using atomized PAA. All surfaces inside the isolator are wetted with 4 percent PAA and the chamber is then sealed under pressure for a specified dwell time of one hour. Surfactant (Nacconal, a sulfonic acid) is added to the PAA (0.1 percent) for spraying of sterility test sample containers.

Table 11.3 shows sterilization cycle parameters for both empty and fully loaded isolators that were estimated to give a

Table 11.2. Barrier Isolator Laboratory Sterilization Using Peracetic Acid Vapor

	2-Suit Isolator 4.2 m^3 / 148 ft^3	Transfer Isolator 0.58 m^3 / 20.5 ft^3
Volume 3.5% PAA	150–250 ml	80–100 ml
Dwell Time[a]	4 hr	1.5 hr
Aeration Time	Overnight	NLT[b] 30 min

[a]Airflow rate 40 ℓ/min (est PAA conc., 0.8–1.0 mg/ℓ); *B. subtillus* var. *niger* D-value ≅ 13 min.

[b]NLT = not less than

Table 11.3. Barrier Isolator Laboratory Sterilization Using Peracetic Acid Liquid Spray

	2-Suit Isolator 4.3 m^3 / 152 ft^3	Transfer Isolator 0.99 m^3 / 32 ft^3	Transfer Isolator Fully Loaded
Volume 4% PAA	400 ml	150 ml	300 ml
Spray Time	16 min	10 min.	15 min.
Dwell Time[a]	1 hr	1 hr	1 hr
Aeration Time	NLT 6 hr	NLT 6 hr	NLT 6 hr

[a]Transfer Isolator loaded with product containers for surface sterilization (Davenport 1989).

probability of survival of 10^{-24} for spores of *Bacillus subtilis* var. *globibii*. It may be seen that the combined sterilization and aeration time is approximately eight hours.

Hydrogen peroxide gas is currently the most widely used sterilizing agent for isolator systems. AMSCO International Inc. developed a fully automated VHP®1000 hydrogen peroxide vapor generator specifically for decontamination of enclosed systems with internal chamber volumes up to 1000 cubic feet (see Figure 11.6). The unit is connected to an isolator using two hoses to form a closed-loop as shown in Figure 11.7. A two-stage drying system inside the generator uses activated alumina and a molecular sieve to dehumidify the enclosure air. The drying agent must be periodically regenerated by a heating and aeration process. Following dehumidification, a patented vapor generator system controls the mass of hydrogen peroxide injected into the moving air stream to give reliable and reproducible sterilization conditions. As hydrogen peroxide vapor returns to the VHP®1000 after passing through the enclosure, it is catalytically converted into water vapor and oxygen, which can be discharged directly into the room without environmental hazard or concern for personnel exposure. A small, plastic tube connected from the isolator to a pressure sensor in the VHP®1000 permits controlled operation of the system under a slightly negative or positive pressure (i.e., atmospheric pressure ±2 inches of water column).

Figure 11.6. VHP®1000 hydrogen peroxide vapor generator attached to a transfer isolator. (Photo courtesy of AMSCO International, Inc.)

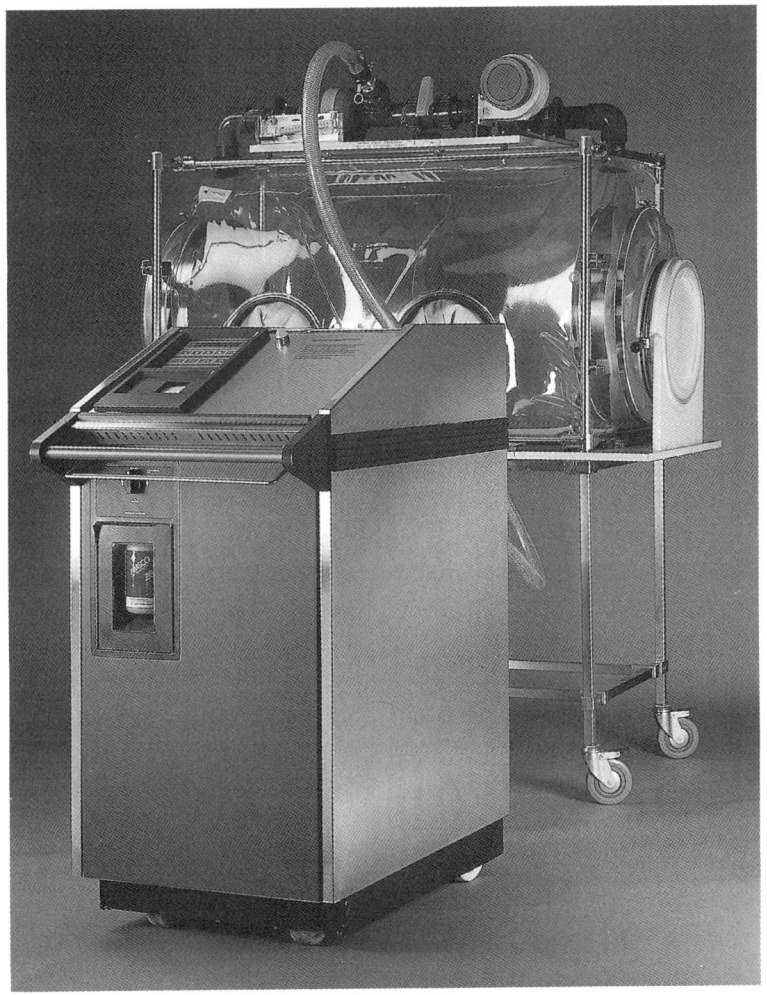

Typical VHP®1000 sterilization parameters for sterility test isolators are shown in Table 11.4. It may be seen that the vaporized hydrogen peroxide sterilization process has four distinct phases. Dehumidification of the chamber space to less than 10 percent RH is required first before hydrogen peroxide vapor can be introduced. If the humidity level is higher than

Figure 11.7. Diagram of VHP®1000 attachment to an isolator for sterilization. (Adapted from Desjardins (1995), courtesy of ISPE)

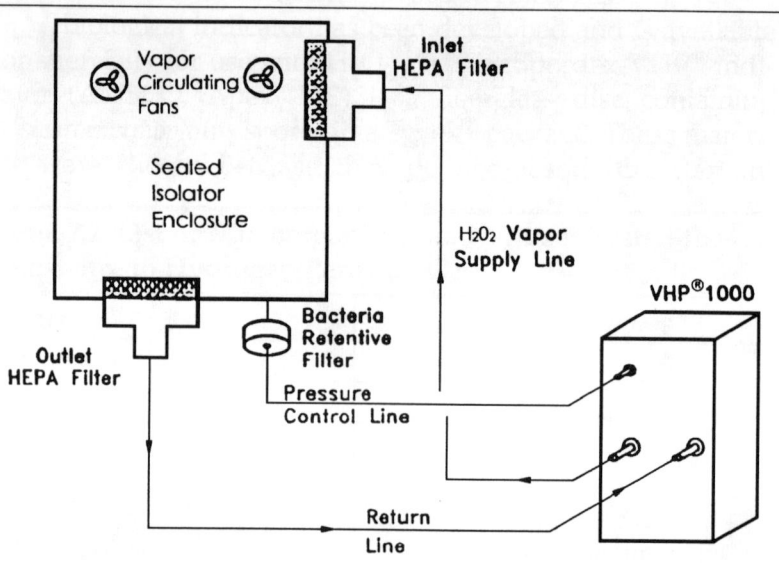

Table 11.4. Barrier Isolator Laboratory Sterilization Using Vapor Phase Hydrogen Peroxide
Time / Injection Rate / H_2O_2 Concentration
@ 20 scfm airflow rate

Cycle Phase	Autoclave Isolator 5.1 m³ / 180 ft³	2-Suit Isolator 4.55 m³ / 160 ft³	Transfer Isolator 0.6 m³ / 21 ft³
Dehumidification	42 min	30 min	5 min
Conditioning	5 min 9.2 g/min 5 mg/ℓ	4 min 9.2 g/min 5 mg/ℓ	2 min 5.4 g/min 4 mg/ℓ
Sterilization	35 min 4.5 g/min 1.5 mg/ℓ	35 min 4.5 g/min 1.5 mg/ℓ	35 min 2.8 g/min 1.7 mg/ℓ
Aeration	NLT 6 hr	NLT 5 hr	NLT 3 hr

10 percent, the peroxide vapor will condense. During the second or conditioning phase, hydrogen peroxide vapor is introduced into the air stream at a relatively high injection rate (e.g., 9.2 g per minute) to reach sterilization concentrations rapidly. Throughout the sterilization phase, hydrogen peroxide levels are maintained at steady state levels in the range of 0.5–2.4 mg per liter. Hydrogen peroxide at these concentrations is not corrosive for most materials. The final phase is aeration to reduce peroxide residues to a low level (typically ≤1 ppm).

Chemical and biological indicators (BIs) are placed inside the isolator during Vsterilization cycle development to measure sterilization effectiveness. The purpose of the chemical indicators, which register a visible color change, is to show that the hydrogen peroxide vapor reaches all areas inside the enclosure. Electric fans are strategically placed inside the chamber to help distribute the gas.

Bacillus stearothermophilus exhibits a relatively high resistance to hydrogen peroxide vapor (e.g., D-value $\cong$ 5.0 minutes at 1.5 mg per liter) and can be used to challenge the sterilization process. Spores of this organism can be inoculated onto stainless steel coupons or fiberglass disks (ca. 10^5 per carrier) that are then used as BIs. The half-cycle approach can be used to establish effective sterilization cycles. In this approach, the exposure time required to completely inactivate all BIs is determined, then the time is doubled to provide a substantial safety factor.

M.D.H. Limited recently introduced the MICROFLOW HyPer-Phase™ 31000 hydrogen peroxide vapor generator for sale outside the United States (see Figure 11.8). This generator operates on the same principle as the VHP®1000, but offers some advanced features. It utilizes a two-stage refrigerant drier with automatic defrost for continuous air dehumidification, and has an exhaust gas monitor that can measure and display hydrogen peroxide concentrations from 0.1 ppm to 1000 ppm. Reportedly, the HyPer-Phase™ generator has a capacity to decontaminate enclosure volumes to approximately 6000 cubic feet.

Monitoring Instruments

The only physical parameter continuously monitored when an isolator is in operation is the internal pressure in the enclosure.

Figure 11.8. The MICROFLOW HyPer-Phase™ 31000 hydrogen peroxide vapor generator. (Photo courtesy of M.D.H. Limited)

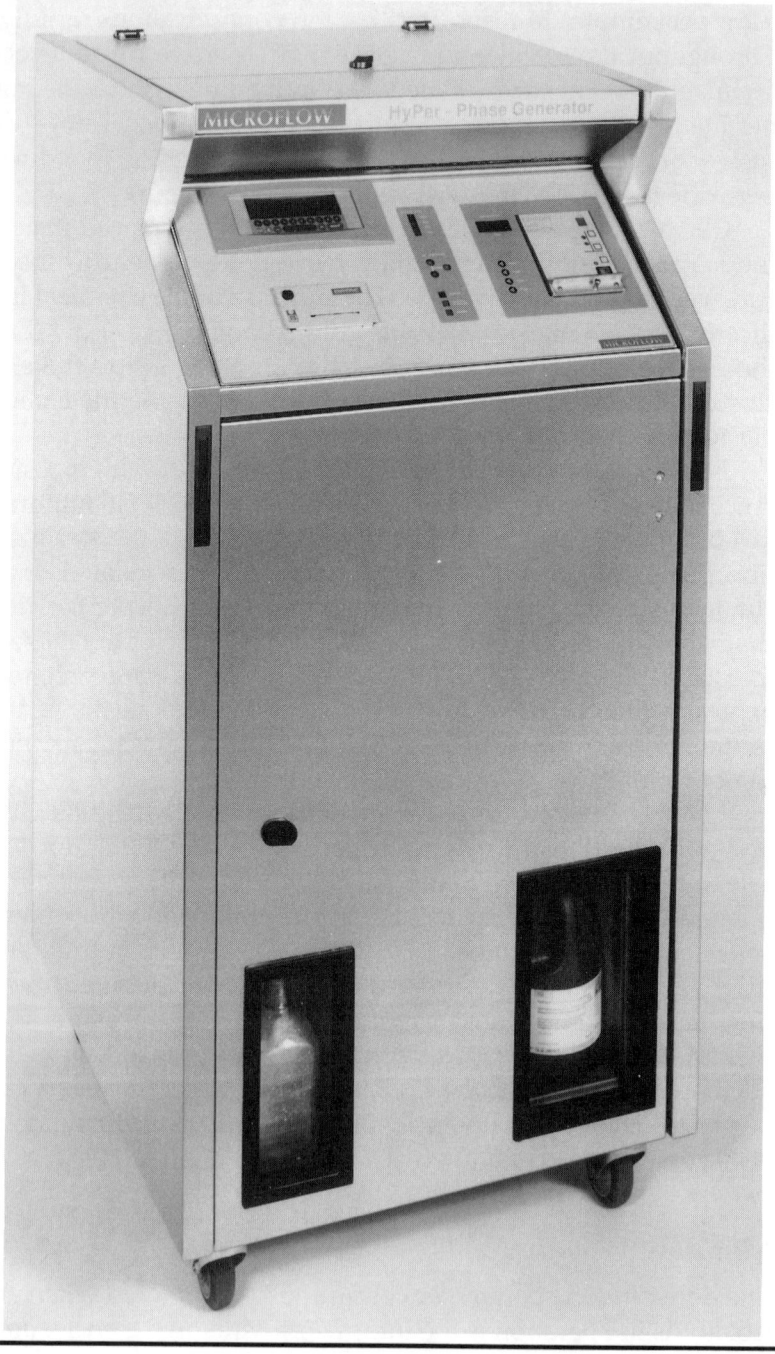

An instrument as simple as an incline manometer is suitable for this purpose. However, more elaborate set ups can be used such as photohelic gauges or sensitive pressure recording devices. Maintenance of a positive pressure at all times is important to protect against small leaks that may occur in the system. Testing is conducted at regular intervals to detect and repair leaks.

Environmental Monitoring

Microbiological environmental monitoring is conducted routinely in sterility testing isolators, and sterility test controls are used to show that the quality of the testing environment is maintained. The information provided by these environmental tests is very important during a sterility test failure investigation. Monitoring methods that can be used include swabbing of surfaces, and exposure of sterile liquid or solid culture media. The most sensitive sampling method appears to be a glove rinse. Gloves are immersed in sterile purified water or saline solution containing a low concentration of surfactant and the liquid is then passed through a microbial retentive membrane filter. The filter disk is either incubated on the surface of a suitable agar medium, if quantitative recovery is desired, or in a tube of broth to detect microbial contamination. While none of these methods are sensitive enough to detect the extremely low bioburden levels that might occasionally be present in an isolator, they will detect a breakdown of the system.

Test Incubators

It is desirable to have the test incubators close to the isolator, preferrably in the same room. Test containers should be tightly sealed (e.g., Steritest™ canisters) or wrapped in sterile plastic bags when they are brought out into the nonsterile environment, especially if these containers must be re-introduced into the isolator as in the case of direct-transfer sterility tests. Alternatively, test containers can be incubated directly in transfer isolators.

Validation

Validation of sterility testing isolators focuses on proving the effectiveness of isolator sterilization and the ability to maintain a germ-free test environment. When an autoclave is interfaced with an isolator system there is the additional requirement to validate the autoclave. The three phases of validation currently practiced in the pharmaceutical and medical device industries are followed—installation qualification (IQ), operational qualification (OQ), and performance qualification (PQ). Validation of an isolator system is not difficult, and it can be done in a practical and cost effective manner.

Installation Qualification

The room in which the isolator is installed does not have to be equipped in any special way, but layout is important. The room should be designed with adequate space surrounding the workstation isolator for access and maintenance, and for docking of transfer isolators, etc. Ceiling lighting should fully illuminate the interior work surface of the isolators or lights can be attached to the framework on top of the isolators. Air conditioning outlets should not open directly over the isolators if hydrogen peroxide vapor sterilization is employed. When cool air blows directly on an isolator it can cause vapor condensation on the inside of the envelope.

Sterilization agents such as peracetic acid and hydrogen peroxide can be hazardous, so protective equipment such as self-contained breathing apparatus and eye wash stations should be available in the room. When a noxious chemical agent such as peracetic acid or chlorine dioxide is used as a sterilant, an exhaust system equipped with a fan is connected directly to the output hose on the isolator, and the exhaust is routed to the outside of the building.

Isolators are supplied by the manufacturer in kit form and are easily assembled on site. A careful inspection should be conducted at each step of the assembly to make sure all parts fit as intended. For example, RTP doors should function properly, and any attachment of an isolator to an autoclave or to another isolator should provide an airtight seal.

Installation of critical isolator systems and controls should be documented. These include: installation and integrity testing of HEPA filters, proper alignment of ventilation fans used to circulate gas during sterilization, and installation and calibration of pressure monitors and controllers. The primary and secondary pressure control systems that are linked to the

VHP®1000 hydrogen peroxide vapor generator during isolator sterilization are also critical control systems.

Gloves and half-suits can be the "Achilles' heel" of isolator systems. They should be carefully inspected and integrity tested before they are installed. The final step in installation qualification is to leak test each fully assembled isolator. A simple way to accomplish this is to release ammonia vapor in a sealed, pressurized isolator and to look for a color change in a sensitive pH indicator cloth as it is slowly wiped across the outside of the isolator.

It is important that an autoclave connected to an isolator be programmed to eliminate practically all water vapor and condensate at the end of each sterilization cycle to prevent moisture from entering the isolator when the door is opened. This can be accomplished by applying cooling water to the autoclave jacket from the bottom up, after decompression cooling has occurred, followed by a purge of the chamber with sterile air until a temperature in the range of 65–75°C is reached. A sliding autoclave door that opens automatically at the touch of a button is ideal for an isolator system, but maintenance of the door mechanism is difficult once the isolator is attached to the autoclave.

All critical instruments that play a role in the operation of isolators and ancillary systems should be identified and calibrated before operational qualification begins.

Operational Qualification

Standard operating procedures (SOPs) for running the isolator laboratory and validation protocols should be available at least in draft form at the start of operational qualification. SOPs should be prepared for cleaning, sterilizing, maintaining, and operating the isolators on a daily basis. SOPs should also be available for microbiological environmental monitoring, for performing sterility tests, and for conducting and evaluating sterility test investigations.

Protocols are needed to validate isolator sterilization cycles. Guidelines for qualifying these cycles are usually supplied with commercial sterilization equipment. For example, both AMSCO International, Inc., and M.D.H. Limited provide cycle development guides with their hydrogen peroxide vapor generators that lead the reader in a stepwise manner through the development of sterilization cycles. Protocols are also required for validating the decontamination of sterility test samples, and for showing that the sterilant used does not penetrate into the samples and interfere with sterility tests.

A software functional specification and qualification report should be supplied with sterilization equipment that is controlled by a microprocessor. Operational qualification involves starting up the equipment and checking the performance of programming and security systems, sterilization cycle sequencing, and cycle alarms and aborts.

Operational qualification of isolators is not very complicated. It involves starting them up and monitoring the performance of chamber and half-suit ventilation systems, VHP ventilation fans, and pressure monitors and controllers. In addition, the performance of ancillary equipment such as vacuum systems for membrane filtration sterility testing, and sterilant exhaust systems are also checked.

Performance Qualification

Isolator sterilization is validated prospectively during performance qualification and it requires a biological challenge. *Bacillus stearothermophilus* is the organism of choice. BIs can either be purchased and used as is (e.g., spores inoculated onto filter paper or fiberglass strips), or they can be prepared by inoculating spores onto other carrier materials such as plastic or stainless steel.

The *D*-value of BIs should be known so they can be used to estimate the lethality of sterilization cycles. *D*-value can be determined experimentally by exposing BIs to specified lethal conditions during a series of short-duration sterilization cycles. *D*-value is the negative reciprocal of the slope of the curve generated by plotting $\log_{10}$ survivors against the corresponding exposure times in minutes.

Proposed sterilization cycles are then conducted in the isolators to determine the times required to completely inactivate all BIs distributed throughout the chambers and/or loads. These times represent half-cycles, and cycle times are doubled to provide a substantial safety factor for routine sterilization.

Another important aspect of isolator validation is determining the time required for outgassing of sterilant vapor. If a hydrogen peroxide generator is used that does not have an automatic exhaust gas monitoring system, the exhaust stream can be sampled manually during isolator aeration, with a device that measures sterilant levels chemically. For example, Dräger detector tubes (supplied by BGI Inc.) can be used for hydrogen peroxide and peracetic acid vapors; they will detect concentrations down to 0.1 ppm.

Tests are also conducted to show that sterilant cannot penetrate into sample containers. Containers are artifically inoculated inside and outside with viable microorganisms and they are exposed to decontamination cycles. The exterior and interior surfaces of the containers are then sampled for surviving challenge organisms. The expected result is that all organisms are inactivated on the outside of the container, while the organisms inside the containers are unaffected.

After it is has been shown that the isolators can be effectively sterilized and that they are impervious to external contamination, they are nearly ready for routine service. However, it is necessary first to gain experience running sterility tests in the isolators. This might include blind studies with sterile and nonsterile materials. Environmental monitoring is also initiated to begin collecting a data base. The final step is to prepare validation task reports and to set up a documentation file.

CONCLUSIONS

The use of isolation technology has revolutionized sterility testing. An isolator is a free-standing, sealed enclosure constructed of impervious material that is ventilated through HEPA filters. Chemical sterilizing agents are used to eliminate microorganisms inside the enclosure, and materials and samples enter and exit in such a way that the sterile environment is preserved. Sterility tests are conducted through flexible rubber gloves or plastic half-suits attached to the enclosure to further prevent the introduction of microbial contamination. Isolators have the potential to eliminate false positive sterility tests, and to greatly increase testing efficiency. Points to consider in the design, validation, and operation of isolator systems for sterility testing were presented in this chapter.

REFERENCES

Akers, J. E., J. P. Agalloco, and C. M. Kennedy. 1994. *Experience in the design and use of barrier isolator systems for sterility testing.* Basel, Switzerland: Parenteral Drug Association International Symposium.

CFR Title 21. 1995. Part 211: *Current good manufacturing practice for finished pharmaceuticals.* Washington, D.C.: Department of Health & Human Services, Food and Drug Administration.

Davenport, S. M. 1989. Design and use of a novel peracetic acid sterilizer for absolute barrier sterility testing chambers. *J. Pharmaceutical Science & Technology* 43:158.

Desjardins, C. 1995. Vapor phase sterilization technologies for isolators. In *Sterilization techniques.* East Rutherford, NJ: International Society for Pharmaceutical Engineering.

FDA 1993. *Guide to inspections of microbiological pharmaceutical quality control laboratories.* 1993. Rockville, MD: The Division of Field Investigations, Office of Regional Operations, Office of Regulatory Affairs.

Harbord, P. E. 1986. Sterility testing and its relevance to sterility. In *Sterilization of medical products,* edited by E. R. L. Gaughran, R. F. Morrissey, and W. Yon-sen. Montreal: Polyscience Publications, Inc.

Olson, W. P. 1987. Sterility testing. In *Aseptic pharmaceutical manufacturing, Technology for the 1990's,* edited by W. P. Olson, & M. J. Groves. Buffalo Grove, IL: Interpharm Press, Inc.

Pharmacopeial Reviews. 1995. Vol 41. <71> Sterility tests. In *Pharmacopeial Forum.* Rockville, MD: The United States Pharmacopeial Convention, Inc.

The United States Pharmacopeia, Vol XXIII. 1990. Easton, PA: Mack Publishing Co.

Wood, R. T. 1990. *Advanced aseptic processing: Barrier technology sterility testing laboratory.* Washington, DC: PDA/PMA Sterilization Conference.

Section III
Applications: The Industry Experience and Perspectives

12

Barrier Isolation Technology: A Systems Approach

Jack P. Lysfjord
Paul J. Haas
Hans L. Melgaard
Irving J. Pflug
TL Systems Corporation
Minneapolis, MN

Clean rooms are bathed in highly filtered air and contain products and processes together with humans garbed in clean fabrics, rubber, and plastic.

Barrier isolators are mini-clean rooms that enclose a process and exclude humans.

Barrier isolator technology is the culmination of a long evolution in pharmaceutical manufacturing. Pharmaceutical manufacturing began with open-manual production (Figure 12.1) and progressed to glove boxes. World War II saw developments of both drugs and blood products as well as clean rooms. Sandia Laboratories (Albuquerque, New Mexico) originated the clean room concept. Clean room applications became common practice for the handling of radioisotopes, the processing of wafers for the microelectronics industry, and the

Figure 12.1. Early, manual pharmaceutical filling (*Note: degree of product protection*). Photo courtesy of The Upjohn Company.

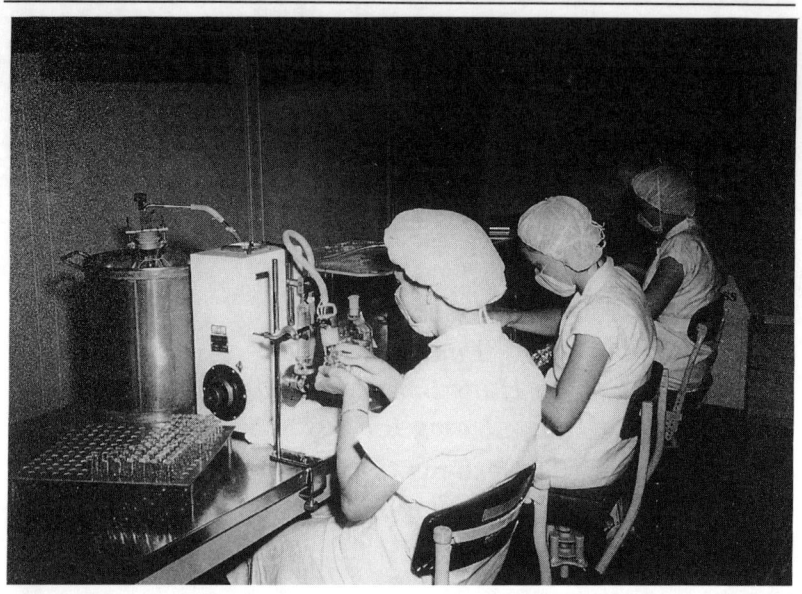

filling and testing of drugs. Clean room applications commenced to become widespread in the 1960s.

One of the first steps taken by the pharmaceutical industry in moving toward barrier isolators for pharmaceutical use was installed by SmithKline Beecham in the mid 1980s. Walls were built through filling lines to separate the clean room from the gray side maintenance area (Figure 12.2). The gray area involves exposure to items or actions that are inherently dirty (e.g., equipment maintenance). Dr. Willie Lhoest of Belgium was one of the original promoters of gray side maintenance such as this. Taking this concept a step further encloses the filling line and removes the operator from the open vial area. Up to this point, the few barrier isolators in use had not been very user friendly.

Barrier isolators for sterility testing have been in use for the past several years. The applications of barrier isolation to production systems for pharmaceuticals have been few, but use is increasing rapidly. The task with production (filling)

Figure 12.2. Clean room pharmaceutical filling with a wall for separating the clean room from "gray side maintenance" area. Photo courtesy of SmithKline Beecham.

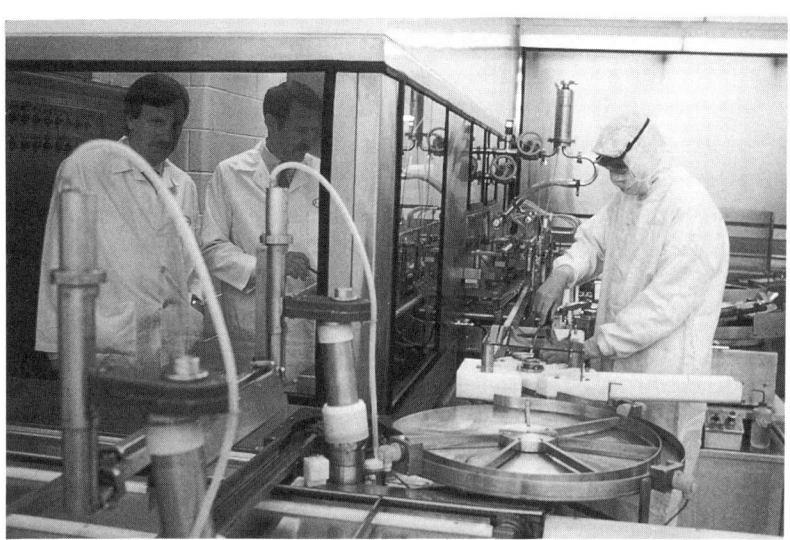

applications is to create a sealed enclosure, sterilize it, bring sterile components (such as vials and stoppers) inside, bring in the sterile product, and fill the product so that the completed package leaves the barrier isolator without contaminating the interior of the barrier isolator. This must be done at a high sterility confidence level (SCL) with the process located in a nonclassified, but controlled, environment. A continuous process system is not sealed, but controlled by overpressure zones. This is a challenge in itself, but validation of the system is an even greater challenge.

People represent the largest source of bioburden or viable particles in the classical clean room operation. The barrier isolator approach separates people from critical processes done with the open vial. A barrier isolator allows for easier monitoring of parameters and provides a consistent environment—an analogy could be made to a product tank or an autoclave. Barrier isolators also separate the operator from hazardous products. Numerous papers have been written demonstrating improved SCL (reduced contaminants) by keeping people away from open vials prior to stoppering. The Upjohn Company presented data at an FDA open forum in October 1993 that showed media fills in excess of 100,000 without a positive (SCL 10^{-5}) were done with an "open" (not sealed) barrier located within a Class 100 clean room.

Reduction in cost, using barrier isolators, is a significant factor given the atmosphere of medical cost containment in the industry. Merck has presented numbers that indicate capital cost savings of 50–70 percent can be achieved over conventional clean room facilities with barrier isolators of the same capacity. Operating cost savings come from energy savings due to reduced volume of sterile area enclosed; reduced gowning expenses estimated at $50,000 per operator, per year; and better utilization of operators. Upjohn expects three times the people utilization when barrier isolators are used since people can cover multiple lines. (Figures 12.3 and 12.4 show comparable facilities, conventional clean room versus barrier isolator approach.)

Operator protection is important when potent compounds are being filled. Barrier isolation is the most cost-effective way of dealing with potent compounds.

In the United States, as in Europe, the objective throughout the pharmaceutical manufacturing industry is to produce product where the SCL is less than 10^{-6} (fewer than one unit in one million units are nonsterile). Only a process that has positive control of the critical points of contamination can be validated to produce a SCL of 10^{-6}. It is impractical to prove a SCL of 10^{-6} by testing the product.

Our processing system has an integrity that actively prevents microbial contamination. Our barrier system is similar to an autoclave sterilization process in that it can be validated. Only product manufactured by a validated process carried out according to an established protocol will have an SCL of 10^{-6}.

Two very important words are *control* and *validation*. *We cannot validate a process where we do not have control of the process variables.* Only barrier isolator systems provide the control necessary to validate the system to an SCL of 10^{-6}.

In the aseptic assembly of pharmaceutical products in the mid 1990s, we are using containment systems and new, small barrier isolators. When we use a containment-type system

Figure 12.3. Layout for four 300-per-minute vial processing lines in a conventional clean room format. Length = 140 ft; width = 80 ft; total area = 11,200 sq ft; total Class 100 area = 2,464 sq ft.

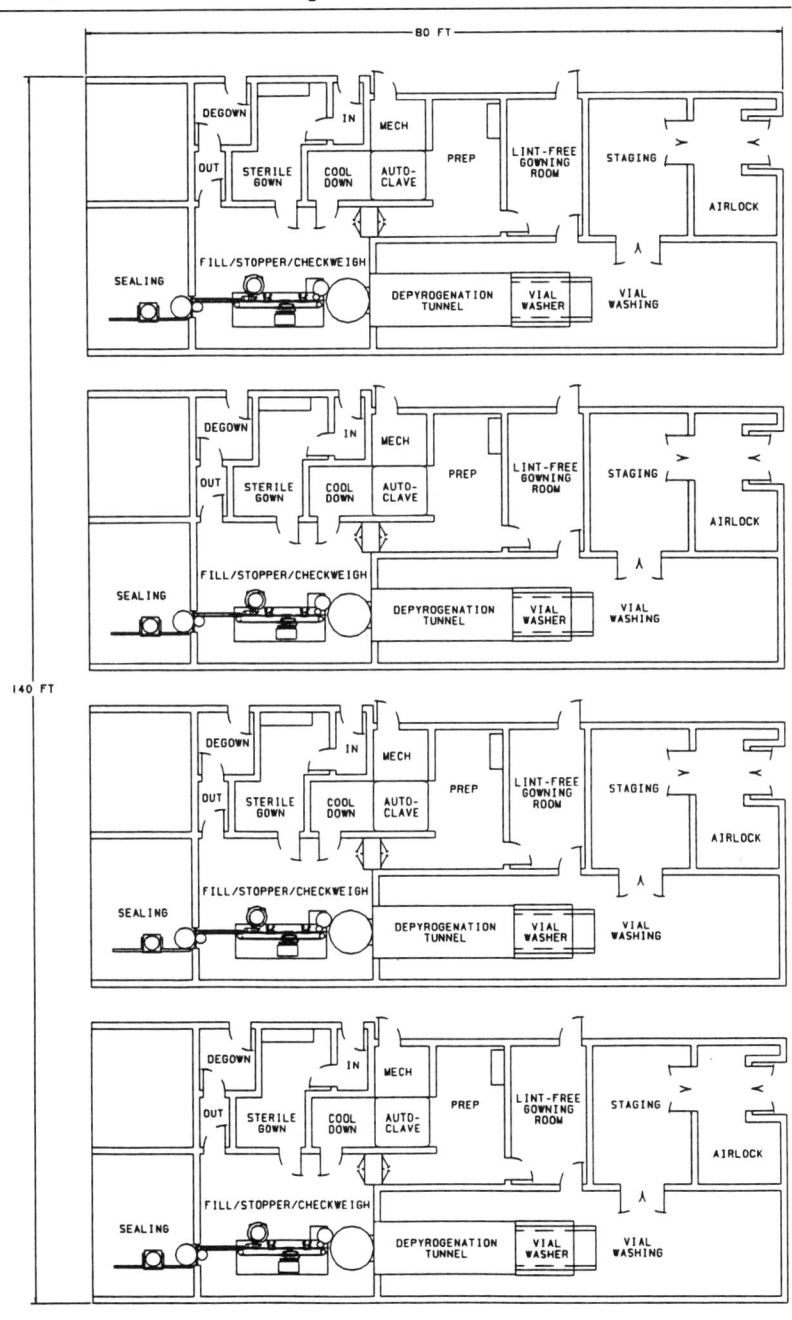

Figure 12.4. Layout for four 300-per-minute vial processing lines utilizing barrier isolator technology. Length = 89 ft; width = 68 ft; total area = 6,052 sq ft; total Class 100 area (prep and barrier only) = 688 sq ft; barrier area only (shaded) = 292 sq ft. (*Note: reduced facility size and reduced Class 100 area compared to Figure 12.3*).

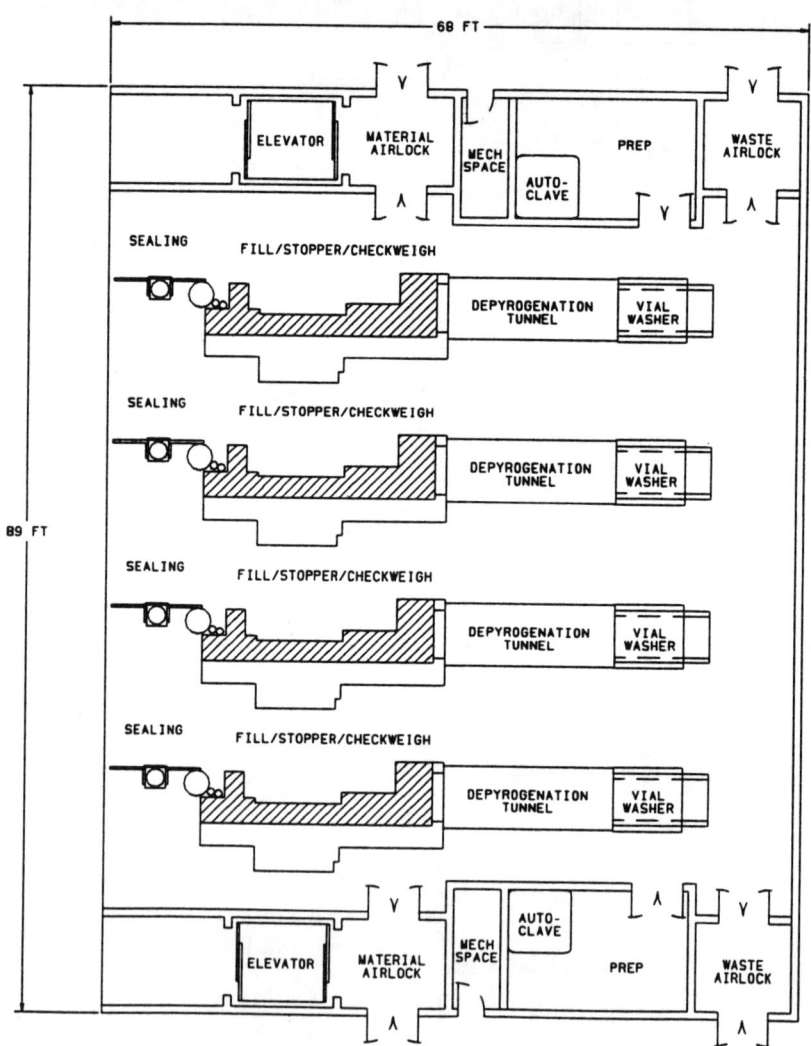

(such as gloves, masks, and bunny suits), we have a structure between the sterile area and the nonsterile person or element that will resist but, in general, will not prevent microorganisms from moving from the nonsterile person to the sterile product. There is general agreement in the industry that we cannot truly validate a clean-room production facility that contains a person in protective clothing (bunny suit) in the way that we can validate an autoclave. To validate to an SCL of 10^{-6}, we must have a true, positive barrier isolator to limit the movement of contamination.

A *barrier isolator system* is a system with a positive barrier between the sterile area and the nonsterile surrounding area. It is necessary to distinguish between different kinds of barrier isolator systems: *flexible barrier isolator systems* have flexible components (for example, gloves, flexible isolators, half-suits, and similar systems) and *rigid barrier isolator systems* have rigid walls to maintain overpressures for an integrity control system.

The general goals for our barrier isolator system are to

1. Protect the product from line operators. We need to remove people from the open-vial filling area and maintain an aseptic assembly environment through the use of HEPA[1]– and ULPA[2]–filtered air that will produce a probability of contamination of a product unit with an SCL of less than 10^{-6}.

2. Protect the operators from new, very toxic, pharmaceutical products. This means that we must have a positive barrier isolator between the toxic product and the people.

3. Reduce the overall costs of producing aseptically assembled products.

4. Design equipment systems that are flexible and user friendly.

---

[1]A HEPA (high efficiency particulate air) filter is an extended-media dry-type filter in a rigid frame having minimum particle-collection efficiency of 99.97 percent for 0.3 μm thermally generated dioctylphthalate (DOP) particles or specified alternative aerosol, and a maximum clean-filter pressure drop of 2.54 cm (1.0 in.) water gauge, when tested at rated airflow capacity.

[2]A ULPA (ultra low penetration air) filter is an extended-media dry-type filter in a rigid frame having minimum particle-collection efficiency of 99.999 percent for particulate diameters >0.12 μm in size.

A parenteral product filling line in a barrier isolator is so designed and constructed that the manufacturing and packaging operation will produce pharmaceutical products with a microbiological SCL of 10^{-6}. To do this, the following three activities must be carried out successfully:

1. The system must transfer and deposit product in the package and close the package so that the SCL of the unit of product is 10^{-6}.

2. There must be an active, continuous control system in place so that if there is a problem, the control system alerts the operators and will cause production to stop if critical control points (necessary to produce or maintain an SCL less than 10^{-6}) fail or move out of specification.

3. There must be an acceptable validation and certification program. Validation is a series of tests that substantiate that the specific process or activity will produce the required result; certification is assembling the results and accumulated reports of the validation program in a package reviewed and then approved or signed off by the responsible persons in the company.

To produce an aseptically assembled product that has an SCL of less than 10^{-6} in a system using barrier isolation technology requires the following parts and inputs to the barrier isolation enclosure:

1. The product, as it arrives for packaging, must have a very low microbial load so that, after packaging, the product unit SCL will be less than 10^{-6}.

2. A rigid isolation enclosure. A rigid unit of stainless steel and glass, with opening lockable doors for assembly and disassembly of equipment; these doors can be sealed so that isolation enclosure becomes, in effect, a low pressure vessel. The inside of the enclosure is sterilized prior to start-up. It will remain sterile because it will be pressurized with HEPA– and/or ULPA–filtered input air.

3. Packaging in Glass Vials.
   a. Glass vials will arrive at the barrier isolator from the discharge end of a continuous flow glass sterilization-depyrogenation unit.
   b. Closures must have an SCL of less that 10^{-6} when they enter the isolator.
4. Microbial Control and Validation of the Barrier Isolator.
   a. Validate that through wipe-down, clean-in-place (CIP), decontamination, and/or sterilization before start-up, the microorganisms inside the barrier enclosure are killed so there is assurance that at start-up there is less than one viable microorganism per 10 square meters of surface. A validated HEPA– or ULPA–filter system must be in place that provides air to the barrier isolator with a very low viable particle count per cubic meter of air.
   b. A validated control system must alert operators and stop production if the barrier isolator integrity is breached during production.
   c. A validated particulate measurement-control system must continuously sample the air at the container opening level, alert operators, and halt production if the particulate count in the air at the filling nozzle/top of open-vial level exceeds the established control point.

When we examine the requirements listed above, we see that item number one is part of the pharmaceutical product manufacturing operation, and we assume that it is being taken care of since, at the present time, the general assumption is that the product has an SCL of 10^{-6} when it enters the manufacturing area.

Item number three above is a given in today's manufacturing system, where glass containers, sterilized in a sterilization-depyrogenation tunnel, arrive at the isolator in a sterile condition. The closures will be presterilized and, therefore, will arrive at the isolator in a sterile condition.

The following major topics now will be presented:

1. The Barrier Filling System
2. Filler Design
3. The Barrier Isolator
   A. Materials Selection and Compatibility
   B. Interface Issues
   C. Handling of Freeze-Dried Products
   D. Particulate Control Considerations
   E. Barrier Isolator Internal Condition Control and Monitoring
4. Clean-in-Place of Barrier Isolators
5. Sterilization of Barrier Isolators
   A. Atmospheric Steam/Hydrogen Peroxide Sterilization System
6. Validation Considerations

THE SYSTEM

A systems approach to barrier isolator technology is comprised of the filler, the barrier isolator, and the sterilization process, along with control of critical parameters that allow the system to be operated under control and validated.

FILLER DESIGN

The filler design forms the foundation for the system and is the basis for potential success of the system from an ergonomic standpoint. The concept for the design of the filler must be resolved first. Whether the line is rotary or linear (Figure 12.5) must be resolved along with whether to use indexing motion or continuous motion. A rotary machine is typically much wider, and has more potential for restricted access when compared to a linear system. Speed usually dictates whether the

Figure 12.5. Top view of rotary versus linear vial processing equipment for ergonomic considerations.

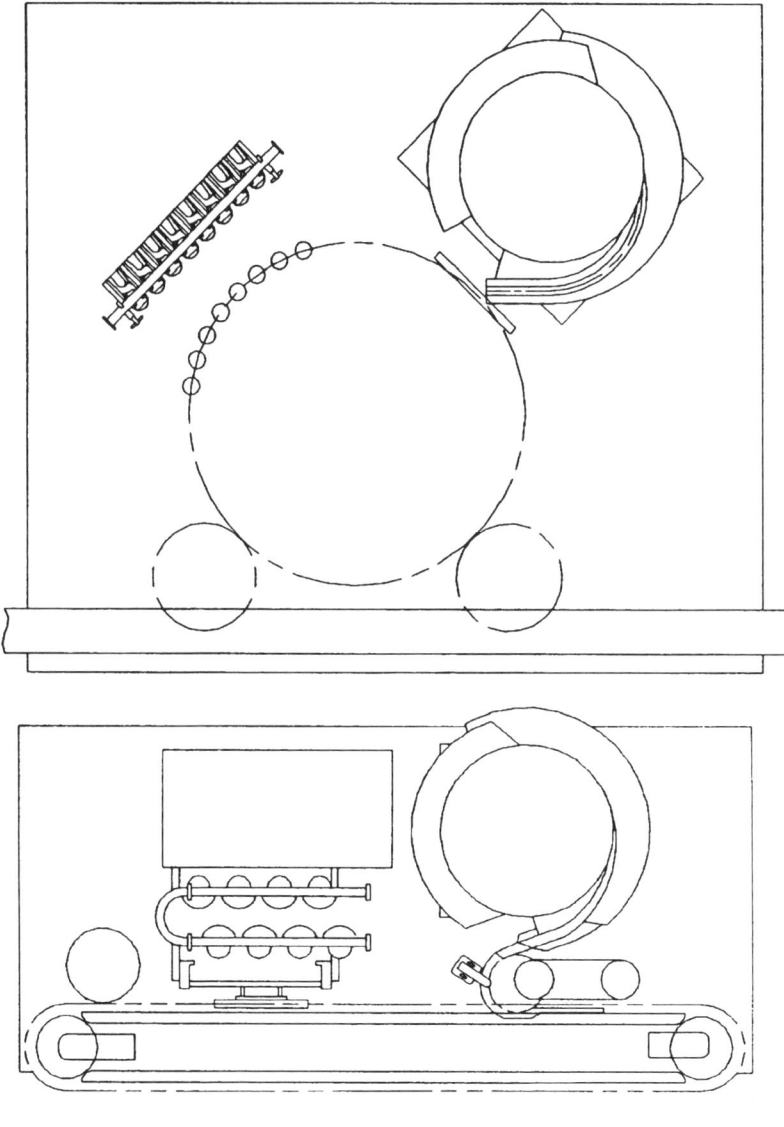

line has indexing or continuous motion. Reliability, redundancy, and particulate concerns increase in barrier isolators at higher SCLs. Continuous motion can be done with a lighter duty machine, is gentler to sensitive protein products, and results in lower particulate generation due to reduced glass vial "clatter." The best approach is a linear continuous motion filling system.

The total system elements need to be considered. A continuously operating production filling line in a barrier isolator, at improved SCLs, must have components (glass vials, stoppers, product) continuously fed to it. The system has difficulty accepting glass in a batch process. An upstream vial washer and depyrogenation tunnel would be utilized upstream from the filler. Often an accumulator disc is utilized as a capacitor between the tunnel and the filler. A disc works well for this function, but does not give first-in, first-out motion of vials. This gives a variable open time for a given vial prior to stoppering or a process that varies from vial to vial. Accumulation is necessary, but it must be done with first-in, first-out flow in mind.

Filling must be done accurately, repetitively, and cleanly without drips. The fill mechanism must operate with low shear to prevent damage to protein-based products. Vials cannot tip and should be separated to prevent glass-to-glass particle generation. The filler should have rinse-in-place and steam-in-place (SIP) capability. At the molecular level, rinse-in-place is a more appropriate term than CIP with rubber or plastic components.

Since there are no people in the interior of the barrier isolator, automated checkweighing is necessary to determine what fill volume each nozzle is actually producing.

A stoppering system capable of running both plug and slotted stoppers in appropriate sizes is necessary. The system should be capable of dealing with stoppers with reduced siliconization levels. This is driven by two items:

1. Silicone is a particulate that transfers to the product.

2. Protein products degrade with silicone.

The overall system must be easy to reach across and must have easy access through doors (with interlocks) for changeover or maintenance in the enclosed area. It is not realistic to enclose a system and never open the barrier isolator.

Other considerations for the system are as follows:

1. Keeping people away from the open vial

2. Desired operating speed

3. Container sizes to be handled
4. Fill volume range in each container
5. Product cost
6. Product characteristics—foaming, viscosity, etc.
7. Unique process for product
8. Minimizing the enclosed volume inside the barrier isolator
9. Minimizing mechanisms inside the barrier isolator
10. For potent compounds, the filler should have CIP capability on the surface interior for the barrier isolator
11. The system should tolerate various sterilization methods
12. Stopper reservoir must hold more stoppers than the time it takes to transfer another sterile batch of stoppers into the barrier isolator
13. Easy maintenance
14. Ergonomics

An example of the evolution of filler development for liquid products is shown in three phases. The first phase is a rigid barrier isolator placed over a conventional fill, checkweighing, and stopper machine (Figures 12.6 and 12.7). Phase II removes many mechanisms from the enclosed volume, and the width of the enclosure drops by 20 inches to 33 inches (Figures 12.8 and 12.9). Phase III (Figures 12.10–12.12) is radically different and leaves only necessary components inside the enclosure. Phase III reduces volume, provides drains for CIP, and again reduces width by another 10.5 inches to 22.5 inches at the glove ports. TL Systems greatly appreciates the input of personnel from Eli Lilly & Company, the Upjohn Company, and Merck Manufacturing Division in this evolution.

THE BARRIER ISOLATOR

The design of the filling machine forms the basis for the barrier isolator that is mounted to it. A rigid-walled barrier isolator is

244 *Isolator Technology*

Figure 12.6. Top view of conventional vial filling, check-weighing, and stoppering equipment with a barrier isolator installed. (TL Barrier Isolator, Phase I, 1991–early 1992)

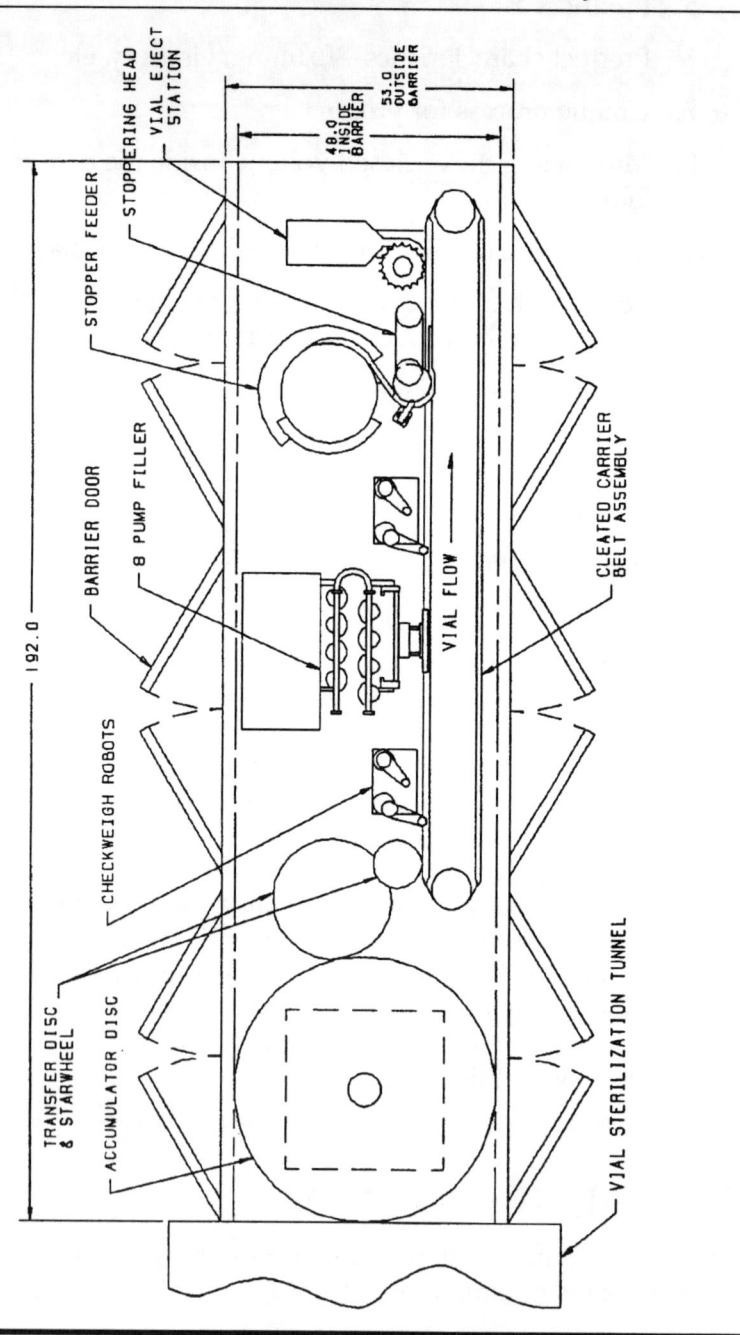

Figure 12.7. Section view of Figure 12.6 through filler. (TL Filler, Phase I) (*Note: outside width is 53 inches*).

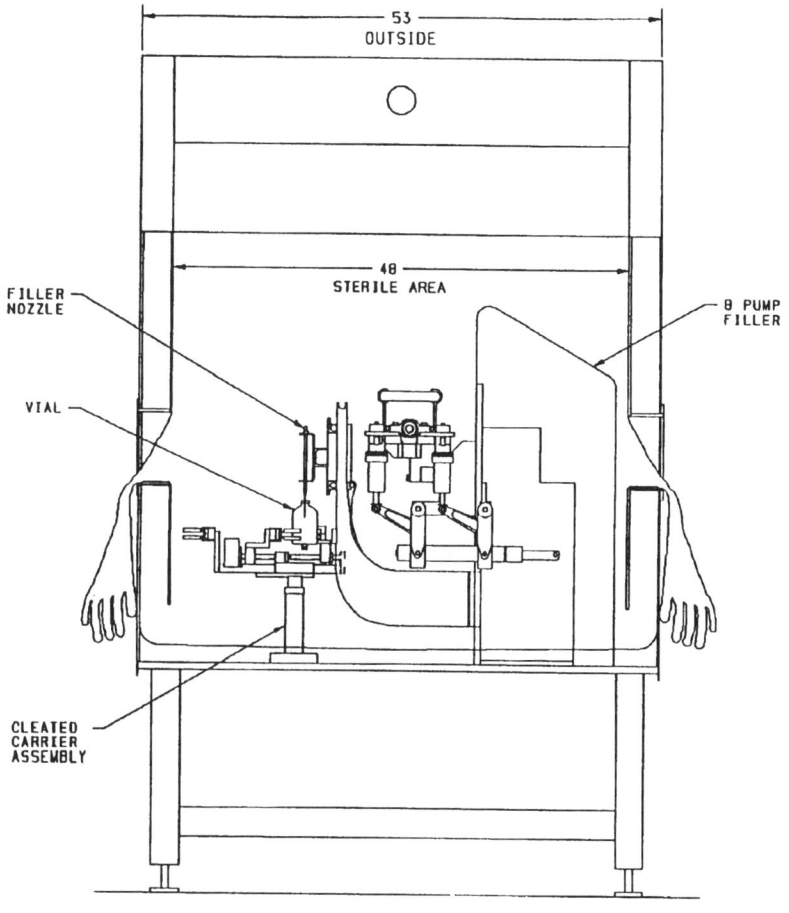

desired with construction of stainless steel and glass to minimize material able to absorb the sterilant. Ergonomic considerations need to be taken into account to allow for easy use by the maximum number of potential operators. The enclosure must be designed to properly interface and provides access to critical filler components. A study between the filler supplier, the barrier isolator suppliers, and the ultimate user is necessary to determine where glove ports or manipulators are needed to allow for reliable operation of the system. Ergonomic modeling with computer simulation is a good place to start this evolution (Figure 12.13 shows a computer model of

Figure 12.8. Phase II top view of improved vial filling, checkweighing, and stoppering equipment that has been redesigned to move most of the fill mechanism below the tabletop and to narrow the equipment for ergonomic reasons. (TL Barrier Isolator, Phase II, mid 1992)

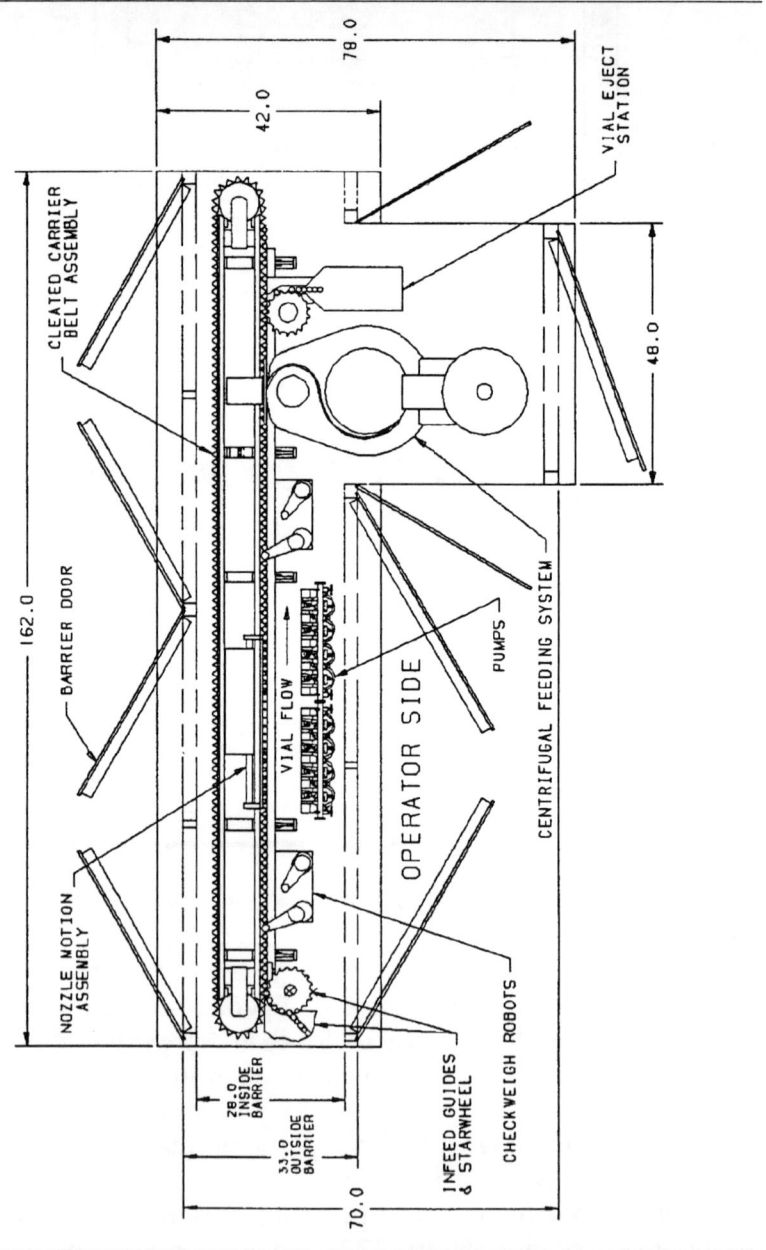

Figure 12.9. Section view of Figure 12.8 through filler. (TL Filler, Phase II) (*Note: outside width is 33 inches*).

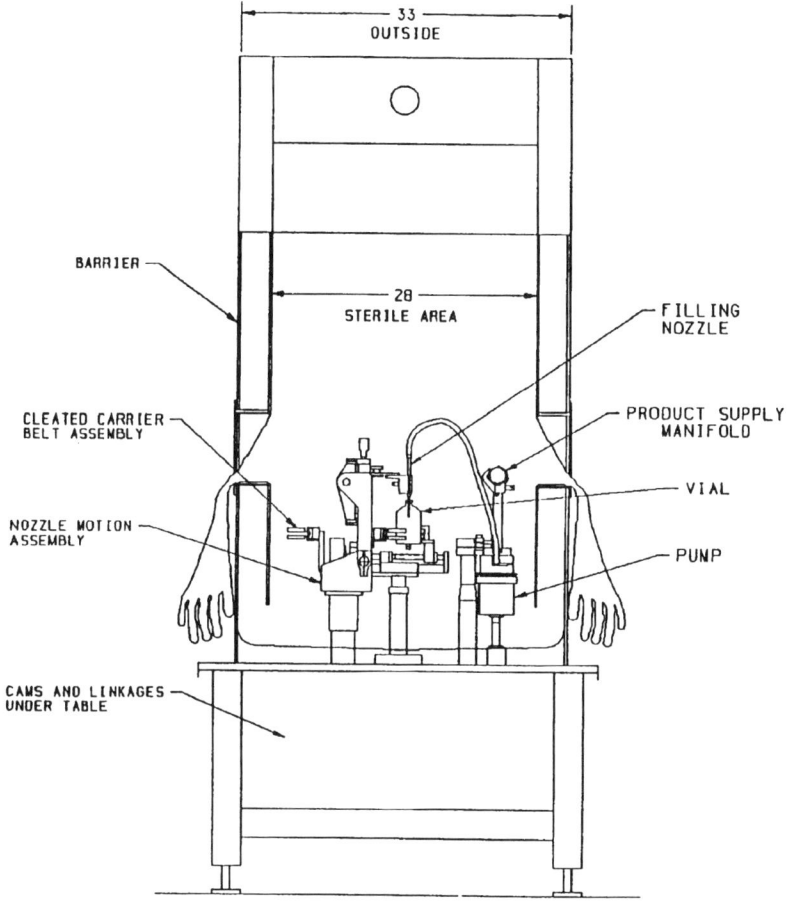

accessibility). A second model is necessary to look at airflow distribution (A computer model of this is shown in Figure 12.14). A third model necessary is construction of an actual mockup system to ensure no oversight occurs. This can be cardboard or plywood and plexiglass. The payback on this effort is manyfold (see Figure 12.15.)

Materials Selection and Compatibility

Filler and barrier isolator materials must be compatible with the CIP/SIP processes. With respect to the use of hydrogen

Figure 12.10. Top view of Phase III. Dramatic redesign with same functions as in Figure 12.6 and Figure 12.8. MAFS (Mini Aseptic Filling System)™ (patent pending).

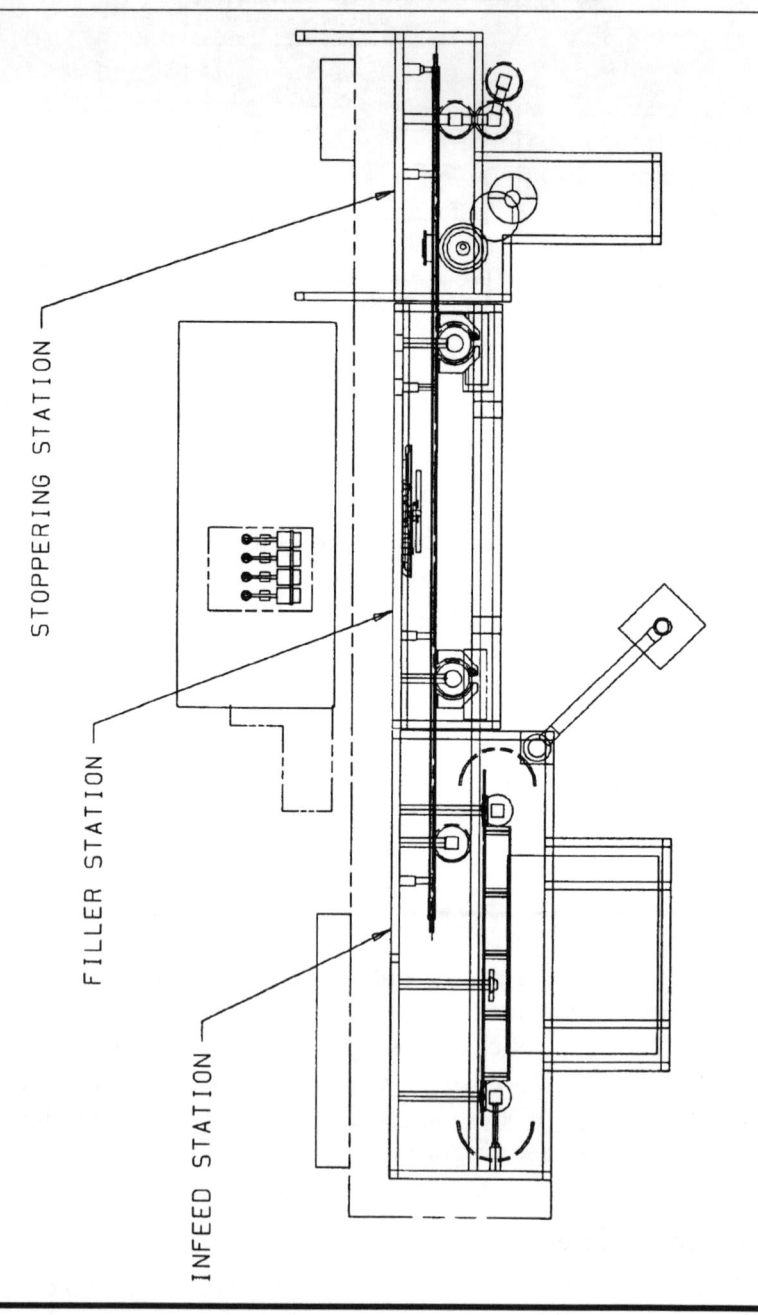

Figure 12.11. Section view of Figure 12.10 through filler. (TL Filler Phase III; MAFS™, patent pending) (*Note: width is 22.5 inches*).

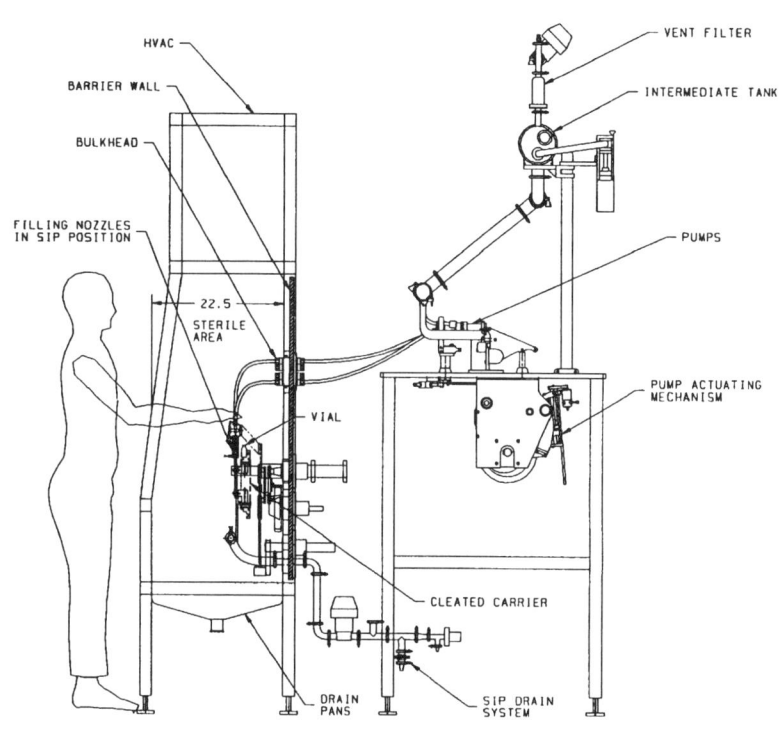

peroxide as the sterilant, either in vapor form or in combination with steam, there are a number of materials fully compatible with the use of the sterilant. These materials are, in most cases, impervious to the penetration of hydrogen peroxide, especially the metals. Plastics and elastomers are normally held to minimal content to avoid any absorption and desorption of the sterilant. In the case of the steam/hydrogen peroxide system, the materials of construction must repeatedly withstand 100°C temperatures and 100 percent humidity conditions. See Table 12.1 for a chart of material compatibility with hydrogen peroxide.

250 *Isolator Technology*

Figure 12.12. View of MAFS™ from operator side without barrier isolator (patent pending).

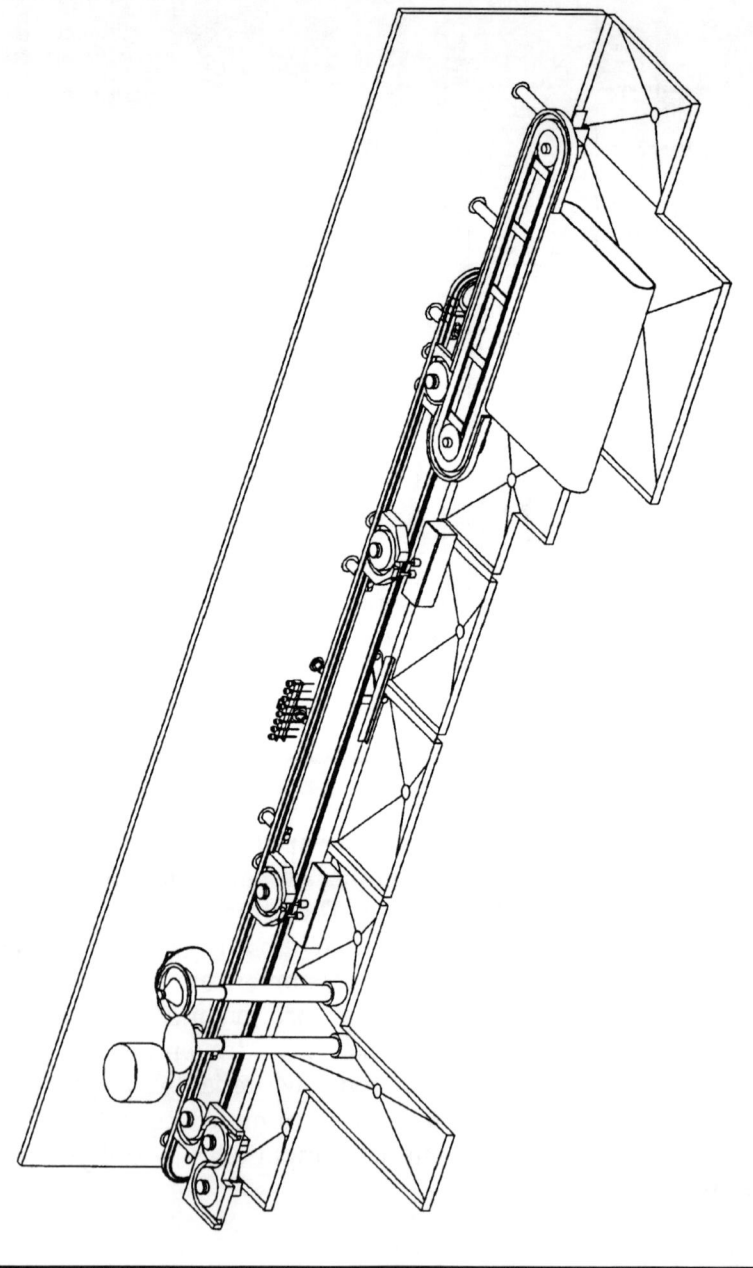

Figure 12.13. Computer simulation of ergonomic aspects of fill area.

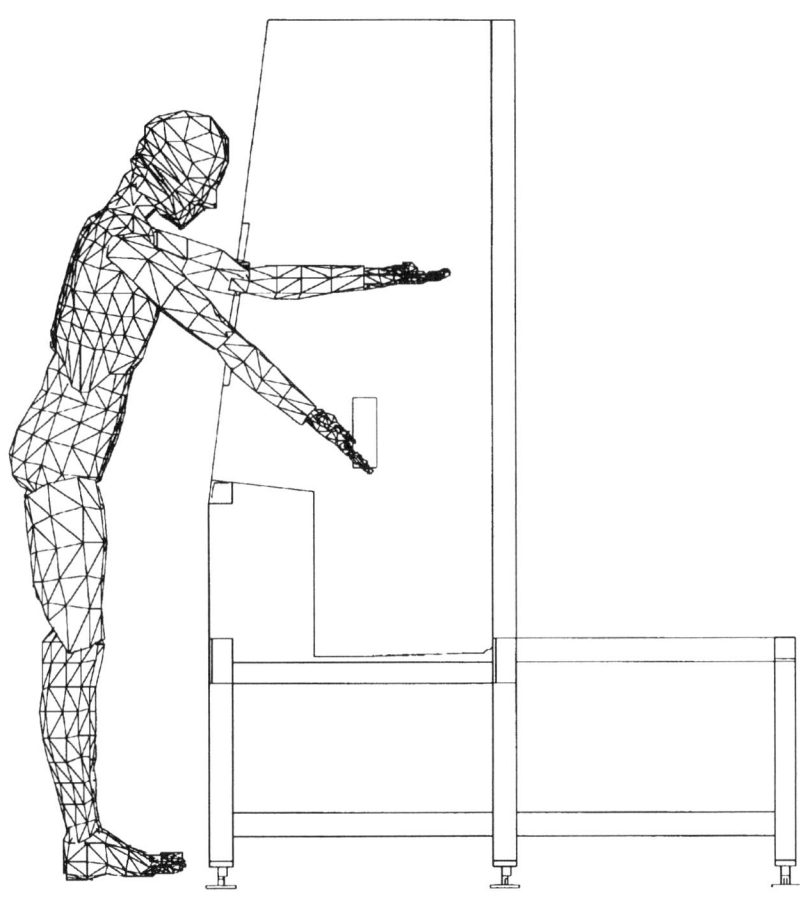

Interface Issues

Several issues need to be addressed with any barrier isolator used with a high speed parenteral filling line. First and foremost, commodity entrance and product exit must be properly engineered. The largest volume of material coming into a parenteral filling line is glass. The glass typically exits a depyrogenation tunnel with a pressure differential between the barrier isolator and the tunnel itself. The opening at the end of the tunnel may be as large as the entire width of the infeed

Figure 12.14. Computer simulation of airflow in fill area.

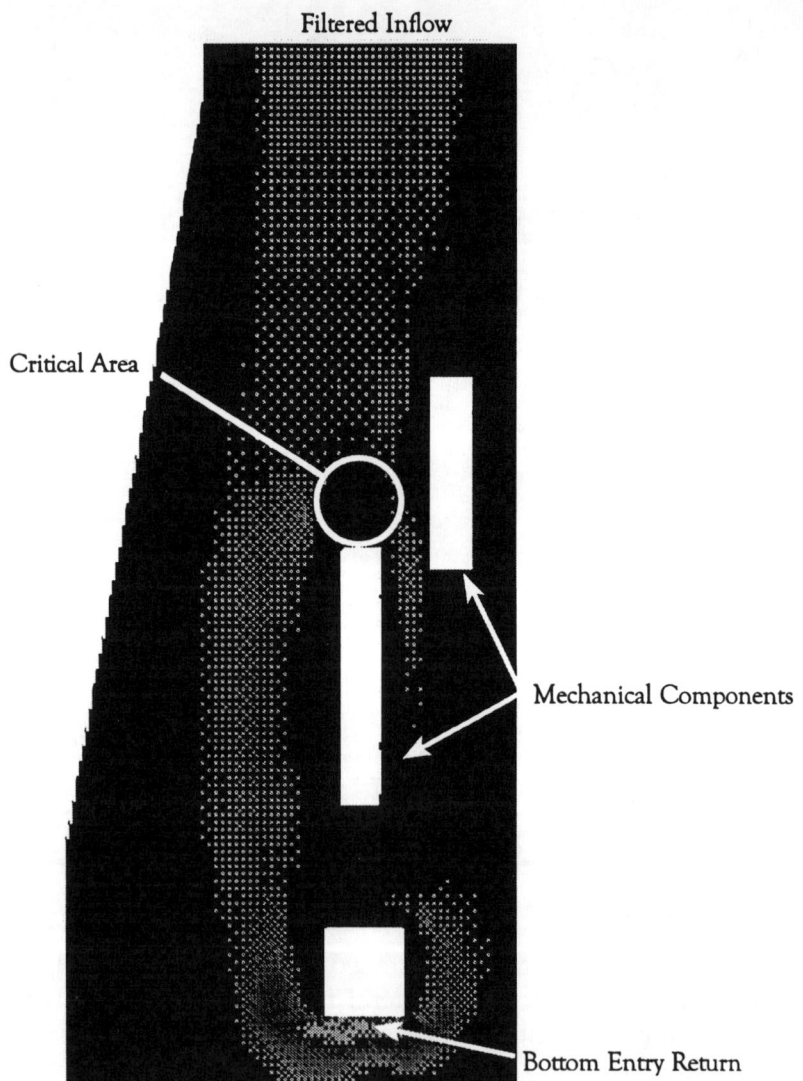

Figure 12.15. Cardboard and Plexiglas™ mockup for ergonomic evaluation.

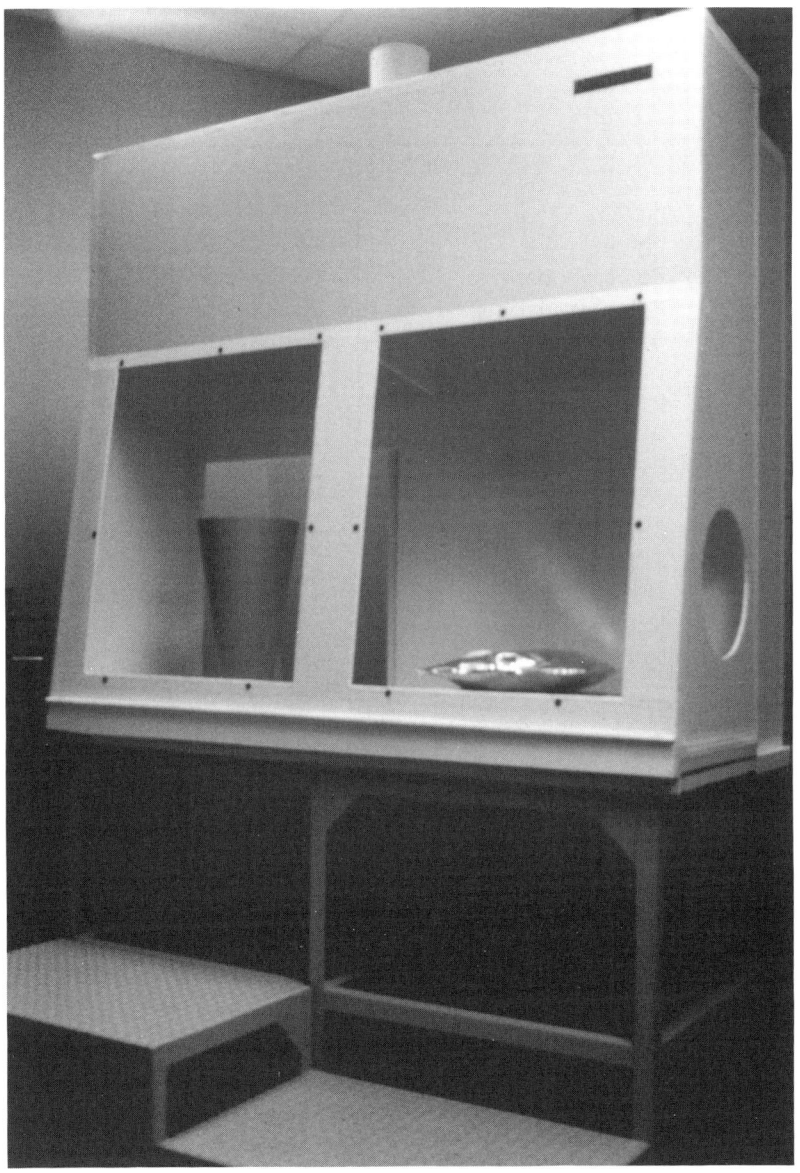

Table 12.1. Material Comparability with Hydrogen Peroxide

	Material	1%	2%	3%
Plastics	ABS Plastic	—	A	—
	Acetal (Delrin™)	C	D	D
	CPVC	—	A	A
	Epoxy	—	C	B
	Hytrel™	—	—	—
	LDPE	—	A	C
	NORYL™	—	A	A
	Nylon	—	C	D
	Polycarbonate	A	A	A
	Polypropylene	A	A	B
	PPS (Ryton™)	—	A	A
	PTFE (Teflon™)	A	A	A
	PVC	A	A	A
	PVDF (Kynar™)	—	A	A
	Buna N (Nitrile)	—	D	D
	EPDM	—	A	B
	Hypalon™	—	D	D
	Kel-F™	—	A	B
	Natural Rubber	—	B	C
	Neoprene	C	D	D
	Phar Med	A	A	A
	Silicone	A	A	B
	Tygon™	—	B	B
	Viton™	A	A	A
Metals	304 stainless steel	B	B	B
	316 stainless steel	A	B	B
	Aluminum	A	A	A
	Brass	D	—	—
	Bronze	—	B	B
	Carpenter 20	—	C	B
	Cast Iron	—	C	B
	Copper	D	—	D

Continued on next page.

Continued from previous page.

	Material	1%	2%	3%
	Hastelloy-C™	—	A	A
	Titanium	—	A	B
Non-metals	Carbon Graphite	—	C	C
	Ceramic Al$_2$O$_3$	A	—	—
	Ceramic Magnet	—	A	A

Ratings: A = No effect—Excellent
B = Minor effect—Good
C = Moderate effect—Fair
D = Severe effect—Not recommended
— = No data

Data from published material and exposure observation.

Trademarks: Delrin, Freon, Hypalon, Hytrel, Teflon, Viton are registered trademarks of E.I. du Pont de Nemours & Co.; Hastelloy-C is a registered trademark of Cabot Corp.; Kel-F is a registered trademark of 3M Co.; Kynar is a registered trademark of Pennwalt Corp.; NORYL is a registered trademark of General Electric Co.; Ryton is a registered trademark of Phillips Petroleum Co.; Tygon and Phar Med are registered trademarks of Norton Co.

---

tunnel, or there may be a transfer within the cooling zone of the tunnel to feed the glass single-file into the barrier isolator. The main concern here is establishing the flow required to maintain a pressure differential between the filling area and the tunnel exit.

The next major consideration is the entry of stoppers and other commodity products. Some lines have been designed to interface the barrier with a batch stopper processing system. These involve the bulk transfer of large quantities of sterilized stoppers into the barrier isolator through a sterilized or decontaminated interface port. Another method of transporting either commodity materials or filler components into the barrier enclosure is through a Rapid Transfer Port (RTP). The RTP allows for an aseptic or sterile transfer of material from the outside environment to the inside of the barrier isolator without exposure to contaminates. (An RTP interface is illustrated in Figure 12.16.)

Recent concern has been raised relative to the line (ring of confidence) interface formed by the inner and outer door seals

Figure 12.16. Rapid transfer port with transfer container.

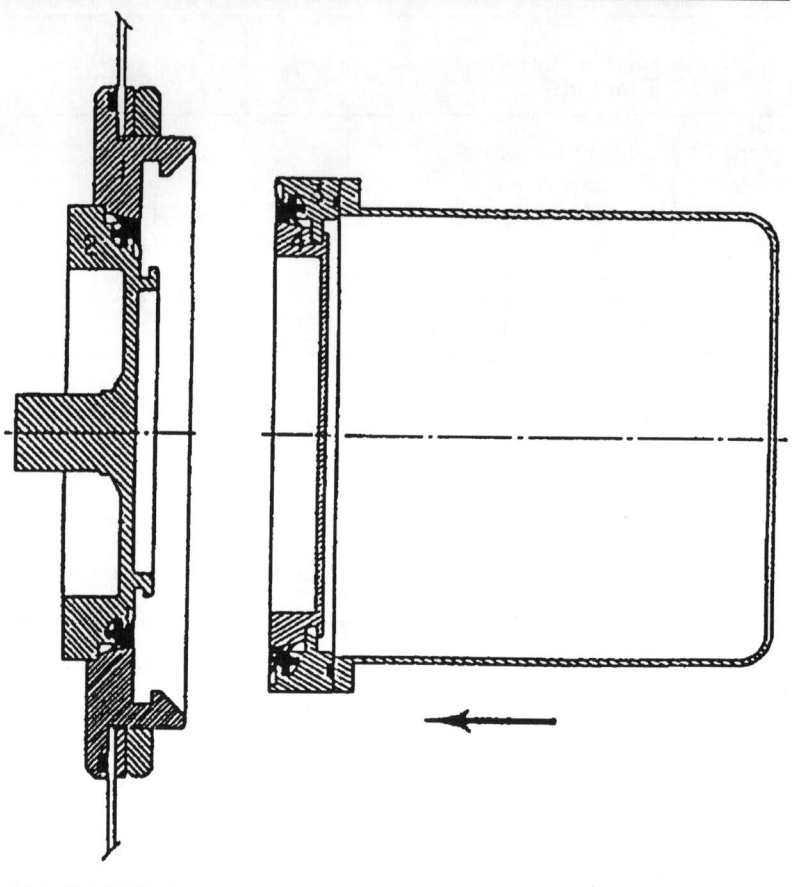

of this type of transfer. Work is currently under way to provide a fully sterilizable line interface between these components. (An example of a fully automated transfer port that can be dry heat sterilized is shown in Figures 12.17 and 12.18.)

Further examples of transfer mechanisms include the double-ended autoclave and the high-intensity ultraviolet pass-through tunnel. The ultraviolet pass-through tunnel allows for surface sterilization of prepackaged components required to be transferred into the barrier isolator. (An example of the UV pass-through is shown in Figure 12.19.)

The product exit is the final consideration for interface with the barrier isolator. The product exit may be through a transfer

Figure 12.17. Rapid transfer port that can be dry-heat sterilized. Illustration courtesy of Central Research Laboratories (patent pending).

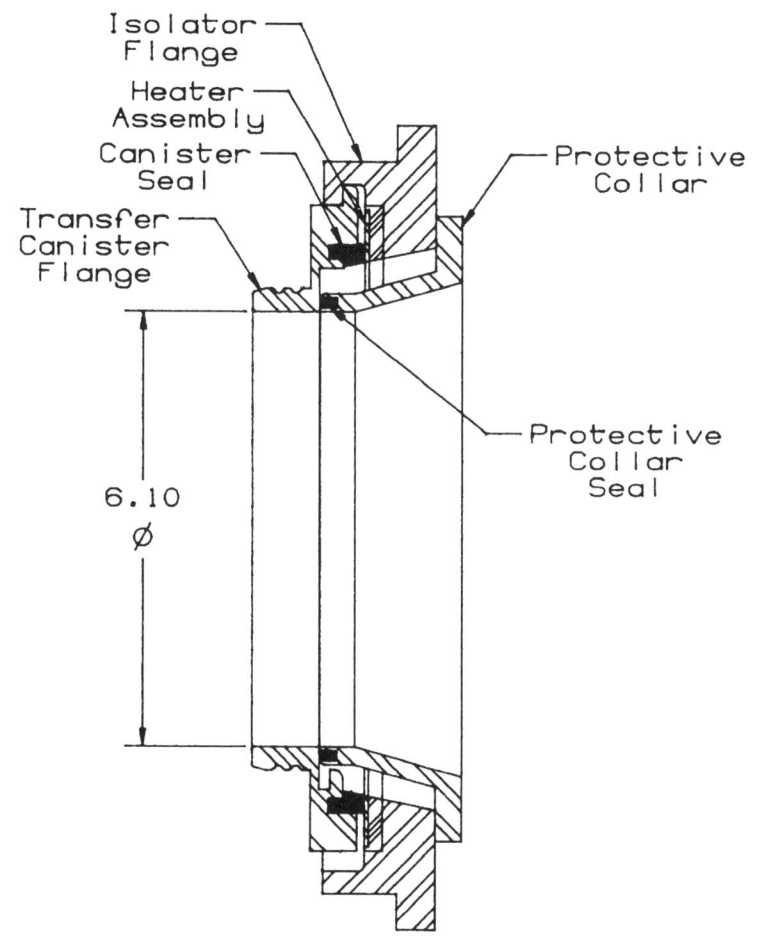

star wheel system, or a small tunnel that feeds the finished product single-file from the isolator into the packaging section of the line.

Handling of Freeze-Dried Products

Products to be freeze-dried (lyophilized) can be handled in two ways. Vials can be tray loaded into special protected carts that

Figure 12.18. Rapid transfer port cycle for connection, sterilization, opening insertion of protective collar, and transfer of components. Illustration courtesy of Central Research Laboratories (patent pending).

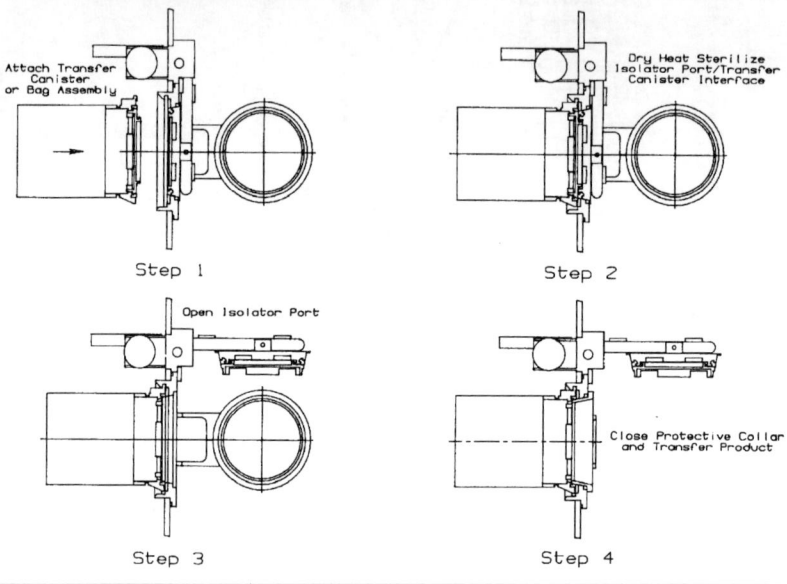

Figure 12.19. UV pass-through for component transfer.

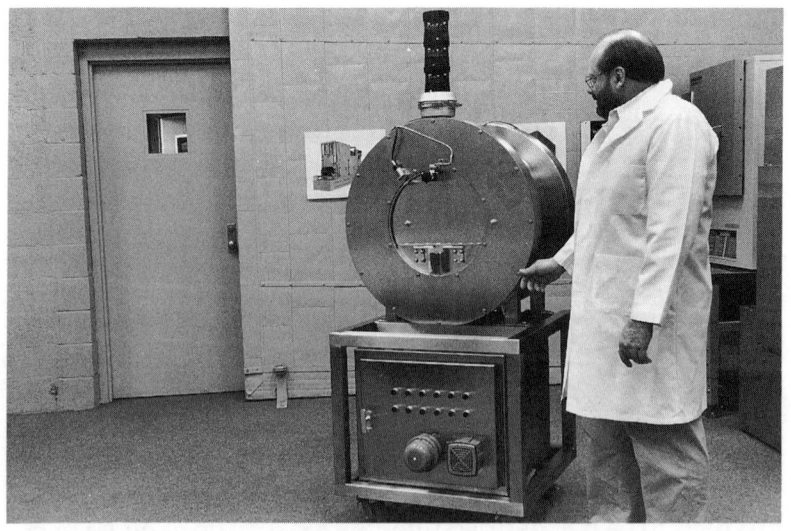

attach to the output end of the barrier isolator utilizing the Standard Mechanical Interface or SMIF Pod concept, as is used in the microelectronics industry. The other approach is to use a freeze dryer with an automated loading system in an uninhabited Class 100 clean room that mates up to the barrier isolator.

In the case of potent compounds and other materials that must be isolated from operators, it is possible to build bidirectional flow tunnels where the pressure inside the initial enclosure is positive with respect to the outside world, yet flows counter to a flow from the outside environment through a higher level negative pressure located in the middle of the entry and exit tunnel. (This is shown in Figure 12.20.) This prevents the potent compounds from exiting through the sterilization tunnel or the vial exit tunnel.

Particulate Control Considerations

Particulate control is critical in barrier isolator design. The most important consideration is the filtration of the outside air used as makeup air for the barrier isolator. All filter banks must have challenge and checking ports available for test. Since

Figure 12.20. Pressure diagram when potent compounds are considered.

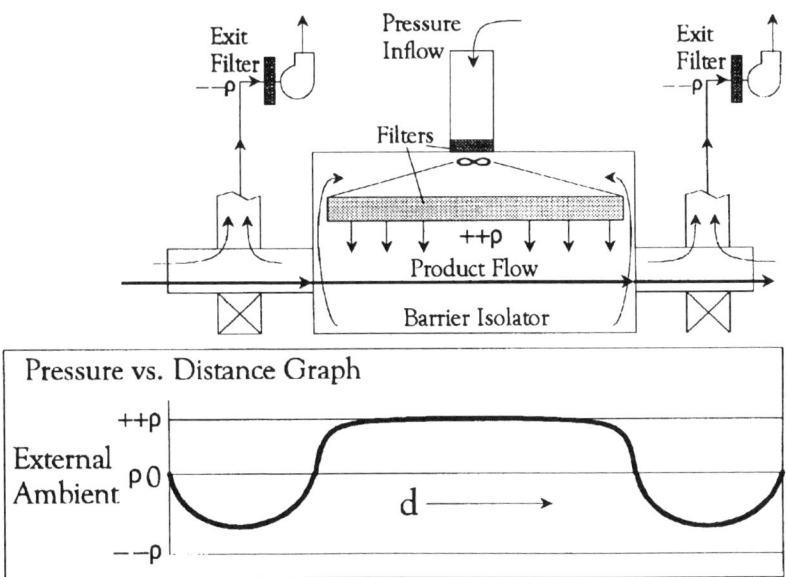

Figure 12.21. The airflow into and inside the barrier isolator.

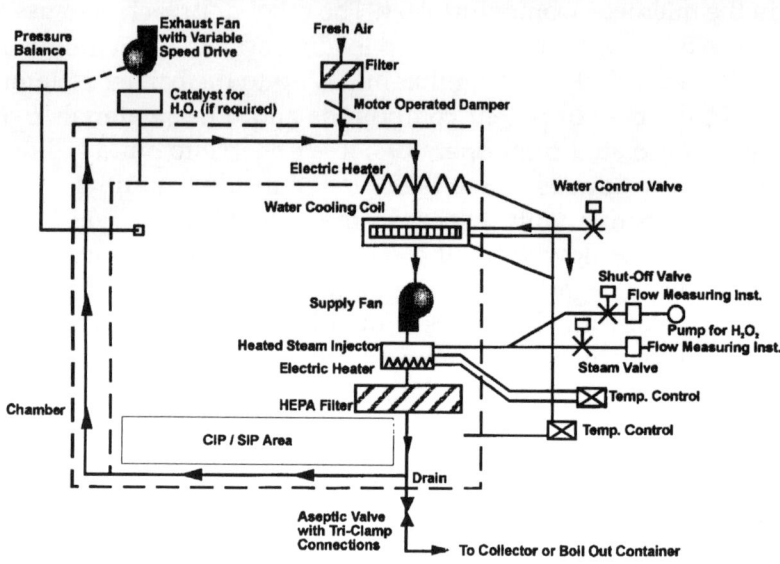

viable particles may be present, the general technique for barrier isolators is to recirculate, through the HEPA filter, the air inside the isolator and to add filtered makeup air as required, to keep the positive pressure inside the barrier isolator (see Figure 12.21).

The makeup air system usually is provided with one or two roughing filters to extend the life of the HEPA or ULPA filter used as the final filter. The probability of a particle passing from the makeup air system into the isolator enclosure, and finally through the recirculation filter on the isolator enclosure to the product environment below, is shown in Figure 12.22. This is not to say that this is the probability of having a particle of any type at the level of the product. This is the probability of a particle making its way through the multiple levels of filters to reach the sterilized, inside critical area. Using the known references, the probability of a viable particle (as opposed to an inert particle) is on the order of 10^{-5}. The probabilities shown in Figure 12.22 must be reduced by that probability to determine the probability of a viable particle reaching the inside of the barrier from its external environment.

Figure 12.22. The level of particulates at different points in the barrier isolation airflow system and associated probabilities.

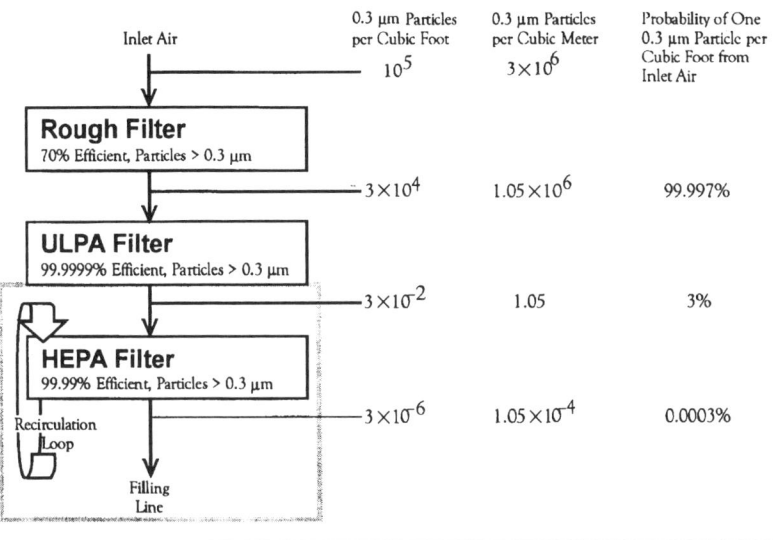

Barrier Isolator Internal Condition Control and Monitoring

The internal barrier isolator conditions are both controllable and measurable. This lends itself to a much higher level of repeatability than those systems that have random human presence and intervention. Key among the internal conditions is the maintenance of internal positive pressure within the barrier isolator. Incoming flow requirements of makeup gas into the system are based upon both a cross-sectional open area and the pressure differential between the barrier inside and its surrounding area. Typically, pressure differentials between filling sites and surrounding areas have been on the order of 0.05 of an inch water column. The following calculations show the flow through an open orifice of large size due to the magnitude of pressure differential.

Calculation of the velocity required to maintain a specified pressure differential across an opening starts with the Bernoulli equation for steady flow:

$$p = \left(\frac{V^2}{2g}\right)\left(\frac{\delta}{5.192}\right) = \left(\frac{V}{1096.7}\right)^2 \delta$$

where p is the pressure in inches of water column, V is the velocity in ft/min, and δ is the density in lb/ft³.

$$V = 1096.7\left(\frac{p}{\delta}\right)^{0.5}$$

Air at standard temperature and pressure is 0.075 lb/ft³, therefore

$$V = 4 \times 10^3 \left(\frac{p}{\delta}\right)^{0.5}$$

$$Q = V \times A$$

Example: If the pressure difference across the wall of the sterile enclosure is 0.05 inches water column and A is 0.25 ft², then:

$$V = 0.05 \times 4 \times 10^3 = 8.94 \times 10^2 \text{ ft/min}$$
$$Q = 8.94 \times 10 \text{ ft/min} \times 0.25 \text{ ft}^2 = 223 \text{ ft}^3/\text{min}$$

This flow (Q) is with containers present and approximates the gross airflow requirements to maintain the pressure differential between the sterile enclosure and the ambient environment.

One of the questions raised with respect to barrier isolators was the ability to stay at a positive pressure condition when gloves are rapidly removed from the enclosure. Figure 12.23 shows an experiment conducted with removal of two full-size gloves from an enclosure with normal makeup air fed into the enclosure. The pressure measurement was made close to the exit hole of the enclosure and shows that at no time, even with rapid removal, was there a pressure reversal for the inside of the enclosure transition from positive to negative.

CLEAN–IN–PLACE OF BARRIER ISOLATORS

Any barrier isolator must be openable. Following the opening of a barrier isolator, a CIP and SIP process must be completed

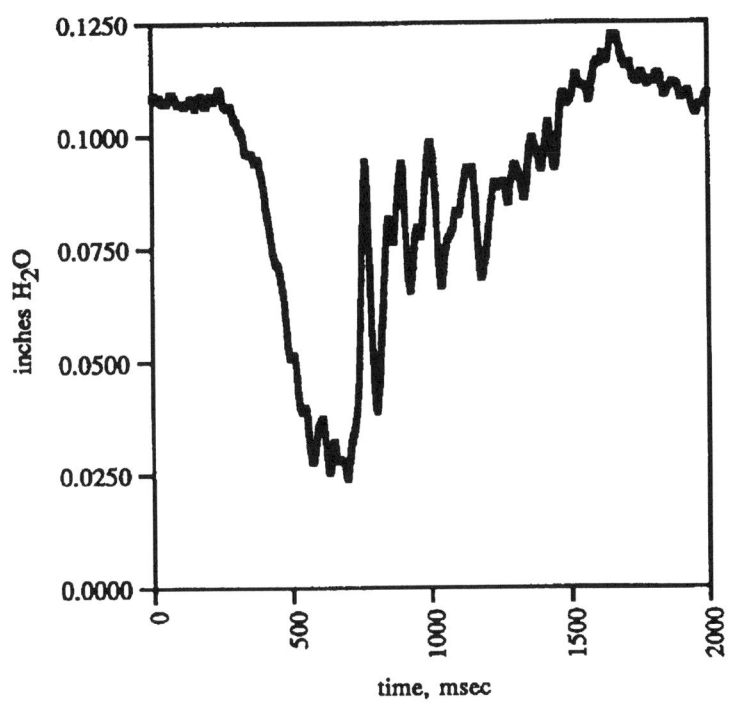

Figure 12.23. The barrier isolator pressure near the exit when two hands were withdrawn from the glove ports. Glove volume = 404 cu. inches; chamber volume = 102,214 cu. inches.

to render the inside of the barrier sterile for filling operations. The CIP cycle may also be done to decontaminate potent drugs prior to opening the barrier isolator.

The CIP process can be operated with several different approaches. The best approach is spray balls with full pattern coverage. Filter protection with some type of screen is required to prevent wetting of the HEPA filters. Rounded corners in all cleanable areas and proper drain location assist in completing the removal of material from within the barrier isolator.

STERILIZATION OF BARRIER ISOLATORS

Sterilization-in-place of the barrier isolator can be accomplished through a number of different methods. The method currently used on sterility test isolators has been a room temperature vaporized hydrogen peroxide sterilant. Despatch Industries and TL Systems recently developed a sterilization process consisting of saturated steam at atmospheric pressure for use in barrier isolators. Other methods, such as ozone, ethylene oxide, or raw steam, have also been used.

Atmospheric Steam/Hydrogen Peroxide Sterilization System

The atmospheric steam with hydrogen peroxide (H_2O_2) sterilization system was developed as part of the systems approach to barrier isolation. Steam/H_2O_2 provides a robust sterilization process that can be completed in two hours or less. The sterilization cycle is described in Figure 12.24.

The test apparatus used to gather basic data on the destruction of microorganisms is shown in Figure 12.25. D-values as a function of hydrogen peroxide concentration are shown in Figure 12.26. D-values for four bacterial spores are shown in Figure 12.27. Figure 12.28 shows the process time with hydrogen peroxide at various concentrations. A prototype barrier isolator of 50 cubic feet in volume was constructed to do thermal imaging and other microbiological tests (Figure 12.29). Planchets of *Bacillus stearothermophilus* spores were placed in the coldest locations to evaluate the process (see Figures 12.30

Figure 12.24. Steam hydrogen peroxide sterilization process cycle.

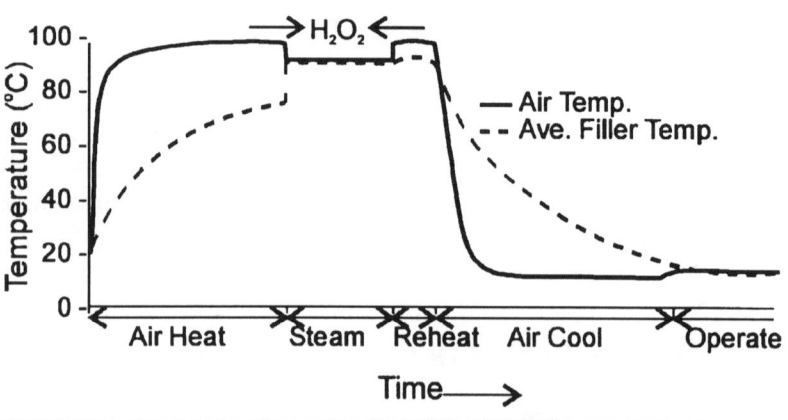

Figure 12.25. Diagram of atmospheric steam hydrogen peroxide test apparatus.

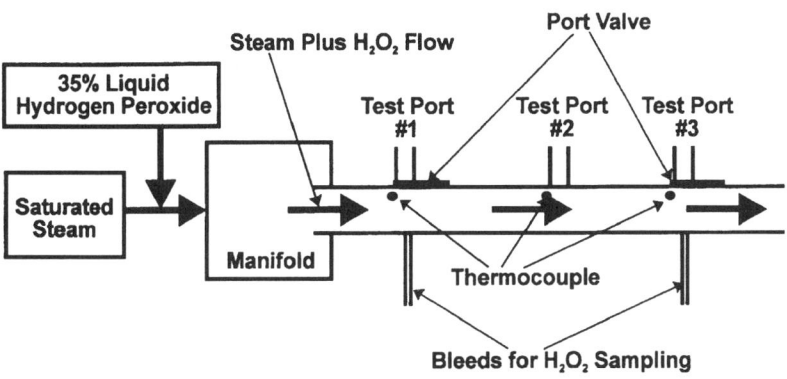

Figure 12.26. D-value vs. hydrogen peroxide concentration for spores on planchets in the steam plus H_2O_2 system: Spore and planchet received heat treatment immediately before testing, which is similar to the condition that will exist when steam plus H_2O_2 is used to sterilize a barrier enclosure.

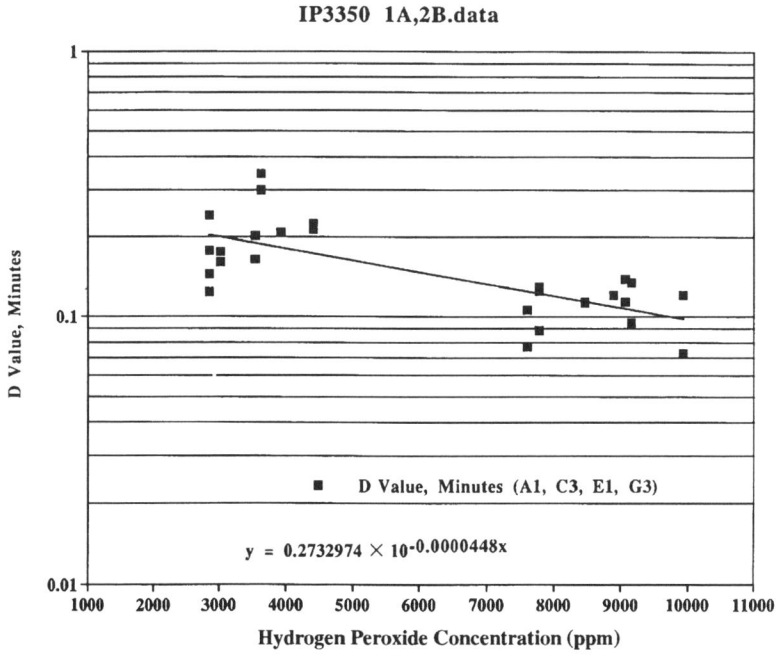

Figure 12.27. D values for four species of spores subjected to steam plus 2500 ppm hydrogen peroxide in the tube system.

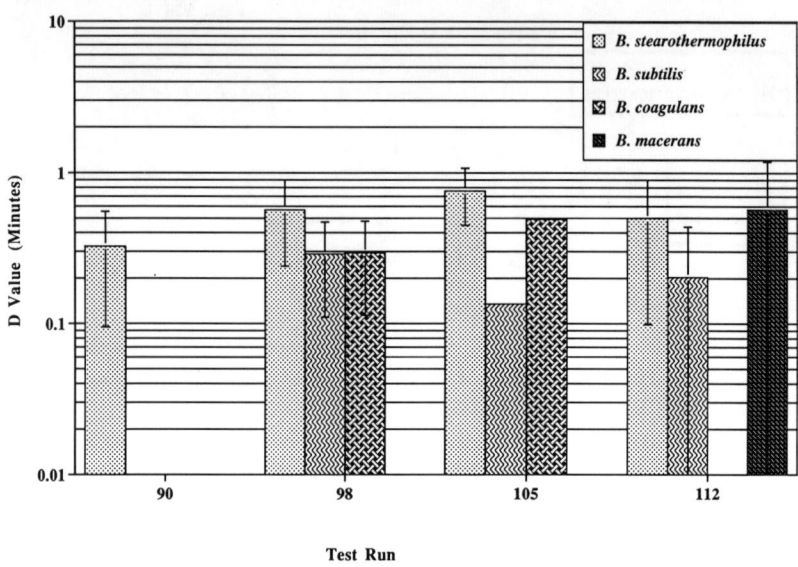

Figure 12.28. Process time for a 12-log cycle microbial control process using atmospheric steam plus hydrogen peroxide at various concentrations.

	Process Time Minutes
750 ppm	2.4
2500 ppm	5.7

and 12.31). With the system cycle (dry preheat, steam, hydrogen peroxide with steam, steam, evaporation, and cooling), total SIP time was two hours or less. Such cycles, with concentrations of hydrogen peroxide from 0.25 percent to 1 percent, killed all *B. stearothermophilus* spores.

It is important as part of the cycle to verify the sterilant concentration. A method provided to do that is shown in Figure 12.32 (patent pending). This method has excellent precision with the steam hydrogen peroxide sterilant. It is also necessary to ascertain residual levels of peroxide. Several pieces of equipment are available to accomplish this. Following the completed sterilization cycle, removal of all sterilant from the enclosure

Figure 12.29. Prototype barrier isolator for thermal imaging and running microbiological tests.

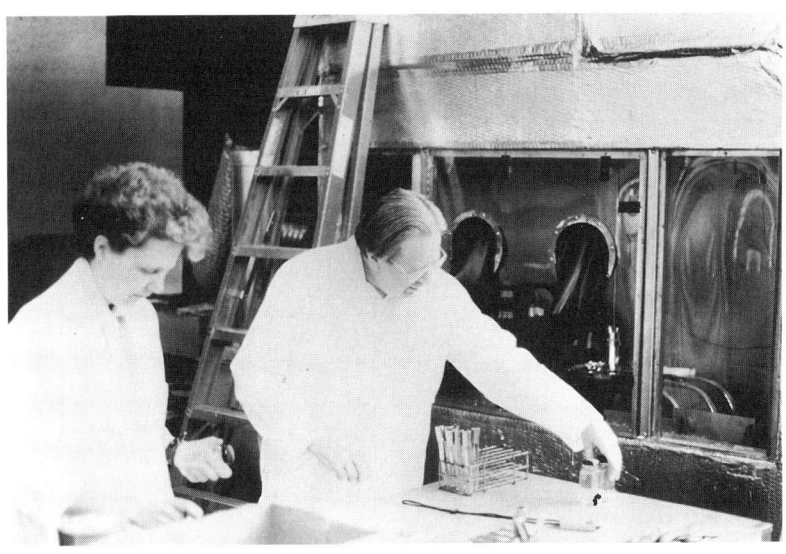

Figure 12.30. Planchet location diagram. Vertical longitudinal cross-section through the prototype barrier isolator enclosure showing the inlet for the steam or steam plus hydrogen peroxide, the HEPA filter bank, the location of the inoculated planchets used in evaluating the system, and the exhaust area.

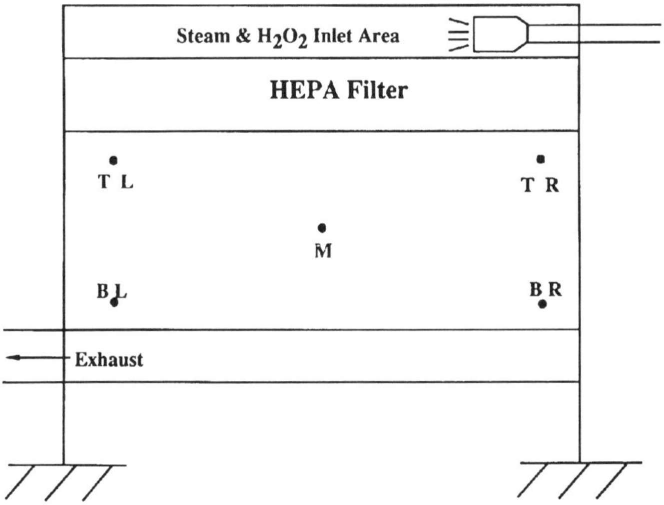

Figure 12.31. Test results on planchets from a prototype barrier isolator.

Results of a series of teste where *Bacillus stearothermophilus* spores PB27CT desposited on stainless-steel planchets were subjected to a steam hydrogen-peroxide (H_2O_2) atmosphere at an H_2O_2 inflow rate of 150 ml/m^2 of isolator cross-section area for 6 and 12 minutes.

In the initial experiments, there were two replicate planchets at each location. Halfway through the project, we increased to three replicate planchets per location. (Empty boxes are conditions not tested.)

Test ID	Initial Number	900 ml H_2O_2/m^2						1800 ml H_2O_2/m^2					
		BL[1]			BR			BL			BR		
		P1[2]	P2	P3	P1	P2	P3	P1	P2	P3	P1	P2	P3
CM2196	5.33E+6	1820	2850		5	453		0	0		0	0	
CM2204	6.00E+6	597	14340		0	0		0	0		0	0	
CM2211	4.92E+6							0	0		2	2	
CM2217	1.49E+7	323	359		0	0		0	0		0	0	
CM2225	1.45E+7	1507	2977		0	27		0	25		0	0	
IP2232[3]	1.15E+6	0	0		0	0		0	0		0	0	

Continued on next page.

Continued from previous page.

Test ID	Initial Number	900 ml H_2O_2/m^2						1800 ml H_2O_2/m^2					
		BL[1]			BR			BL			BR		
		P1[2]	P2	P3	P1	P2	P3	P1	P2	P3	P1	P2	P3
IP2240[4]	1.54E+7	0	2251		0	0							
IP2245[4]	1.39E+7	7152	11474	17860	280	3895	6885						
IP2253A[5]	1.27E+7	3	5	535	0	1	54	0	12	0	0	0	0
IP2253C	1.27E+7	1	1	19	1	29	304						
IP2260	1.34E+7	63	1911	5615	359	1089	1214						

[1] Data are for the bottom of the barrier isolator column. BL is the bottom left and BR is the bottom right. See Figure 12.5.
[2] P1, P2, and P3 are replicate planchets.
[3] In Experiment IP2232, the N0 was 1.15E+6, whereas in adjacent experiments N0 was one log higher.
[4] In Experiments IP2240 and IP2245, the 900 ml of H_2O_2 was delivered in 12 instead of 6 minutes.
[5] In Experiment IP2253, the 6 minute experiment was repeated two times: A and C.

must be well documented. The normal level to be reached before initiation of filling, using hydrogen peroxide would be less than 1 ppm residual.

Figure 12.32. The hydrogen peroxide concentration measuring system (patent pending).

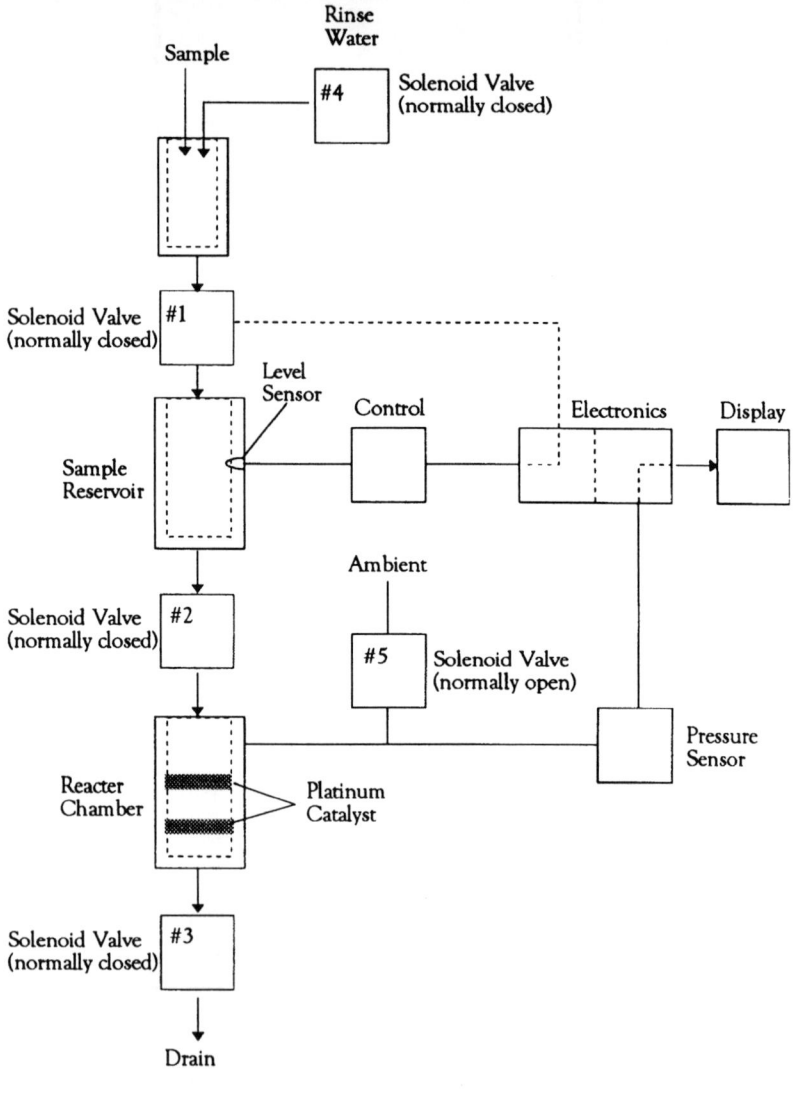

VALIDATION CONSIDERATIONS

In order to ensure that the conditions seen by the process lines are repetitive, conditions must both be controlled and monitored. The controlled conditions include the pressure differential between the inside of the barrier isolator and the outside. This can be done by utilizing a pressure transducer feeding to a variable frequency drive package, as illustrated in Figure 12.33.

The barrier isolator CIP/SIP cycle must be controlled. The CIP cycle control includes the length of time and fluid volume passed into the enclosure during the spray operation. The SIP cycle depends on which sterilant is used. Most sterilants require preconditioning (i.e., temperature or humidity control, or both). Following the preconditioning, sterilant flow and time require control. The sterilant removal cycle also must be a controlled parameter.

The physical locking of the access doors into the enclosure must be assured during and following the sterilant cycle. Verification of enclosure integrity can be accomplished through air pressurization and decay testing, with all openings closed. The measured variables during the operation of the barrier isolator enclosure include pressure differential to the outside environment, sterilant flow, quantity and duration for the sterilization cycle, and sterilant concentration.

For the sterilant concentration, Despatch Industries developed an instrument for monitoring the concentration of

Figure 12.33. The pressure balance control system.

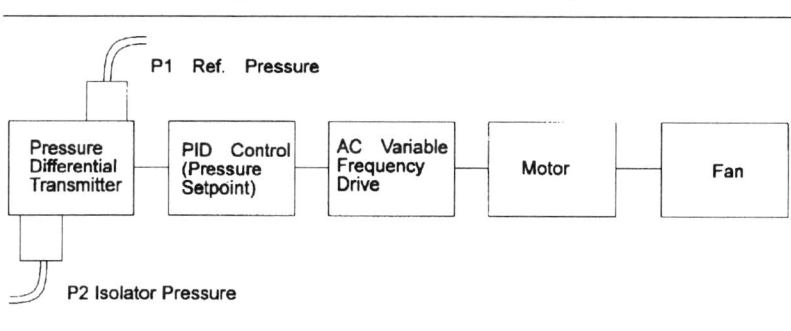

peroxide during the steam/peroxide cycle. This instrument is consistent with titration measurements and data are reported in under one minute (Figure 12.32).

Measured variables include particulate levels at the filler elevation. Experiments have shown that after opening and then reclosing a barrier isolator system, the makeup and recirculation air brings the particulate level at the filler elevation to within Class 100 conditions in less than 10 minutes of sealed operation. Class 10 levels are achieved within 30 minutes of closing the system. These measurements were made while operating the barrier isolator in an uncontrolled environment with particulate levels of 10^{-5} 0.5 micron particles per cubic foot. Figure 12.34 shows the barrier isolator on which these tests were conducted.

OVERVIEW

It is a giant step from the present Class 100 clean room technology to the new system shown in Figures 12.35–12.38. The major issues are ergonomics, particulates, and increasing the product SCL from 10^{-3} (current technology) to 10^{-6} (barrier isolators). Simply placing a barrier isolator over an existing conventional filler does not achieve the goals. A holistic approach is required in designing a pharmaceutical product filling line with a barrier isolator. The goals of barrier isolator technology are as follows:

1. A product SCL of 10^{-6}.
2. Reduced overall costs.
3. Protection of operators from potent compounds.
4. A system that is flexible and user friendly.

It is a paradigm shift to design, build, control, validate, and operate a system such as this with no human exposure to the open vial.

Figure 12.34. The barrier isolator operating in the unclassified environment.

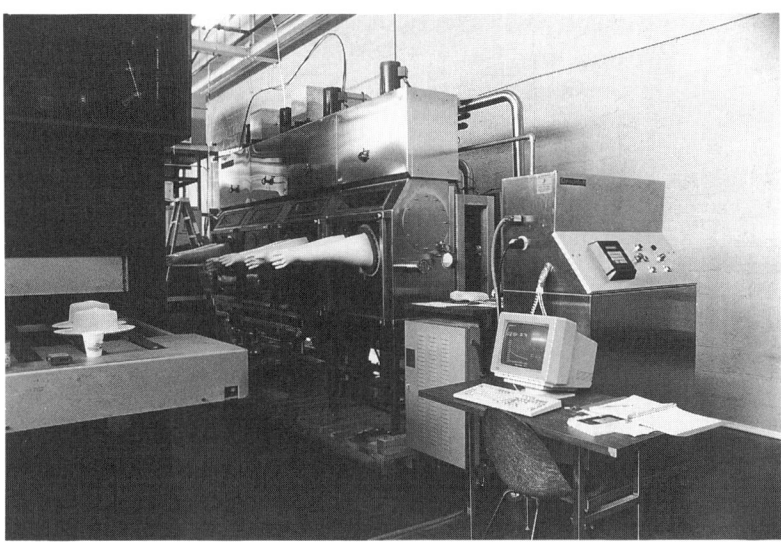

Figure 12.35. The complete system: washer, tunnel, and barrier isolator with filler, checkweighers, and stoppering.

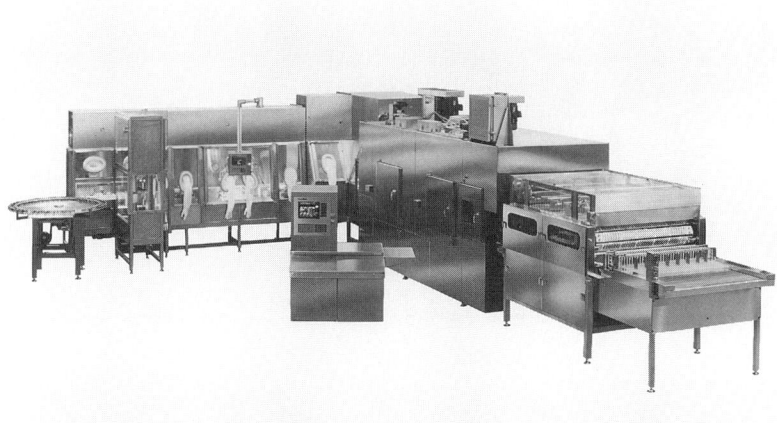

Figure 12.36. Tunnel exit accumulation into infeed tunnel.

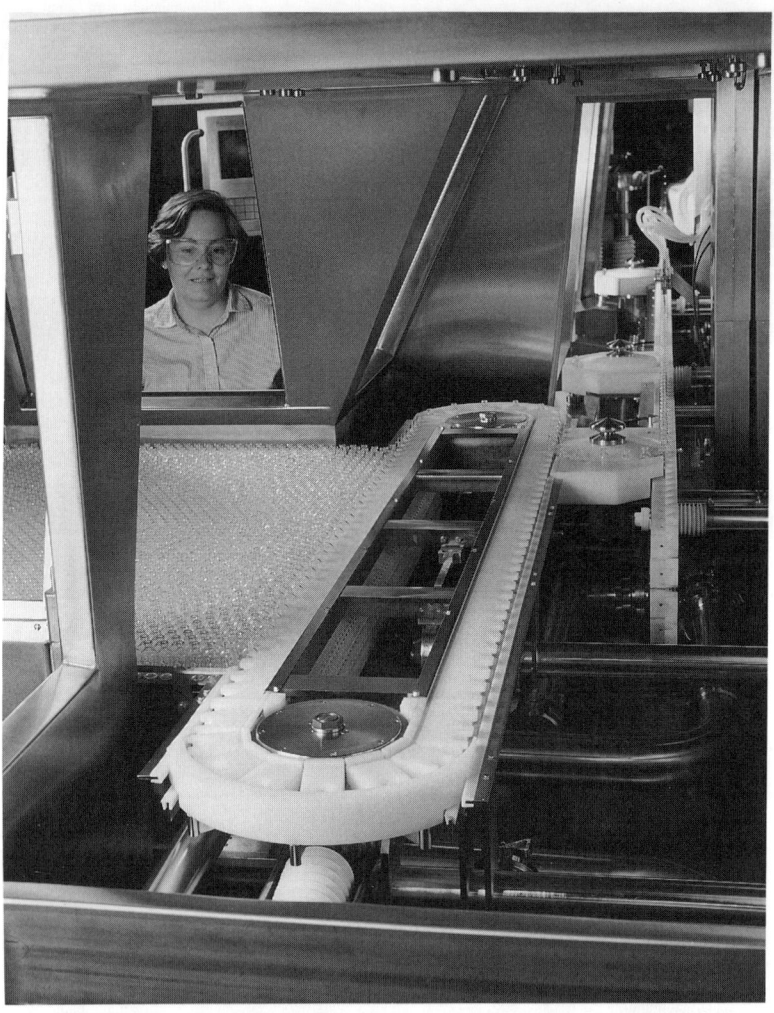

Figure 12.37. Stoppering area.

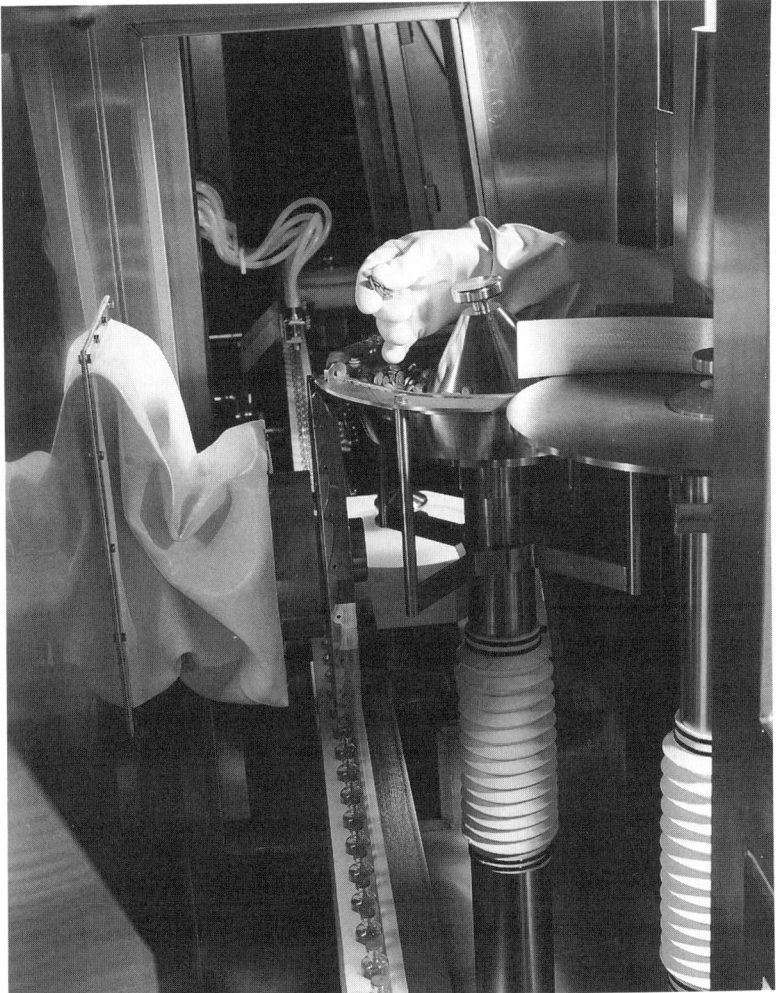

Figure 12.38. Mechanical access for maintenance from back side of barrier isolator.

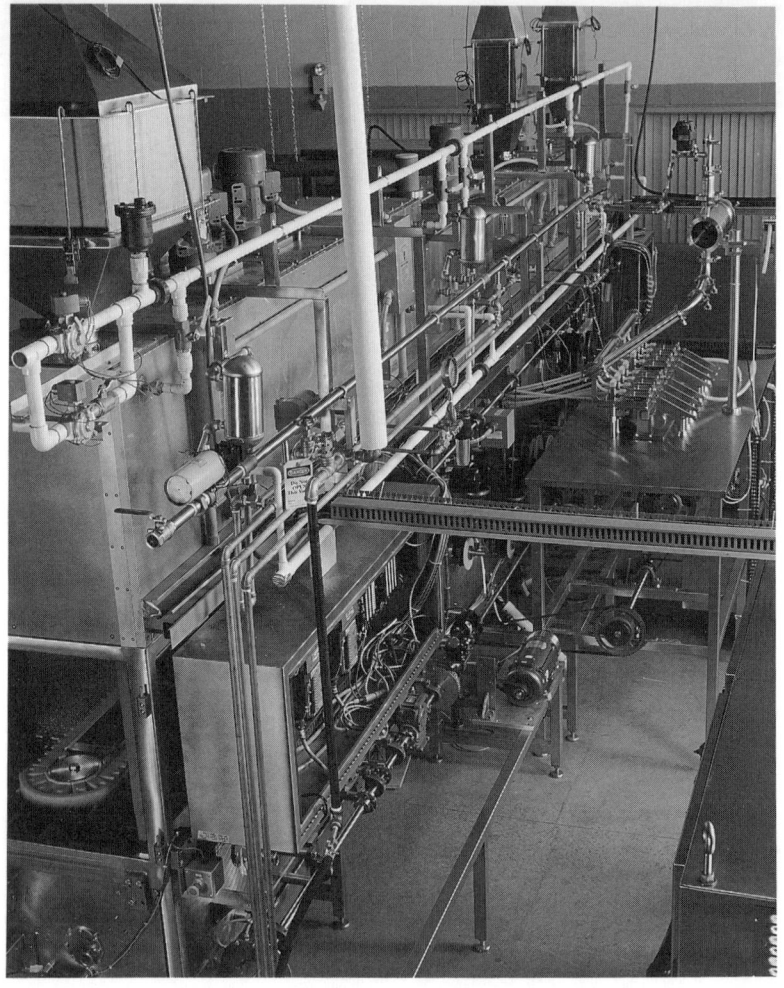

RECOMMENDED READINGS

Akers J. E., and J. P. Agallaco. 1993. Aseptic processing—a current perspective. In *Sterilization technology: A practical guide for manufacturers and users of health care products.* New York: Van Norstrand Reinhold.

Akers, J. E., and C. Wagner. 1994. *Barrier technology.* Third International PDA Congress and Workshops, 14–18 February, in Basel, Switzerland.

Block, S. S. 1991. *Disinfection, sterilization and preservation,* 4th ed., pp. 85–128. Philadelphia: Lea and Febiger.

Bradley, A., S. P. Probert, C. S. Sinclair, and A. Tallentire. 1991. Airborne microbial challenges of blow/fill/seal equipment: A case study. *J. Paren. Sci. Technol.* 45 (4).

Casamassina, F. J., J. W. Hulse, and R. P. Tomaselli. 1993. Controlling medical product contamination. In *Sterilization technology: A practical guide for manufacturers and users of health care products.* New York: Van Norstrand Reinhold.

Curran, H. R., R. R. Evans, and A. Leviton. 1940. The sporicidal action of hydrogen peroxide and the use of crystalline catalase to dissipate residual peroxide. *J. Bacter.* 40:423–434.

Federal Standard 209D. 1988. *Clean room and work station requirements.* Washington, D.C.

Farquharson, G. 1994. Aseptic filling in network of rigid isolators. Third International PDA Congress, 14–16 February, in Basel, Switzerland.

Frieben, W. R. 1993. Presentation at FDA Open Conference on Sterile Drug Manufacturing, 12 October, in Bethesda, MD.

Haas, P. J., H. L. Melgaard, J. P. Lysfjord, and I. J. Pflug. 1993. Validation concerns for parenteral filling lines incorporating barrier isolation techniques and CIP/SIP systems. PDA Second International Congress, 22–27 February, in Basel, Switzerland.

Hoffman, G. 1992. Presentation at Barrier Isolation Technology Conference, 26–27 August, in Minneapolis, MN.

Killick, P. F. 1992. Facility design—Isolation technology. Fourth International Congress of Pharmaceutical Engineering, 8–10 September, in Vienna, Austria.

Klapes, N. A., and D. Vesley. 1989. Vapor-phase hydrogen peroxide as a surface decontaminant and sterilant. *Appl. Environ. Microb.* 56:503–506.

Leaper, S. 1984. Comparison of the resistance to hydrogen peroxide of wet and dry spores of *Bacillus subtilis* SA22. *J. Food Technol.* 19:695–702.

Lewis, J. S., and J. R. Rickloff. 1991. Inactivation of *Bacillus stearothermophilus* spores using vaporized hydrogen peroxide. Unpublished paper, presented at the 1991 ASM Meeting, in Dallas, TX.

Loy, L. H., and J. F. Melanhn. 1993. Current stopper processing methods and handling techniques. Barrier Isolation Technology Conference, 19–20 August, in Minneapolis, MN.

Lysfjord, J. P., P. J. Haas, H. L. Melgaard, and I. J. Pflug. 1993. The potential for use of steam at atmospheric pressure to decontaminate or sterilize parenteral filling lines incorporating barrier isolation technology. Presented at PDA Spring Meeting, 10 March, in Philadelphia, PA. (To be published in the *Journal of Parenteral Science and Technology*.)

Melgaard, H. L. 1994. Barrier isolation design issues. ISPE Barrier Isolation Technology Seminar, 12–13 May, in Philadelphia, PA.

Melgaard, H. L. 1989. The historic and current atatus of dry heat sterilization and depyrogenation. Presented at ISPE EXPO '89. (Unpublished report by Despatch Industries, Minneapolis, MN.)

Melgaard, H. L., and I. J. Pflug. 1993. Nature and quality of the air leaving the filters at the top of a barrier isolator. Unpublished.

NASA. 1968. *Standard procedures for the microbiological examination of space hardware.* National Aeronautics and Space Administration Document No. NHB 5340.1A. Washington, D.C.: Government Printing Office.

Peck, R. D. 1988. What will the new federal standard 209C mean? *Pharm. Eng.* 8 (2):17–21.

Peterson, A. 1994. Barrier isolator filler design issues. ISPE Barrier Isolation Technology Seminar, 12–13 May, in Philadelphia, PA.

Pflug, I. J. 1992. Microbiological testing program of the TL/Despatch barrier system. Barrier Isolation Technology Conference, 26–27 August, in Minneapolis, MN.

Pflug, I. J. 1990. *Microbiology and engineering of sterilization process*, rev. 7th ed. Minneapolis, MN: University of Minnesota.

Pflug, I. J., A. B. Larson, and H. L. Melgaard. 1992. Barrier isolation system. (US Patent Pending.)

Pflug, I. J., H. L. Melgaard, C. A. Meadows, J. P. Lysfjord, and P. Haas. 1993. Rigid isolation barriers: Decontamination with steam and steam hydrogen peroxide. In *Sterilization of medical products*, Vol. VI, pp. 115–132. Somerville, NJ: Johnson & Johnson.

Pflug I. J., H. L. Melgaard, S. M. Schaffer, J. P. Lysfjord. 1994. The microbial kill characteristics of saturated steam at atmospheric pressure with 7,500 and 2,500 ppm hydrogen peroxide. Presented at PDA Spring Meeting, 10 March, in Chicago, IL. (To be published in the *Journal of Parenteral Science and Technology*.)

Rickloff, J. R. 1988. The development of vapor phase hydrogen peroxide as a sterilization technology. A report presented at HIMA Conference on Sterilization in the 1990's, 30 October–1 November, in Washington, D.C.

Rickloff, J. R., and P. A. Orelski. 1989. Resistance of various microorganisms to vapor phase hydrogen peroxide in a prototype dental handpiece/general instrument sterilizer. Presentation at the 89th Annual Meeting of the ASM, in New Orleans, LA.

Sinclair, C. S. 1993. Predictive sterility assurance for aseptic processing. Presented at the Kilmer Memorial Conference on the Sterilization of Medical Products, 13–15 June, in Brussels, Belgium.

Toledo, R. T., F. E. Escher, and J. C. Ayres. 1973. Sporicidal properties of hydrogen peroxide against food spoilage organisms. *Appl. Microb.* 26:592–597.

Whyte, W. 1994. The influence of clean room design on product contamination. *J. Paren. Sci. Technol.* 38 (3).

13

The History and Future of Barrier Isolation Technology at Merck & Co., West Point, PA

Michael E. Porter
Merck & Co.
West Point, PA

Leslie M. Edwards
Advanced Barrier Concepts
Cary, NC

The implementation of barrier isolation technology for sterile production applications was contemplated at Merck through the late 1980s and early 1990s. At that point, the traditional clean room and Class 100 laminar flow hoods were being used for sterility testing. The sterile processing of pharmaceuticals and biological products was performed in an aseptic core environment in which operators were fully gowned and the process resided in a Class 100 area, buffered by air locks and rooms of lower classification levels.

The development of barrier isolation technology offered an opportunity to increase the sterility confidence level for the products bring produced, thereby increasing product quality to Merck's customers. Other advantages included decreasing the system size, decreasing capital and operational expenses, biologically removing the operator from the process, and eliminating the need to construct "brick and mortar" facilities for product testing and processing.

In 1991, Merck completed the installation and start-up of an isolation based sterility testing system. This facility houses numerous flexible wall isolators, including an autoclave interface unit, transfer isolators, one and two half-suit workstations, and sterile incubation isolators. The isolators are sterilized using hydrogen peroxide gas and operate at least two shifts per day. This facility processes a large number of sterility tests with an impressively low false positive test rate.

In 1995, Merck will take delivery of their first full-scale, high speed barrier isolation technology vial processing line. After over a year of prototype testing, both with a small-scale Merck prototype system and with the full-scale prototype at TL Systems, Merck has defined the major physical and microbiological characteristics of the isolation system and processing equipment. Also, Merck has explored the steam/hydrogen peroxide sterilization process and has defined a system for use in their production vial filling system.

In the future, Merck plans to continue increasing capacity for the production of sterile pharmaceuticals, vaccines and other biological products utilizing barrier isolation technology. The fundamental advantages of increasing sterility confidence in the process, thereby improving product quality, will remain the driving force for implementing barrier isolation technology. At the same time the decrease in size, capital expenditures, and operational expenses will allow this higher quality product to be provided to the customer at the best price.

14

Use of Isolation Technology for Production of a Sterile Anti-Cancer Drug

Paul Martin
Aquitane Pharm International
Idron, France

Aquitaine Pharm International (API), a French pharmaceutical company dedicated to the manufacturing of injectable products for the Pierre Fabre Laboratories, evaluated the application of isolation technology in order:

- To improve its aseptic processing facilities.
- To successfully receive FDA approval for a new anti-cancer drug called Navelbine.

OBJECTIVES

API had three major objectives:

- To protect people by completely separating personnel from the work area.

- To ensure product sterility by isolating the product from human or airborne contamination.
- To protect the environment by containing the process within the isolator.

To Protect People

The high toxicity of this product was a great concern to our management. In order to improve employee protection, it was important to build a facility that would emphasize:

- No direct contact with the cytotoxic active ingredient and the solution during the preparation and the manufacturing of the product.
- No direct contact with contaminated air or atmosphere during the manufacturing.
- No contamination possibility during vial manipulation after manufacturing, such as during inspection, during packaging, or at the hospital.
- No human contact with the cytotoxic waste effluent and no contact with contaminated equipment or parts during maintenance intervention or adjustment of operation steps.

In order to meet these objectives, API decided:

- To use a physical barrier between the product and the people, while maintaining enough visibility to facilitate manipulation of the process.
- To use rigid isolators equipped with rapid transfer ports.
- To use negative pressure where the cytotoxic powder was to be manipulated.
- To transfer the contaminated effluent by way of an automatic safety system.
- To design an air conditioning filter that could be removed with no risk to the maintenance operator.
- To include a vial decontamination step to ensure decontamination of the vial external surface as it exited the filling line.

To Ensure Product Sterility

The second major consideration was to ensure the sterility of the product. The high cost of the drug substance made it imperative to take extreme caution with the aseptic process to avoid loss of product at any stage of production. Thus, the facility and the process were designed to ensure that:

- Human or airborne contamination could be completely avoided.
- Facility could meet Class 100 or M 3.5 standards from start to finish.
- Filled vials would be closed as quickly as possible.
- Aseptic conditions could be achieved easily and could be maintained throughout the process.
- Manipulation and transfer of materials could be done without compromising the integrity of the production environment.

To meet these objectives, it was decided:

- To have isolators directly connected to the depyrogenation tunnel.
- To maintain positive pressure in the the isolators containing the sterile product.
- To keep the stoppering operation close to the filling station, inside the same isolator and under a laminar flow equipped with HEPA filters.
- To reduce the isolator's volume and to have complete accessibility to all parts of the aseptic zone.
- To install an automatic monitoring and alarm system to measure the air pressure and the particulate level inside the isolators, on a continuous basis.
- To include a clean-in-place/steam-in-place (CIP/SIP) system to clean and sterilize the solution tank.
- To connect a flexible wall isolator to the autoclave.
- To use a mobile, flexible wall isolator to transfer the sterile accessories and components.
- To sterilize the system with H_2O_2 (hydrogen peroxide).

To Protect the Environment

Protecting the environment was also a very important goal since toxic contamination could be primarily propagated through the air and the liquids. Thus, objectives included:

- To have no contamination to other parts of the plant.
- To protect the people and other products.
- To guarantee that the air conditioning system or the rejected air would not contaminate the atmosphere.
- To ensure the contained recovery and neutralization of all the liquids used decontamination, cleaning of accessories, equipment, and the walls of the isolators.
- To incinerate the solid waste.
- To allow no contamination to exit the cytotoxic area in emergency situations.

MEETING THE OBJECTIVES

To meet all these objectives, API decided to build a dedicated area to manufacture all cytotoxic products. Isolator technology was chosen because it builds an effective barrier, much better than any other conventional system. The new manufacturing area, with isolators, has been equipped with a dedicated air conditioning system that is never in contact with the product. The isolators are connected to a central exhaust system equipped with special filters. All the cytotoxic effluents are recovered and transferred to a neutralization station by the use of a seal draw off system.

The Facilities

This facility (Figures 14.1 and14.2) has 10 different isolators designed to meet the criteria of specialized tasks within the process. Figure 14.1 represents the manufacturing area with:

- preparation
- manufacturing

Use of Isolation Technology for Production of . . . Drug 287

Figure 14.1. Layout of isolation facility at API. E, F, and J are flexible isolators used for the transfer of components and accessories. Other isolators (A, A', B, C1, C2, D1, D2) are rigid wall isolators that house equipment and other machinery.

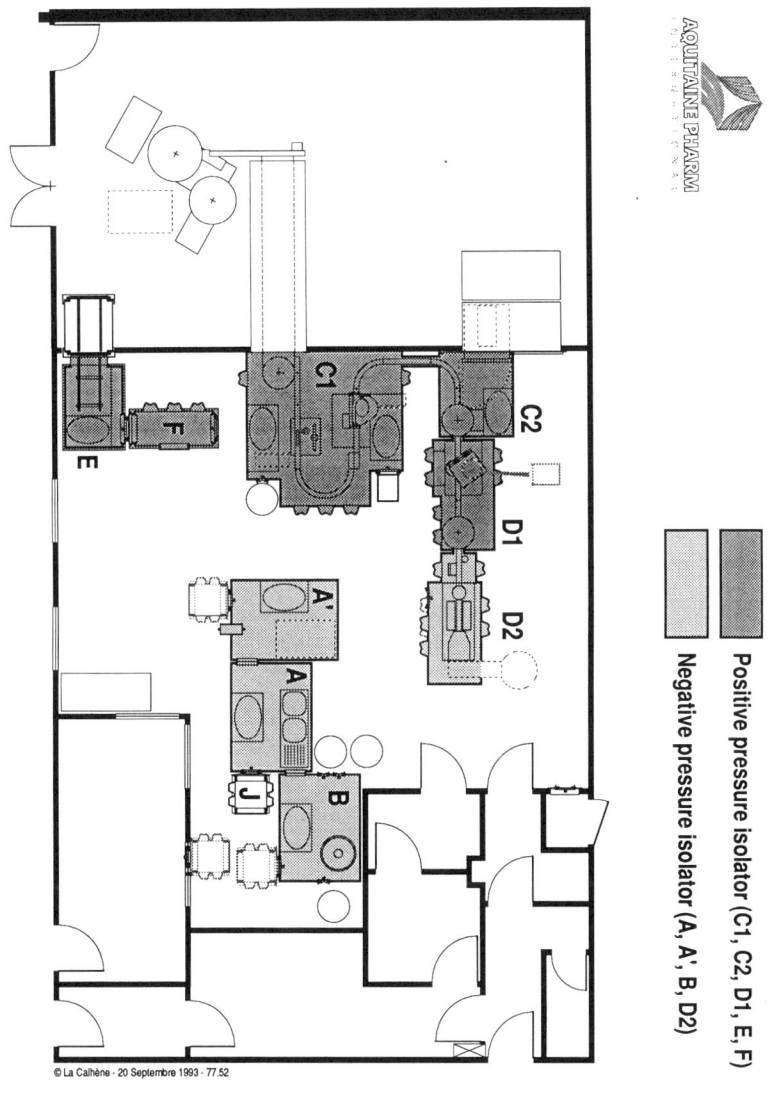

Figure 14.2. Illustration of production flow.

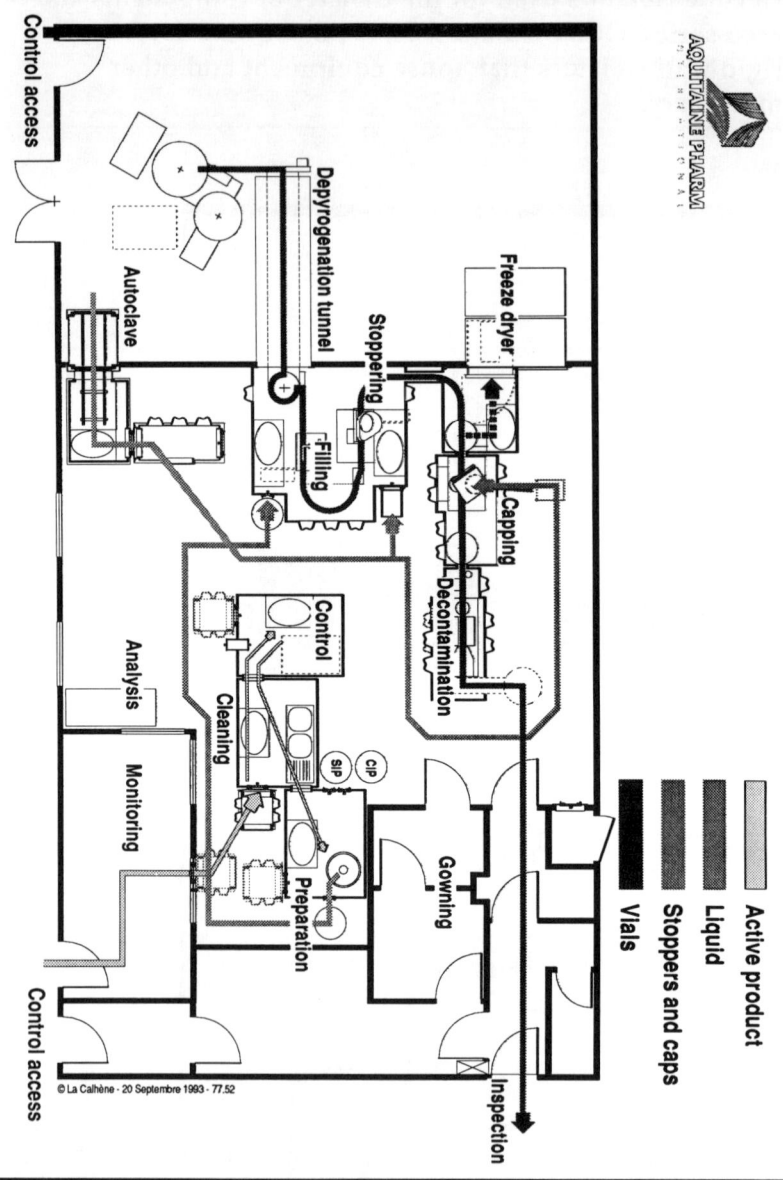

- intermediate storage
- visual inspection
- final packaging

- laboratory control
- effluent treatment

The isolators are identified by letters (A, A', B, C1, C2, D1, D2, E, F, J). We used flexible wall isolators for the transfer of components or accessories (E, F, J), and rigid wall isolators for housing equipment and other machines. Isolators are under positive pressure where it is important to guarantee and maintain the sterility, and to protect the product. Where there is a risk of contamination for the operators, the isolators are maintained under negative pressure.

Environment Classification

The manufacturing room around the isolators where people work is Class 10,000 or M 5.5. The negative pressure isolators are Class 10,000 or M 5.5. The isolators in positive pressure are Class 100 or M 3.5. The other parts of the shop are Class 100,000 or M 6.5. Isolators C1, C2, D1, E, and F are maintained sterile.

The filling and stoppering isolators are monitored on a continuous basis for particulates at three different points. We have Class 0 when the machines are not running. During production runs, under dynamic conditions, we have observed results between Class 0 and 100 at the filling and stoppering points. The average value recorded with the three sampling points, during 90 days of filling operations is thirty-one (31) 0.5 micron particles.

Regarding pressure, we continuously monitor a dynamic cascade of air between the depyrogenation tunnel and the outlet of the line through all the isolators. The cascade of pressure is between + 4 mm and – 3 mm of water column. We regulate the differential pressure between isolators at 0.5 mm of water column. This continuous monitoring method for barrier technology was designed by API specifically for this facility.

VALIDATION OF ISOLATORS—STERILITY

We use the La Calhène SPRAM system to generate a fog of hydrogen peroxide. The SPRAM system is a sterilant spray equipment that uses the nebulization principle to generate a sterilizing mist. The sterilization process includes two phases: sterilization and rinsing. Exposure is based on a validated contact time for the sterilant. For the filling isolator, due to its geometry, the laminar flow is stopped during sterilization.

Methodology

During validation a 15 percent solution of H_2O_2 was injected through nozzles installed on the isolator's wall. Isolators were rinsed afterwards. We used *Bacillus stearothermophilus* on strips at 10^6 spores. Strips were located at the most difficult places to ensure complete sterilization of enclosures. For the 8 m^3 filling isolator, we used 11 strips.

Strips were incubated for 7 days between 55°C and 60°C. The acceptable criteria was a 6 log reduction on all the strips. The validation was acceptable if we succeeded on three different successive tests. For revalidation, the same approach is taken and these tests are performed twice a year.

For routine production, the validated volume of H_2O_2 and the rinsing time are each increased by 10 percent over the validation parameters. Under normal working conditions, residues are measured with a dragger pump. Our specification is less than 1 ppm.

Regarding the validation of the process, Media Fill Tests (MFTs) were carried out following guidelines similar to the ones used in a conventional clean room facility. Three MFTs were performed on three different days. Media fill samples were incubated for 7 days between 30 and 35°C, and 7 days between 20 and 25°C. Vials were incubated upside down. A growth promotion test was performed with 4 microorganisms, as recommended by the United States Pharmacopeia (3 aerobes and 1 anaerobe). For the initial validation the following critical operations were tested:

- change of filling pump
- glove replacement
- check valve change on the filling line
- gauntlet change
- filling speed at low and high speeds

- stop of laminar flow
- pressure cascade reversed remaining positive to the room
- nitrogen and air blanketing

More than 10 MFTs, with more than 3000 vials/run, were performed during validation, and no positives were identified. The same MFT method is used for routine process monitoring. Following the use of the isolator for one month, three (3) MFTs are conducted. Based on our current experience, our sterility assurance is guaranteed, without resterilisation, for a period of over one month. Environmental monitoring is performed daily and no out-of-limits results have been obtained during routine use of the isolators.

Monitoring

We use an alarm system to monitor the over-pressure between each isolator and the outside environment of the working shop, on a continuous basis. Before each production run, we check if the over-pressure has been maintained since the last sterilization operation and if we had no particle contamination. The particle level inside and outside the isolators are recorded. Bacteriological monitoring is performed each shift. Four Reuter Centrifugal Sampler® (RCS®) measurements are taken at the beginning and at the end of the run. Settling plates are used on a continuous basis, including:

- 1 settling plate at the filling station.
- 1 settling plate at the stoppering station.

CONCLUSION

For the last three years we have used this dynamic barrier technology system to manufacture Navelbine, a product of Pierre Fabre Laboratories to be shipped all over the world. API was successfully inspected and the Food and Drug Administration (FDA) approved shipment of Navelbine to the U.S. on December 23, 1994. The product was launched in the U.S. on January 17, 1995. The U.S. supplier for this product is Burroughs Wellcome.

Navelbine is the first French anti-cancer drug approved for the U.S. market by the FDA. It is also the first new drug licensed for this treatment in the U.S. in 20 years. API is excited to be the first company ever approved by the FDA to produce a sterile product in isolators.

15

Aseptic Filling in a Rigid Isolator at Evans Medical

Julian Wilkins
Total Process Containment Ltd.
Elstead, Surrey, United Kingdom

Isolators provide a cost effective and environmentally benign alternative for filling in aseptic conditions. Isolator and total containment systems using barrier technology protect people, the environment and the product or process and reduce capital and running costs. Total Process Containment at Evans Medical (Figure 15.1) is a good example of isolator technology in use. It provides an alternative to clean rooms for the aseptic fill of a vaccine into pre-sterilised syringes. The filling environment and incoming pre-sterilised syringe packs are sterilised by means of vapour-phase hydrogen peroxide (VHP) surface sterilisation. This approach minimises the opportunity of product contamination, improves the safety of the operation, increases output from 40,000 to 120,000 units/day using an existing filling machine and reduces capital and unit operating costs. In use it has reduced to zero the number of colony forming units directed in the filling zone compared with occasional

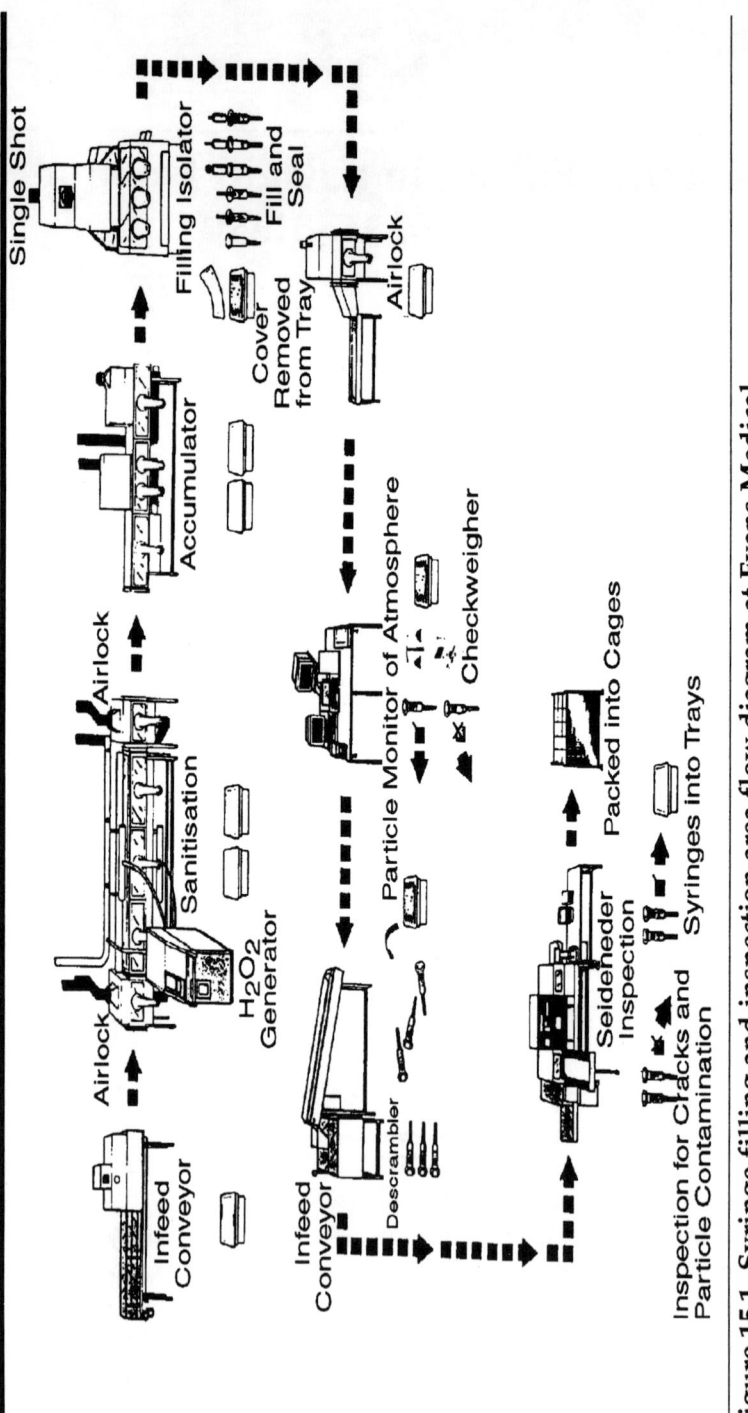

Figure 15.1. Syringe filling and inspection area flow diagram at Evans Medical.

incursions of colony forming units in the conventional clean room.

PROJECT REQUIREMENTS

The goals for the project were to continuously sanitise Hypak syringe packs for vaccine filling and to upgrade and expand the capacity of a filling line for a human flu vaccine using an existing filling machine. Total Process Containment (TPC) was invited to explore the best route using novel isolation or barrier technology.

The process involves bulk vaccine suspension produced in a separate part of the plant and stored in 25 vessels. The vessels are transported to the aseptically connected filling machine and the contents are transferred for filling into Becton Dickinson SCF Hypak barrels on a syringe filling machine. The syringe barrels and plugs are pre-sterilised by the vendor and placed in outer wraps. These then are surface sterilised as part of the filling line process.

THE TRADITIONAL APPROACH

Within the 'core' of the cleanroom suite, aseptic filling conditions are required and microbiological and particulate cleanliness levels of the highest order must be achieved. At Evans, the operators entered the aseptic zone through a three stage changing complex with segregated entry and exit and with fresh garments required for each entry.

The external surface of the vessel containing the vaccine required surface sanitisation using a manual spray or fumigation process. The vessel itself was introduced into the filling room through a controlled airlock. Empty vessels passed out in the reverse direction. The entry airlock exposed batches of bagged packs to fumigation or gaseous disinfection. Filled and plugged syringes left the aseptic filling room either by conveyor or through an airlock.

The traditional formaldehyde disinfection of the syringe pack was a process limiting step and difficult to control in terms of reliability and repeatability. It presented safety problems and consumed expensive sterile room space for the disinfection stage.

TPC concluded that by its very nature, the traditional approach was hazardous and difficult to control. For instance the packs enclosing syringe packs also require surface disinfection but due to the large number, and the need for a safe, validatable process, manual spraying or formaldehyde gassing is not practical or effectively repeatable.

ISOLATOR NETWORK

Once this conclusion had been reached TPC looked at an alternative solution based on isolator technology. The aims were to remove hazardous processes such as fumigation, reduce manufacturing costs and improve quality assurance with particular emphasis on sterility. Other objectives included the establishment of surface sanitisation, lower capital investment compared to a clean room option and reduced manual handling.

A number of concepts were considered and rejected, including individual fixed isolators with a mobile transfer isolator for transport between process steps. Finally a route based on a continuous fixed line of directly connected functional modules was selected. This avoids multiple isolator-to-isolator docking and transfer requirements. The continuous VHP process is a TPC patent.

DETAILED DEVELOPMENT

Once the isolator technology approach had been identified by the feasibility study, detailed design and ergonomic studies were carried out. The detailed design stage involved considerable engineering input into construction techniques. Hygiene considerations were critical and surface cleanliness and ability to sanitise inside the line were examined.

The ergonomic study was one of the most important technical evaluation activities in TPC's eyes. With isolation technology human intervention becomes constrained and limited by the necessity to use glove ports. It is particularly important to consider how the operator will carry out the manual manipulations and to recognise that it will be performed by individuals with different height and reach capabilities.

Ergonomic evaluation was essential to satisfy the requirements of GMPs to ensure that the process was secure and repeatable. The operation of the filling machine is important to assure sterility.

ERGONOMIC MODELLING

Computerised ergonomic modelling (Figure 15.2) is very effective when exploring either the anthropometrics of actual individuals or a statistically valid range of individuals. Using a base range of 5 percentile female to 95 percentile male, the extremes of size were explored while intended operators at Evans Medical were also identified.

Further evaluation of the most critical modules was carried out using a physical mock-up of the filling process. This confirmed the findings from the computer modelling and enabled tests on particular manipulations to be carried out.

A process line was developed with the use of VHP for surface sanitisation to 10^{-6} sterility assurance level (SAL) of the bagged packs, and also the sanitisation of the whole isolator network on a strategic basis.

SEPARATED OPERATIONS

In the final design, the continuous sanitisation and filling operation was divided into seven compartments: line feed area, pass-in airlock, sanitisation tunnel, pass-out airlock, accumulator, operations isolator for the filling machine, and exit airlock.

Wrapped packs containing 100 ml barrels of plastic sealed with Tyvek® panels are taken to the line feed area. The packs are removed from their carton, unwrapped from their outer protective layer and fed by a conveyor to the pass-in airlock using laminar air flow (LAF) protection to reduce environmental contamination.

Figure 15.2. Computer Aided Ergonomics Design System.

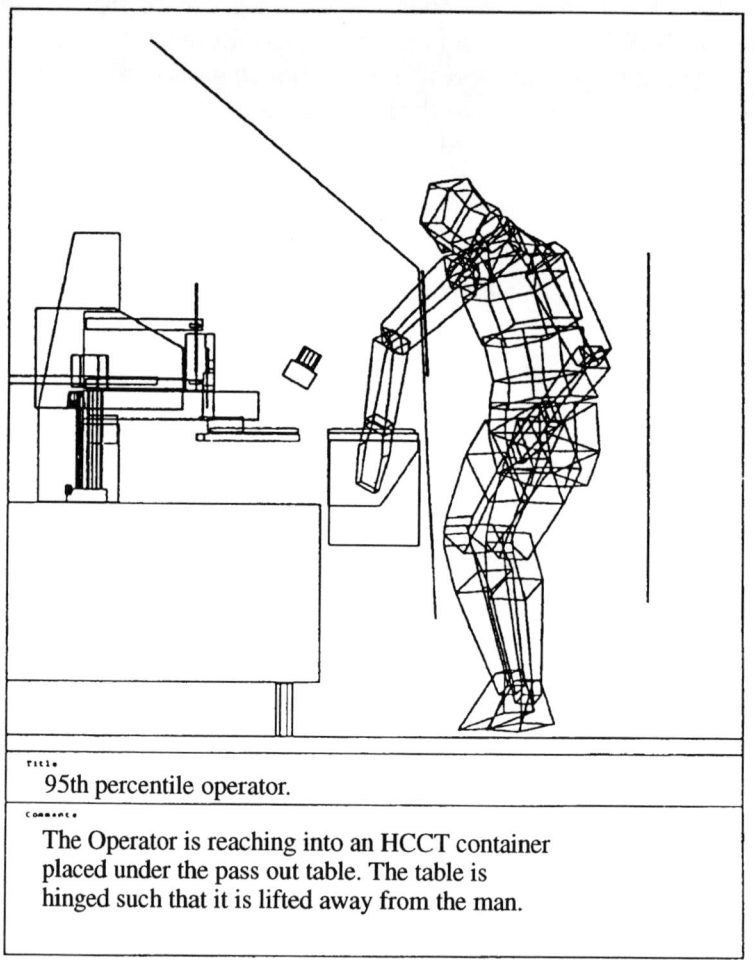

95th percentile operator.

The Operator is reaching into an HCCT container placed under the pass out table. The table is hinged such that it is lifted away from the man.

The primary function of the pass-in airlock is to maintain separation between the unpacking area and sterilisation chamber. The packs are exposed in this conditioning zone to a warmed, dried air stream to improve the efficiency of the hydrogen peroxide sanitisation and remove any surface particulate contamination.

Each pack moves automatically through a door into the sanitisation tunnel where it is exposed to a fixed concentration of VHP for a predetermined time. When the programmed sterilising cycle is completed, the pack passes through another door into the pass-out airlock which separates the sanitising tunnel from the accumulation line. An air stream is used to reduce hydrogen peroxide residuals to a minimum.

The accumulation zone provides a store of packs for the operator and allows any remaining hydrogen peroxide residuals to dissipate. The filling isolator then facilitates the insertion of the packs into the filling machine and provides a unidirectional air flow over the filling head to protect against particulate contamination.

In the filling isolator the operator takes a pack and peels back the Tyvek® panels through glove manipulation. The exposed syringe barrel trays are in turn loaded onto the filling line, removed after filling and plugging, then re-tubbed manually and advanced to the airlock for the pack to pass out.

CONTROL AND INSTRUMENTATION

The continuous sanitisation and filling system is controlled by a dedicated panel covering line operation, environmental control, alarm system diagnostics and production data. A 486SX 33mHz computer with 10mb ram hard disk controls a bit-buss loop which integrates the control mechanisms of the system.

The selection of the control system was important in order to satisfy validation requirements. The system chosen has a proven and traceable operating system with a high level working environment. This enabled the instruction sets to be written in plain language by a TPC process engineer and avoided the need to employ specialist software programmers unfamiliar with the processing needs.

BUILDING INTEGRATION

A fundamental objective of the project was to take maximum advantage of being able to install the isolator network of equipment in a socially clean, unclassified working area. Throughout the project, discussions were held with the Medicines Control Agency and advice taken to ensure a smooth formal acceptance of the installation. Subsequently the line has received FDA approval for aseptic manufacture under unclassified conditions.

Admittance of personnel is restricted to operators with key card access to help maintain the integrity of the system and reduce any unnotified incidents. A materials transfer area is provided to ensure designation of batches of dispensed components and only classified operators can effect material entry and exits.

Although isolator technology is being used, essential GMP concepts such as batch control and environmental monitoring still have to be considered. In particular, tests are required to prove the effectiveness of the barrier at the material entry and exit points to allow the equipment to be housed in an unclassified room. Hence LAF protection was adopted at the inlet point and a fully interlocked airlock employed at the exit. The impact of VHP sterilisation, such as the prevention of VHP penetration and residuals in the glass syringes also had to be examined.

REDUCED WORK VOLUME

The environmental process validation still requires all stages of the validation programme to be carried out in the same way as with a cleanroom. However, the enormously reduced working volume, the exclusion of operators and the intimate relationship between the process and environmental control significantly reduces the amount of test work and volume of data to be assimilated. This saves time and has on ongoing benefit in a re-evaluation.

From acceptance of the feasibility study, the project at Evans Medical was completed in seven months, a shorter timescale than estimated for an equivalent clean room option. TPC was given turnkey responsibility from inception to detailed design, fabrication, factory testing, delivery, assembly, commissioning, qualification and handover. The line is now two years old and has filled in excess of 9 million fills. The line has both FDA and EEC product license (Figure 15.3).

In the two years since it commenced operations, a large amount of data has been collected. Key factors applicable to the Evans facility are as follows:

Figure 15.3. A view of the filling line at Evans Medical.

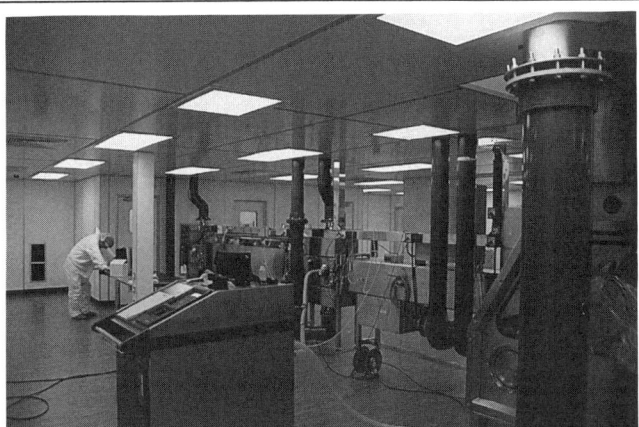

- Reduction in capital cost versus a conventional facility (40 percent).
- Reduction in revenue cost compared to the previous operation of the filling machine in a conventional area (60 percent).
- Increase in unit rate efficiency of the filling machine in an isolator (15 percent).
- Lost production due to colony forming unit incursion (zero).

The client had some positive samples on settle plates and glove swabs and as a result sterility testing procedures have been reviewed. The line provides a 10^{-6} filling environment.

16

Isolation Technology for Sterility Testing at Burroughs Wellcome Co., Greenville, NC

John Shirtz
Burroughs Wellcome Co.
Greenville, NC

The use of isolator technology at Burroughs Wellcome (BW) in Greenville, NC started in the mid-1980s shortly after the technology first became commercially available. At that time, BW was using a conventional clean room for the sterility testing of batches of sterile product but it was apparent that a system upgrade was necessary.

During this same period, the Food and Drug Administration (FDA) and United States Pharmacopeia (USP) developed a stricter policy on sterility retesting. For a pre-1985 sterility failure, most pharmaceutical companies initiated a double unit retest of the batch (or fill day) in question. If the retest result was satisfactory, an investigation was performed to make sure there were no flagrant production problems, and then the batch was usually determined to be acceptable. The USP Sterility Test allowed acceptance based on the retest: "If evidence of growth is found, the article fails to meet the requirements of the test for Sterility, *unless it can be demonstrated by retests or by other means* that the test was invalid for causes unrelated to the article...."

Recognizing the inherent problems with the limited statistical probabilities of detecting low level contamination with the recommended sample sizes, USP in 1980 (USPXX) introduced stronger language relating to sterility retesting by their description of the "First Retest" and "Second Retest." In 1985 (USPXXI), this was further tightened to "First Stage" and "Second Stage." In essence, USP drew the line on simply accepting the test results and began to include other conditions before a sterility test failure could be considered "invalid" and the batch released based on the results of a retest. It became extremely important to minimize all risks associated with sterility testing. It also became important to investigate the production and testing documentation and determine a cause of the failure.

At about this time, FDA recognized that the sterility testing environment played a critical role in the proper conduct of the test. Their *Guideline on Sterile Drug Products Produced by Aseptic Processing* (1987) stated that "... the testing laboratory environment should employ facilities and controls comparable to those used for filling/closing operations...." The argument that a positive sterility test was caused by inadequate laboratory facilities simply would not be considered.

BW decided it was time to upgrade the sterility testing facility to minimize the possibility of discarding production batches due to failures in the sterility test. Like many companies that made products by aseptic means, BW occasionally suffered a substantial loss of revenue from the unnecessary destruction of a batch which failed the sterility test for causes unrelated to the aseptic production facility. This was because BW, like many other ethical pharmaceutical manufacturers, chose to be conservative and rejected batches despite a direct connection of the failure to the sterility testing environment.

Isolator technology was barely out of its infancy when BW first applied the technology to routine sterility testing. Faced with a compelling need to improve the sterility testing conditions, BW evaluated the concept of using isolator technology as opposed to upgrading the facility. After careful evaluation of the alternatives, Quality Assurance (QA) management decided to commit resources to the isolator technology.

The first unit included an autoclave isolator, a principal isolator, two transfer isolators, and two peracetic acid sterilizers. The unit was purchased, validated, and put into routine service within a few short months. Later, another identical set-up became necessary when QA relocated to another building. The new set-up was installed and validated during building construction and the original was relocated to stand side-by-side with the second purchase. The identical set-ups allow for revalidation and maintenance at a reasonable pace on one unit while the other is in service and provides for an alternative "facility" in the event of an unplanned work interruption on the primary unit.

Installation of the first units was not without problems. Sterilizing the cavity for the sliding door of the autoclave, within the autoclave isolator, required installation of a fan to circulate the peracetic acid. Biological Indicators (BIs) used in the validation of the isolators were difficult to place in specific areas until an ingenious technician came up with the idea of attaching the BIs to monofilament fishing line and suspending them on magnetic stirrers held in place by corresponding magnetic stirrers outside the canopy. The importance of the wipedown of the transfer isolator with peracetic acid and the rotation of the load became apparent with some of the first sterilization cycles. Several positive BIs demonstrated a necessity. Container/closure integrity testing of the numerous product combinations was performed to examine for the presence of peracetic acid inside the simulated product containers. Detection of the sterilant inside the product containers would have invalidated this as a sterilization process for the sterility testing system.

Converting to isolators for sterility testing required significant modifications to simple tasks. A learning curve is associated with the operation of an isolator whose exterior is not quite as durable as plastered or stainless steel walls. Numerous leaks occurred from punctures in the canopy not caused by carelessness, but by mishandling. Modifications to the laboratory AC system were necessary when an autoclave was added to the testing area. Resolution of these problems was facilitated because employees preferred working in the isolator versus working in a conventional sterile room.

Included after the initial set-up were the purchase of cold spray peracetic acid sterilization and evaluation of vaporized hydrogen peroxide (VHP) equipment. The success of isolator technology for this sterility testing application led to its consideration for being included in the design for a new sterile products facility recently constructed at the Greenville site. This facility includes Double Porte Transfert Etanche (DPTE) ports in each of the aseptic production rooms as well as the aseptic laboratory area used for the preparation of sterile environmental monitoring plates. After preincubation in the aseptic laboratory area, the plates are transferred through the DPTE port into a transfer isolator and then wheeled up to the aseptic production area DPTE port. These plates are transferred from one aseptic area to the other without exposure to the non-aseptic environment. They need not be wiped down, put through a pass-through, etc.

The new facility also provides for protection of the production samples for sterility testing. A portable isolator, which includes a 350 mm port at one end and a 270 mm port at the other end, will be used to transfer the sterility test units from the aseptic production area to the aseptic isolator where the sterility test will take place. Like the environmental plates, the sterility test units will not be exposed to the nonaseptic environment prior to testing, thereby greatly minimizing the risk of inadvertent contamination.

Despite the routine maintenance required by the isolation system, this alternative has definite financial advantages over the conventional aseptic room concept. Loss of revenue from rejected batches and the numerous man-hours involved in sterility reject investigations can quickly increase start-up expenses. These costs have been eliminated by the use of isolators. The increased productivity of the operators due to the elimination of multiple gown-up sessions and the elimination of the expenses associated with the sourcing and supplying of sterile gowns, masks, and gloves, have contributed to the technological and cost-containment success of the isolation system being used for sterility testing at Burroughs Wellcome Co.

REFERENCES

FDA. 1987. Guideline on sterile drug products produced by aseptic processing. *Federal Register* 181–332:60360.

17

Experience in the Design and Use of Isolator Systems for Sterility Testing

James E. Akers
Colleen M. Kennedy
Akers Kennedy & Associates, Inc.
Kansas City, MO

James P. Agalloco
Agalloco & Associates
Somerville, NJ

Abstract: The use of isolator systems for sterility testing is on the increase. Prior to installation and validation careful consideration must be given to the type of isolator to be used, and the design of the facility which will house the isolator system. The validation of these systems requires development and testing of the sterilization cycle. Vapor phase hydrogen peroxide has proven to be efficacious in this application, and examples of sterilization cycle development are presented in this paper. Also of concern is the penetration of sterilant into test articles, media and supplies.

Copyright © 1994 Parenteral Drug Association, Inc. Reprinted with permission.

Since the mid-1980s, so called isolator systems have come into wide use as clean spaces in which compendial sterility tests are conducted. For the purpose of this presentation, isolator systems are defined as free standing enclosures equipped with integral HEPA–filtered air supplies that allow employees to manipulate test articles using either flexible sleeves and gloves, or special flexible suits that comprise part of one wall of the isolator. These isolator systems are sterilizable to a high sterility assurance level using such chemical agents as peracetic acid, vapor phase hydrogen peroxide, or another cold sterilizing agent.

The isolator system used for sterility testing may be attached to a pass through autoclave for convenient supply of media and testing articles. Alternatively, the system may consist of isolators alone with media and fluids sterilized separately and then transferred into the isolator system. In our experience, sterility tests can be conducted in systems that are not directly connected to autoclaves with a high level of reliability. The use of transfer isolators or specialized transfer canisters can provide a high degree of flexibility in moving supplies and test articles into the test isolator. Transfer canisters are available either for gas sterilization or steam sterilization. These units are docked with transfer ports and their sterile contents can be moved into the test isolator without breaking containment. The integration of autoclaves into test systems can provide advantages in speed and efficiency, but there is no evidence that they provide a greater level of safety against false positive tests. Systems that are not directly connected to autoclaves are typically less expensive to install and easier to validate.

As with any pharmaceutical system, quality and reliability must be considered from the very beginning in the design and layout of an isolator system. The following general areas should be addressed by the prospective users during the conceptual design phase of a project:

1. *The size of the testing isolator and how it should be designed.* Most systems we have seen, and worked with, use two side-by-side half-suit assemblies. However, other configurations are available and may afford operational advantages to some users. For some smaller firms or

facilities that conduct relatively few tests, a single suit isolator may be sufficient.

2. *The flow of materials and supplies must be given careful consideration.* Proper utilization of isolator systems requires that all supplies and test articles are sterilized before entry into the test isolator. Space requirements for docking and storing transfer isolators, storage and hookup of sterilization equipment, and access to the half suits must be considered. Ample space must be left around the perimeter of the isolator system to allow easy traffic flow and movement of transfer isolators. Proximity to incubators must also be considered. Direct inoculation sterility tests that require subculturing will require reintroduction of test articles to the work station isolator. Consequently, some users choose to incubate sterility tests inside a transfer isolator. Here, movement of the transfer systems into and out of the incubator must be well thought out.

3. *Utility service requirements for many sterility testing isolators can be quite simple.* The ability to exhaust sterilization gas directly to a roof stack is important. In some cases, it is possible to vent this exhaust directly to existing ducts for laboratory fume hoods. The prospective user should consult with the vendor they have selected for the sterilization system with respect to exhaust requirements. As you will see later in this chapter, aeration of isolators after sterilization can be an important validation issue. In our experience removal of the sterilizing agent down to safe levels can take significantly longer than expected from air exchange calculations. Obviously the presence of an autoclave will impose a requirement for steam, although in the case of sterility testing clean or WFI steam is not required.

4. *Interfacing of the isolator directly with an autoclave requires an interface isolator.* This interface must be tailored to the specific autoclave that will be used. It is important to assure that the autoclave can be equipped with a proper bioseal so that a safe airtight seal exists between the interface isolator and the autoclave. Pass through

double door autoclaves are typically used. It is tempting to select an autoclave with a sliding or pocket type door. These autoclaves make design of the interface isolator relatively simple since the space for a swinging door does not have to be accommodated. However, the pocket door autoclave is typically more expensive and may require a custom plenum to allow for movement of the door. Care must be taken to avoid "dead spaces" where sterilizing concentrations of sterilizing agent cannot be reached.

Consideration must also be given to the inevitable maintenance on the door system or replacement of the inflatable gasket. Since interface isolators are typically equipped with half-suits, consideration should be given to locating the half-suit so that simple adjustments to the door or replacement of the gasket can be accomplished without a complete disassembly of the system. Swinging door autoclaves have been successfully used with interface isolators, and we think have the virtues of simplicity and economy. Whatever autoclave design is chosen, they must have a door interlock system that prevents both doors from opening simultaneously.

5. *Isolators have no special power system requirements, and since they are usually equipped with both inlet and exhaust HEPA filters, power is not required to maintain isolation.* In fact, one could argue that the more air forced through the HEPA filters the greater the likelihood of a microorganism breaking through. Thus, we do not require that isolators be constantly powered up, and an uninterruptible power supply is unnecessary.

6. *There has been some debate about the classification of the room(s) in which isolator systems for product filling are located.* Most isolators for sterility testing are located in standard unclassified laboratory space. Some of these isolators have functioned without a false positive sterility test for years. We are aware of systems located in unclassified laboratory space in which hundreds of media control or negative control tests have been done

without a single failure. Also, it is exceedingly rare to find any microbiological contamination in an isolator system through environmental monitoring. Where we have heard of such instances, they have been the result of glove failures or contaminated media. We see no need to place a sterility test isolator in a classified area. Consistent with this view, we also do not believe that aseptic gowning is required.

Control of temperature and humidity within the room can be very important, particularly if sterilization using vapor phase hydrogen peroxide is employed. We have had to bring additional dehumidification capacity to some facilities during validation studies.

7. All of the sterility testing systems we have worked with have been turbulent flow units constructed of heavy duty polyvinyl chloride. We think these units are completely satisfactory for sterility testing. Rigid wall isolators and laminar flow isolators are now widely available. Rigid wall isolators have the advantage of affording better optical properties, but may be significantly more expensive. Laminar flow units offer no real advantage for sterility testing, and are typically more costly to purchase, and to operate, than turbulent flow units. Certainly, the rigid wall laminar flow units appear more substantial, but experience has shown the flexible wall turbulent flow units to be both reliable and inexpensive to operate and maintain. The prospective user can make this decision knowing that whatever design they choose, provided that it is built to remain leak free, will provide the same level of performance.

Careful consideration of these matters before purchase can result in cost savings in construction, installation, validation, maintenance and operation. As with many technical issues in our industry, spending more money does not correlate directly with enhanced performance or convenience of operation. In fact, spending more often results in more complexity, which can increase both maintenance costs and downtime.

SPECIFIC VALIDATION TESTING

After installation and commissioning of an isolator system, the next step, at least according to the United States validation system, is the so called installation qualification (IQ) and operational qualification (OQ). We have expressed concern that in the United States the cost benefit ratio with respect to IQ, OQ testing is heavily biased in the direction of cost. Whenever organizational conditions allow, the IQ and OQ should be combined into a single protocol and pared to the essentials. After all, the purpose of these "phases" of validation is to demonstrate the equipment is capable of meeting design parameters. In actual fact this requires only a modest amount of data. The key operational points are:

1. The HEPA filters must pass certification testing.
2. The system must be free of leaks.

The rest of the IQ/OQ qualification is pro forma and holds no surprises.

STERILIZATION

The conditions required for an isolator system to provide a germ-free environment are really quite simple.

1. The isolator system must have physical integrity. That is, it must function as an "isolator" to the introduction of contaminating microorganisms, and it must maintain conditions which "isolate" the system's contents from the environment.
2. The interior of the isolator must be sterilizable to a high level of sterility assurance.

As you will see from the data that we are going to present, the sterilization of isolator systems, supplies, and test articles to a high level of sterility assurance is readily achievable. Selection of a sterilization method is very important. We are familiar with two systems, both of which have proven to work well for the purpose of sterility testing. These are peracetic acid and vapor phase hydrogen peroxide. There is a firm in the United

States developing a combination of steam and hydrogen peroxide as a sterilization system for isolators. Formaldehyde had been used in some early isolator applications, although we know of no systems currently using this agent. We understand that some development work is underway on the use of ozone as a sterilizing agent for certain isolator applications.

In recent years vapor phase hydrogen peroxide (VHP) has become the most frequently used sterilizing agent for isolator systems. All the systems we have tested over the last two years have used VHP as the sterilizing agent. In our experience VHP is efficacious and as safe as any sterilizing agent can be. It has the further advantage of breaking down into water and oxygen which are innocuous to the environment. The data we are presenting will be based upon our experience with VHP.

STERILIZATION CYCLE DEVELOPMENT

Sterilization cycle development for isolators is very similar in concept to the development of steam sterilization cycles. As with validation of an autoclave, the first step in the development of VHP sterilization cycles is identification of fixed loading configurations. In sterility testing applications a surface sterilization of test articles, supplies and tools occurs in the transfer isolator. The work station isolator and interface isolators (if used) are usually essentially empty during sterilization. Thus, it is important to keep a few key issues in mind as you develop loading configurations:

1. *VHP in the isolator behaves as a gas, and it cannot sterilize items which it cannot reach.* Items should be placed upon shelves which raise them off of the floor of the isolator. Stainless steel racks which are readily available commercially work well to support heavy materials for sterilization. Bottles, culture tubes, etc. must be placed in a manner which allows free circulation of gas around them. We have found that hanging wrapped supplies such as spare gloves, tubing, and needles from supports or wire stringers permits good circulation of the gas.

2. *The half-life of H_2O_2 gas becomes shorter as the mass of material in the load to be sterilized increases.* According to

studies conducted by AMSCO, half-life of VHP in a heavy load can be two to three times shorter than in a light load in a work station of approximately 6 m^3 internal volume. However, in a typical transfer isolator with an internal volume of less than 1 m^3 half-life decreases much less as the mass of the load increases. In practice, we have found that quite heavy loads can be sterilized in a transfer isolator.

3. *Loads which consist of primarily metals, hard plastics, and glass tend to absorb less hydrogen peroxide.* We have found that goods wrapped in tyvek, or sterilization papers readily absorb H_2O_2 and can take a very long time to outgas. In one sterilization load we found that an average H_2O_2 concentration of approximately 1.75 mg/ℓ aeration down to a level of 1ppm within the transfer isolator took about twelve hours. This is about three times longer than would be anticipated based upon the ratio of air flow rate to isolator chamber volume which was 0.9. This is because the absorption of VHP by the materials being sterilized did not allow removal of gas to behave as a simple dilution phenomenon. Our recommendation is to avoid paper and plastic bags as much as possible.

TEMPERATURE MAPPING

After the loading configuration has been developed, the next step is to conduct temperature mapping of the isolator to determine heat distribution. We conduct temperature mapping with the hydrogen peroxide generator in the dehumidification phase. We begin our mapping evaluation with studies done on the empty isolator. Many sterility testing operations have only one loading configuration to sterilize. If more than one load is to be sterilized then the heaviest load should be selected as it will be worst case. Thermocouples are placed throughout the load to monitor both temperature penetration and distribution. Sixteen to twenty thermocouples should be adequate for the typical transfer isolator.

The purpose of heat distribution analysis is to determine that cold spot within the isolator or load. This is not done because VHP is more efficacious at high temperatures, but rather to enable us to calculate the maximum safe concentration of VHP which can be used without observing condensation. We have used relative humidity set points of 10–20%. Generally 20% is a good choice, as achieving set points lower than 20% in many climates can add considerable time to the total sterilization cycle. We have found that in rooms with an ambient temperature of 20–22°C, the temperature range observed at the conclusion of dehumidification is typically about 23°–27°C. A conservative assumption should be made unless the seasonal variations in temperature within the room are known to be small.

DETERMINATION OF VHP CONCENTRATION

An estimation of the proper VHP concentration for sterilization is determined from standard tables. These tables indicate the maximum allowable concentration of VHP for enclosures of various sizes. These tables take into account temperature, relative humidity, mass of load, and flow rate of the air/VHP mixture. The users should base their initial estimate on the coolest temperature observed during the mapping studies. For example, the VHP enclosure concentration for a 0.67 m^3 transfer isolator containing a massive load and minimum observed temperature of 22°C at a flow rate of about 0.67 m^3 is about 1.5 mg/ℓ. This value corresponds to an injection rate of 3.6 g/min. VHP sterilizers allow for a conditioning period in which the sterilization concentration can be reached quickly. For the example, in a unit with 1.0 exchanges per minute, a preconditioning injection rate of about 6.5 g/minute for two minutes would be a reasonable conditioning phase set point. The user should view this value as a starting point only.

The efficacy of these parameters is evaluated by running test cycles containing a full worst case load. This load is monitored by both thermocouples and chemical indicators (CIs). CIs are qualitative only, but can be used to make a general evaluation of gas distribution. CIs typically change from a white to gray–violet color in about five minutes upon exposure to VHP. We have placed CIs in some very difficult locations for VHP penetration, including under end cap gaskets, and have observed color change in 15 minutes or less. These gas concentration test runs are closely observed for the formation of condensate. Condensation of VHP is indicative of an enclosure concentration which is too high for the temperature within the isolator. Published studies indicate that the D-value of *B. stearothermophilus* in the example we have chosen with a VHP concentration of 1.5 mg/ℓ would be between two and seven minutes. Our practice is to assume the worst case D-value of seven minutes, and to use an "overkill" type sterilization cycle. In this example we would select an exposure period of 84 minutes to achieve a 12 log kill of the most resistant organism.

BIOLOGICAL INDICATOR CHALLENGE STUDIES

The purpose of any sterilization cycle is to kill microorganisms. Therefore, the challenge of the sterilization cycle with biological indicators is the only way in which the efficacy of the cycle can be verified. There are several studies in the literature describing D-values for various microorganisms. Studies performed by investigators such as Rickloff, Klapes and Griego have shown that VHP is an effective sterilizing agent, which can destroy spore bearing bacteria. In addition, studies have been conducted on a wide variety of molds, viruses, and vegetative bacteria. Evidence indicates that *B. stearothermophilus* is the most resistant organism.

In conducting sterilization challenges we use biological indicators at the highest available titer which is approximately 10^5 spores per strip. Special spore strips for use with VHP are available commercially. The titer and purity of these biological indicators should be verified independently by the user's laboratory. If the user so desires, fraction negative studies can be conducted to confirm D-value. We use a half-cycle approach to demonstrate the reliability of the sterilization cycle we have designed. We also eliminate the conditioning period to create worst case conditions.

For the validation of the transfer isolator we place approximately 20 biological indicators (BIs). We have placed BIs throughout the load, including under glass containers, within baskets of supplies, and under round bottom culture tubes in metal racks. We have never observed a non-sterile BI in a validation test run in transfer isolators.

We have validated the sterilization of combined work station and autoclave interface isolators up to approximately 425 ft^3 or 14 m^3. The autoclave plenum, interface isolator, and work station isolator were sterilized as a single unit to increase the user's convenience and flexibility. This system had a double-door autoclave connected to the interface isolator by a plenum which sealed the movement of the vertical pocket door in an airtight chamber. The plenum assembly had two gas inlets and was equipped with a fan to enhance circulation. We routed the VHP to the two isolators and autoclave plenum as indicated. We configured the system so that VHP passed through all HEPA filters during sterilization. This required us to return VHP through the inlet HEPA of the interface isolator. The autoclave control was interfaced with the VHP control system and the rear or clean side autoclave door opened and closed at approximately 15 second intervals throughout sterilization. Sixty BIs were placed throughout the combined system including the plenum and autoclave chamber. A total of three validation studies were done and all BIs were killed. The total exposure period was 96 minutes, and the total time required for the entire sterilization cycle was approximately 10 hours. This allows for sterilization of the system overnight.

We have created conditions during development studies in which BIs have survived sterilization. We inverted the sleeves and gloves of the half-suit and found that VHP did not reach sterilizing concentration. To assure that folds do not exist in the half-suits, which would prevent sterilizing, we use "dummys" to lift the half-suits and extend the sleeves. We have placed BIs in a variety of areas around the half-suits, and with them properly extended we have observed destruction of all BIs.

OTHER VALIDATION ISSUES

Space does not allow a detailed description of other key elements of the validation program for sterility testing isolator systems. However, we do want to emphasize two points which must be considered.

1. *Container integrity.* It is essential that the user demonstrate that VHP does not penetrate product containers, supplies, dilution fluids, media, environmental control plates or other sensitive items. We have found that containers with positive seals such as threaded bottles (glass or plastic) with gaskets, pharmaceutical vials, and other sterile dosage forms are not penetrated by VHP. This has been confirmed by measurements of the head space with Dräger tubes, or the use of commercial test kits. Of course, this must be further confirmed by growth promotion and bacteriostasis/fungistasis tests if appropriate.

   We have observed the penetration of materials wrapped in thin, flexible plastics. For example, in tests performed on triple bagged petri dishes we found levels of greater than 3 ppm inside the innermost bag after greater than 10 hours of aeration at a F/V of 0.9–1. We obtained similar results when we exhausted the gas through 100 cfm exhaust ducts rather than using the VHP sterilizer in its aeration mode. In at least two cases we have observed inhibition of microbial growth. The organisms which would not grow were *B. subtilis* and *S. epidermitis.* In one study inhibition was observed in both standard trypticase soy agar, and the same media supplemented with lecithin and Tween 80.

   Wrapping the bags with aluminum foil prevents VHP penetration, but also prevents sterilization of the surface of the bags. It should be noted that these problems occurred with environmental microbiological plates only.

2. *We have found that a halo of VHP gas can be detected around the isolator systems during sterilization.* We have observed hydrogen peroxide concentrations of about 1 ppm about 10 cm from the surface of the isolator. Hydrogen peroxide is detectable one meter from the isolator at concentrations of 0.1 ppm. We did not observe higher concentrations near entry points, seals or valves. We have seen concentrations reach 3 to 5 ppm in half-suits during sterilization, and values as high as 3 ppm after aeration. This concentration is reduced by running the

half-suit blowers after completion of the sterilization cycle. We have seen the hydrogen peroxide concentration drop to undetectable levels in 30–45 minutes. As mentioned earlier, aeration times can be lengthened dramatically if porous materials are sterilized within the isolator. We suggest that the area be restricted from personnel entry during sterilization, and that careful consideration be given to the development of aeration cycles. The efficacy of aeration must be confirmed by testing, and should not be left to chance.

CONCLUSION

We believe that isolator systems are the safest and most reliable facilities for conducting sterility tests. We have found that they can be readily sterilized using VHP. The ability to sterilize large and complex enclosures such as the one we have described in this paper indicates that sterilization of isolators for production operations holds no special problems. In fact, because production isolators will be rather lightly loaded, and are likely to contain little if any porous material, validation of sterilization cycles should be straightforward.

It is critical in the validation of isolators for sterility testing that container/closure integrity is established in the validation testing program. The users of these systems must demonstrate that the sterilization of sterility testing supplies does not adversely affect media growth promotion or bacteriostasis and fungistasis test validation. It is also essential that the user prove that exposure of test articles to the sterilizing agent does not interfere with the ability of the sterility test to detect low levels of potentially contaminating organisms.

RECOMMENDED READINGS

Akers, J. E. Simplifying and improving process validation. In press.

Griego, V. Validation of vapor phase hydrogen peroxide sterilization. *Proceedings of the PDA/PMA Symposium on Sterilization in the 1990's.*

Haas, P. J., I. J. Pflug, and J. Lysfjord. 1993. Validation concerns for parenteral filling lines incorporating barrier isolation techniques and CIP/SIP systems. Proceedings of the Second International PDA-Congress, in Basel, Switzerland.

Klapes, N. A., and D. Vesley. 1990. Vapor-phase hydrogen peroxide as a surface decontaminant and sterilant. *Applied and Environmental Microbiology* 56 (2).

Rickloff, J. R., and P. A. Orelski. 1989. Resistance of various microorganisms to vaporized hydrogen peroxide in a prototype tabletop sterilizer. Proceedings of the 89th Annual Meeting of the American Society for Microbiology.

Thorogood, D. 1993. Physical and biological validation of a sterile rapid transfer system. Proceedings of the Second International PDA-Congress, in Basel, Switzerland.

Wagner, C. et al. 1988. Antifungal properties of 0.1% to 3% hydrogen peroxide in neutral buffer. Proceedings of the 88th Annual Meeting of the American Society for Microbiology.

18

Isolation Technology: A Consultant's Perspective

James Agalloco
Agalloco & Associates
Somerville, NJ

The 1990s have witnessed the emergence of isolation technology as a viable option for the production of sterile materials. Recent advances in sterilization technology and regulatory pressures for increased sterility assurance have combined to make isolation a subject of enormous interest in the parenteral industry. The opportunity to eliminate personnel from the environment in which sterile materials are handled, along with the ability to fully sterilize that environment holds enormous promise. Virtually all aspects of sterile drug manufacturing are being looked at with a view towards integrating isolation concepts with existing equipment, facilities, and processes. Only the passage of time will reveal whether the current groundswell of enthusiasm for isolation concepts will permanently change the way in which sterile products are produced.

HISTORY

To those new to the industry it might seem that isolation is a concept just recently introduced. The origins of isolation are nearly as old as sterile products technology. Recognition that personnel are the greatest single source of microbial contamination in an aseptic processing area is not new. Before the advent of high efficiency particulate air (HEPA) filters made conventional clean room technology feasible, many firms utilized glove boxes to handle sterile materials. With the perfection of HEPA filters, the ability to place high speed equipment in a clean environment seemed to be far preferable to the inherent limitations of glove box operations. Over the next 30 years, the majority of sterile drug products were produced in specially designed suites in which gowned personnel performed a wide range of tasks. Glove boxes were still in use for certain specialized tasks where either manual intervention was extensive, or the scale of production extremely small. The isolation demands of the nuclear industry and specialized applications in health care fostered continued refinement of glove box technology and resulted in several advances in the areas of component in-feed and discharge construction materials; ergonomic design; inclusion of HEPA filters; confirmation of integrity; and probably most important, sterilization technology. The design elements utilized in isolators have reached a state of maturity where they must be given serious consideration as a universal replacement for the conventional aseptic processing area (APA) which nearly rendered the isolator's ancestor, the glove box, extinct several decades ago.

DEFINITIONS

Discussion of isolators in the parenteral industry has been hampered by the use of many seemingly similar terms in an inconsistent manner. Without a common basis for understanding, it is easy to discern why there is so much confusion in the industry and regulatory agencies regarding isolation concepts. The following definitions are provided in an attempt to bring some degree of order to the subject, at least within the context of this book.

Isolate (v)—To set apart from others.

Isolator (n)—A piece of equipment which provides for complete and total separation between one environment and another.

Bar (v)—To obstruct or prevent passage, progress or action.

Barrier (n)—A material object which separates, demarcates, or serves as a barricade.

The distinction between an isolator and a barrier may appear subtle, yet it is significant. Isolation affords a degree of separation which is far more effective than a barrier. A parallel can be drawn to the difference between a pane of glass and a window screen. The pane of glass isolates the environments on either side, while the screen serves as a barrier to objects larger than a certain size, yet permits smaller objects to pass. Isolation is total separation of the two different environments. A barrier is an impediment between the two environments without the degree of absoluteness inherent in isolation. The two terms are not interchangeable and the distinction between them should be maintained to avoid further confusion. Their appearance in the same sentence is commonplace, and only adds to the general confusion over terminology. The parenteral industry is currently using both concepts (and sometimes both in a single installation) as replacements for conventional aseptic processing areas.

Closed System—A system which does not exchange air or contaminants with an adjacent environment, i.e., an isolator system.

Open System—A system which can exchange air or contaminants with an adjacent environment, i.e., a barrier system.

These terms provide a much clearer distinction between the different design concepts. A closed system is clearly isolated from its surroundings, while an open system has some opportunity for exchange with an adjacent environment. A closed system is opened only infrequently for maintenance or similar activities. Many open systems are closed only during sterilization and open during normal operation.

Isolation—The use of an isolator where the primary objective is to execute the process in an isolated environment free of contamination, i.e., maintaining a sterile environment through the exclusion of personnel.

Containment—The use of an isolator where the primary objective is to execute the process in a manner that prevents the discharge of contamination to the outside environment, i.e., the handling of a biohazardous material.

Isolation technology can be employed to provide a complete barrier to either the items within the isolator or to the personnel located outside. The only difference between isolators used for isolation and containment is the relative pressure difference between the interior and exterior. Isolation employs internal pressures greater than external, while containment systems employ lower internal pressures than external. Regardless of the operating mode, the ability to maintain the isolator in a closed mode during all parts of the process (sterilization, operation, and cleaning) will afford greater confidence in the performance of the system.

There are of course applications where the intent is to achieve both isolation and containment simultaneously, i.e., the preparation of an oncological injection where operator safety and product sterility are equally desirable.

ADVANTAGES

The increased interest in isolation technology in recent years is due in large part to the numerous operational advantages associated with its application (ITUG meeting 1993). Among the more commonly cited benefits resulting from its implementation include:

- Increased sterility assurance levels (SALs)
- Elimination of personnel from aseptic area
- Sterilization in lieu of sanitization
- Reduced facility costs
- Reduced operating costs

- Reduced time for facility start-up
- Containment of toxic materials
- Reduced environmental monitoring
- Elimination of gowning
- Increased labor efficiency

LIMITATIONS AND OBSTACLES

The advantages cited above might lead one to believe that the universal application of isolation technology is imminent. In reality there are still significant negatives associated with the implementation of the technology and it may be many years before the full potential for it can be realized (ITUG meeting 1993). Some of the negatives include:

- Poorly informed industry
- Lack of continuous feed and discharge for components
- Changes necessary in operational philosophy
- Chemical activity of sterilizing gases
- Existing facilities designed for conventional clean rooms
- Difficulty in removing residual sterilant
- Non-industrial appearance of isolators
- Expected FDA skepticism
- Proprietary appearance of technology
- Conflicting vendor claims

APPLICATION

Isolation technology appears adaptable to virtually any process or equipment type. While this may eventually be true, at the present time applications appear to fall into several major categories.

Sterility Testing

The renaissance in isolation appears to have started with sterility testing. The restrictive nature of the FDA stance with regard to sterility retests defined in the 1987 "Guideline on Sterile Drugs Produced by Aseptic Processing," prompted many firms to re-evaluate their sterility test capabilities. The ability to perform testing in an environment which could virtually eliminate false positives has proved almost irresistible in recent years. Sterility testing appears to be one area where the employment of isolation technology is proceeding swiftly.

Filling

The impetus driving sterility testing into isolators is certainly germane to sterile filling. In the production of injectable drugs by aseptic methods, the presence of personnel in close proximity to sterile surfaces and equipment is anathema. The implementation of isolation concepts for this purpose is under consideration or active execution at many firms. Adapting fill room equipment and developing material interfaces capable of accommodating rapid transfer of components into and out of the isolator are the key obstacles to be overcome before the use of the technology can be more widespread.

Manufacturing

The application of isolation to aseptic manufacturing offers the same advantages with regard to the elimination of human intervention with sterile materials and surfaces applicable for filling operations in isolators. The range of application for isolation in manufacturing is considerably more diverse than in other settings, i.e., sterility testing, aseptic filling. Isolation systems must be adapted to fit the equipment and process activities carried out within them. Manufacturing and compounding operations are usually able to operate with slower feed and discharge rates than filling procedures making the adoption of isolation technology less difficult. The ability of isolators to provide containment for potent or toxic materials is significant as the quantity of potent material being handled is usually substantial. This is another major impetus for the use of isolators in manufacturing. Other than in containment applications, the use of isolators in aseptic manufacturing will increase more slowly than use in aseptic filling. This is partially attributable to the added design requirements and costs associated with adaption to existing equipment.

Clinical Manufacturing

The production of clinical materials is particularly well suited to isolation systems. The low production volume necessary means that the lack of high speed material transfer capability for isolator filling systems is of little consequence. The ability to contain potent materials makes isolation a real advantage when the product being processed is not well characterized.

Manual Procedures

The promise of isolation technology to enhance sterility assurance for aseptic procedures is most evident with predominantly manual processes. It is virtually impossible to argue that a manual procedure carried out in a conventional clean room with gowned personnel is not markedly improved when the process is carried out in an isolator. As a general rule, the more invasive or manipulative the aseptic process the stronger the motivation should be to locate the process in an isolator where the potential for human borne contamination is minimal.

STERILIZATION

Many advantages associated with isolation technology are attributable to the increased sterility assurance provided through the elimination of personnel from the working environment. That elimination would not be exceptional if that environment could not be sterilized. The ability to sterilize the interior of isolators makes the attainment of increased SALs for aseptic processing in isolators a reality. If the interior could only be sanitized, the current enthusiasm for isolation technology would be severely diminished.

Commercially available sterilization modes use either vapor phase hydrogen peroxide or aerosolized solutions of peracetic acid. Under active development is a system which employs hydrogen peroxide and atmospheric steam simultaneously. The use of other gases and gas/steam combinations seems likely given the commercial promise of isolators and what seems to be an equally promising market for sterilization systems fitted to them. The demand for additional sterilization methods is driven by a desire to find a "magic bullet" which will sterilize rapidly, be compatible with a wide range of materials, and degrade into non-toxic components more effectively than the current sterilization methods.

REGULATORY PERSPECTIVES

No discussion of isolation technology would be complete without some consideration of the regulatory view with regard to their application. At the publishing of this book, there is still some controversy regarding regulatory expectations with this technology. The obvious advantages of isolators appear to be held hostage to some eagerly anticipated regulatory clearance. This paralysis appears to be an outgrowth of the confusion between barriers and isolators. When discussion of "barrier technology" was first mentioned in Europe, representatives of the UK Medicines Control Agency (MCA) were asked to comment on the type of environment in which a barrier system should be installed. As the installations in question excluded personnel, they were barrier systems, yet because they exchanged air with the surrounding environment, they were not true isolators. The MCA quite properly indicated that such barrier systems should be installed in controlled environments with classified air, microbial monitoring, and gowned personnel. The distinction between barrier systems and isolator systems is only recently emerging. Many individuals on both sides of the Atlantic continue to use the two terms interchangeably (and unfortunately incorrectly). Because the MCA has taken a clear stance on the definition of a barrier system, there are seemingly similar expectations with regard to the definition of an isolator system. The U.S. Food and Drug Administration (FDA) has been reticent to take a definitive stance, perhaps fearing that the industry as a whole cannot yet distinguish between a barrier and an isolator. The result is a general reluctance on the part of many in the industry to utilize isolation technology for any process other than sterility testing. Many of the operational advantages of isolation technology will be lost if there is a regulatory requirement to install these systems in a classified environment. The industry is playing a waiting game. Until a real distinction is made between barrier technology and isolation technology, the implementation of either technology will proceed slowly. A clear regulatory position by either the MCA or FDA would speed the adoption of these clearly superior technologies.

OTHER SUBJECTS

Retrofitting Isolation Technology to Existing Facilities

One of the issues which firms desiring to utilize isolation technology in their operations must overcome is the adaption of existing facilities and equipment to the isolation concept. A facility in which gowned personnel perform a range of activities in a controlled environment to produce sterile materials represents a sizeable investment. Modification of the facility and equipment to accommodate isolation techniques is a further expenditure whose return on investment is not at all clear cut. In a facility which employs conventional aseptic practices, the conversion to isolation technology imposes additional costs with only modest financial benefits. The real economic advantages with isolation technology accrue when the majority of the facility construction costs associated with conventional clean room design can be avoided. The savings in operational cost alone may be insufficient to justify the incremental expense in the addition of isolation concepts. It appears that the industry will continue to use its existing clean rooms for some time to come and that isolation concepts will be adopted only where the contamination control issues are so critical that a retrofit, regardless of expense, is justifiable. Applications most likely to be converted over are those with a high degree of personnel interaction with sterile materials, e.g., sterile bulk drug production, roller bottle processes, and other manual processes. Another driver in the retrofit of facilities will be applications where a toxic material is processed.

Environmental Monitoring

Isolation technology provides a marked increase in the microbial quality of the enclosed environment. The enclosure is not only sterilized using a validatable procedure, it operates in the absence of personnel. Proper maintenance of the system focuses on the transfer ports, gloves, half-suits, and HEPA filters. This focus assures that the interior remains sterile over long periods. There have been reports of isolators utilized for sterility testing which have been microbially monitored on a regular basis for over 5 years, and the firm has yet to isolate a viable organism from the interior. In light of such results, the identification of a single viable organism inside an isolator should be cause for immediate concern. Despite the impressive viable profiles evidenced to date in isolator installations, there is no justification for not monitoring the environment. An isolation system, however sound conceptually, is subject to contamination as a result of the failure of a part of the physical system or through the inability of a sterilization process to access a contaminant on an item introduced into the system. Any sterilization system is subject to compromise if an organism is located in a area inaccessible to the sterilizing medium. Vapor phase hydrogen peroxide or peracetic acid are not exempt from this limitation, and an investigation into the sterilization procedures should be a part of the investigation into the isolation of an environmental contaminant.

Process Validation

Whether an isolator is utilized for containment or aseptic processing, the underlying pharmaceutical (or biopharmaceutical) process must still be validated. Issues with regard to potency, uniformity, efficacy and purity must still be established. The presence of an isolator changes the validation of these processes only minimally if at all.

Pharmaceutical Process

The process itself will likely have only minimal changes as a result of its operation in an isolator. The most significant concerns are those associated with the effect of residual sterilizing agent on product contact surfaces which could carry over into the final material. Care must be taken in the selection of materials, components and containers exposed to the sterilizing agent to minimize uptake of the gas. Proper aeration of the enclosure before materials are exposed to the environment must also be provided. Aside from these considerations, validation of the procedures carried out inside the isolator should be accomplished in a manner identical to that where the isolator is not present.

Aseptic Processing

Where the isolator is utilized in an aseptic process, that procedure should be validated in accordance with industry norms. For aseptic filling, this entails the performance of a series of media fill trials. The approaches and methods utilized will mimic those employed in ordinary clean rooms and have been well defined in the literature. The only unique aspect associated with the use of the isolator should be in the acceptance criteria utilized for media fill contamination. It is this author's opinion (shared by several of my colleagues) that a media fill performed in an isolator is acceptable only if no contamination is detected in any of the filled units.

Cleaning Procedures

The execution of a pharmaceutical process within the confines of an isolator presents some unique cleaning issues not present in conventional clean rooms. The proximity of the isolator walls and ceiling may result in product residue on those surfaces which might not reach their more distant counterparts in a conventional room. Many isolators do not utilize laminar flow during their operation. While laminar flow is not necessary in the majority of isolators to maintain asepsis, its absence means that deposition of product residuals is possible anywhere within the isolator. If an isolator is maintained in a closed state at all times, then cleaning must be performed via the gloves and half-suits. These items must have sufficient reach for the accomplishment of the process but may not be adequate to allow access to all of the internal surfaces for cleaning purposes.

CONCLUSION

Isolation technology holds enormous promise in the preparation of sterile materials. Fulfillment of that promise will be the objective of those who design, construct, install, operate, and maintain these systems in the next several years. Successful implementation of isolation concepts in a range of applications should lead to additional installations. The installed base of isolators is not large enough to predict with confidence that isolation will become the technology of choice for sterile production activities. In the opinion of many who have been exposed to the technology, it has so many advantages that its eventual replacement of ordinary clean rooms is nearly certain. While the conventional aseptic processing area is certainly not extinct, isolation technology appears to have made it an endangered species.

REFERENCES

Presentation at the ITUG Meeting, 1 December, 1993, in Raleigh, NC.

FDA. 1987. Guideline on sterile drug products produced by aseptic processing. *Federal Register* 181–332:60360.

19

Isolation Technology Issues from an Engineering Company Viewpoint

Dimitri P. Wirchansky
Fluor Daniel, Inc.
Marlton, NJ

Today, many companies are investigating isolation technology for use in a variety of applications. As the technology is investigated for each application, many common questions arise. The following presents several common questions and answers.

Question: From an engineering company perspective, where do you see the technology going?

Answer: When we first started to get inquiries about isolation technology, it was almost always for applications involving the production of cytotoxic materials or for sterility testing. Many isolators used in the United States are involved in sterility testing. Isolation technology has been applied very successfully in sterility testing as a way of reducing false positives to levels approaching zero. Isolators have also been used to protect people from toxic drugs.

The next phase of interest in isolation technology involved packaging sterile products for product development batches. Where highly potent or cytotoxic materials were involved, compounding and filtration were also included within their own isolation systems. Much of this work was small scale production. During this phase, the application of isolation technology involved fitting various machines with isolation systems. Monoblock type machines with a clean tabletop and a minimum of mechanical equipment above the table were used. In some cases minor modifications were made to accommodate functioning within the isolation system. Ideally, the machine would have weight adjustments outside the isolation enclosure and penetrations to the enclosure would be sealed. Some machines were more suitable for use with isolation systems than others. In some cases, the entire machine would be placed within the isolator.

The use of isolator systems has also brought improvement in the sterilization of the controlled aseptic space. Because the small aseptic spaces could be closed and sealed, fumigation with formaldehyde or peracetic acid could provide a higher level of environmental cleanliness than possible in a conventional sterile suite. Most recently, sterilization of these aseptic spaces can be accomplished using hydrogen peroxide. One equipment manufacturer has even introduced a cart mounted system to implement and control the sterilization of small closed systems using hydrogen peroxide.

Recent developments in filling equipment for production of sterile products involve the design of equipment specifically for use with isolator systems. Output rates for the new equipment range from small scale production to high output lines. These machines are longer and narrower to allow for easier access to the various parts of the machine through glove ports. All unnecessary mechanical equipment has been relocated outside of the clean zone. Adjustment to fill weights (or volumes) is accomplished from outside the clean space. In many cases the fill check function has been automated to minimize human intervention in the clean space. Because many of the mechanical functions have been relocated outside the clean space, much of the maintenance can be performed without intruding on the isolator contained part of the machine. A person planning the installation of a filling line today can choose from an increasing number of machines specifically designed for use with isolation systems.

Question: What has our experience shown?

Answer: It is important for users to think through their application to define what they wish to accomplish with isolation technology. This allows for design decisions that provide the right amount of safety, without increasing costs unnecessarily. Planning the integration of an isolation system with the rest of the line or production train is critical to providing a smoothly working system. Interface points between the critical space and the environment are potential sources of problems. The mechanism for transferring material between the critical and non critical space must receive careful attention, since these transfers may introduce contamination. In many cases, the better approach is to contain the material within the process equipment; this is particularly true for aseptic bulk and solid dosage form manufacturing.

Consider how the isolation units will be used from a process and ergonomic standpoint. If the design makes it difficult for operators to do their work, problems will surface in validation or later when it is usually more expensive to correct them. User buy-in is critical to the acceptance and successful operation of isolation systems.

Consider what procedures will be used in the set up mode, the operational mode, the maintenance mode, and the upset condition mode. This will determine how safety features and alarms will be configured. Preplanning maintenance procedures will lead to ways to safely return the unit to service. Advance planning for upset conditions will help determine the scope of the validation effort and minimize risk to product.

Question: **What area do you see as receiving the most attention?**

Answer: Transfer technology. Many people use alpha/beta ports to introduce and remove materials from the isolator. Some people have reported results that indicate the possibility of contamination in the ring area where the port seals to the isolator and the two lids lock together.

Suggestions for overcoming this problem range from placing a sterilized insert over the ring area and wiping the ring area with germicide to protecting the sealing surfaces in the ring area with ultraviolet light. One equipment vendor is working on the development of an alpha/beta connector with a heating element in the ring area. The heating element would allow dry heat sterilization of this area (with about a ten minute cycle time) prior to opening the alpha/beta connector. This is an area of considerable importance for users, and considerable effort is being spent by both suppliers and users to find a solution to this problem.

A related area is the continuous transfer of components in and out of the isolator that would occur during an aseptic fill process. Many applications transfer sterilized, depyrogenated containers from the cooling zone of a tunnel into the isolator. In this case, the pressure balance of the system is important to safeguard the integrity of the isolator and avoid pressure and temperature excursions in the tunnel. On the discharge side, the filled and closed product is transferred out of the isolator for sealing. In this case it is necessary to take precautions to avoid backflows of air into the isolator, since the quality of the area outside the isolator is substantially less than inside. Pressure differential alone is not sufficient to prevent backflow into the isolator, since eddy currents may exist. Some applications use a small tunnel around the discharge of the isolator with reduced opening size, just sufficient for the product to pass out. Some applications may use an intermediate isolator for capping before passing the product to the external environment.

Question: From an engineering perspective, what are some of the issues that still need to be addressed?

Answer: On-line leak detection. This is particularly critical for containment of toxic or superpotent materials.

Guidelines for classifying the room that the isolator is placed in need to be developed. This may also depend on how the isolator will be used and the claims being made for the process. Having to put an isolator in a Class 10,000 aseptic area removes many of the cost and operational advantages that provide the incentive to use this technology.

The development of CIP systems specifically designed for use with isolation systems where multiple products are produced is needed. It would also be useful to see the development of hydrogen peroxide sterilization for larger spaces.

The application of isolation technology to pharmaceutical manufacturing is growing rapidly. As people gain experience with the systems and identify trouble spots, solutions will be attempted and the technology will move forward. Careful planning when selecting the system and application will minimize difficulties as the systems are validated and put into use. It is an exciting time to be working in the pharmaceutical industry and participating in the technological advances.

Section IV
Resources

Glossary

Absolute Barrier—**1.** An isolator (barrier) system which completely eliminates the possibility of external contamination reaching the interior of the isolator. The term *absolute* conveys perfect air filtration and infallible physical integrity. An absolute barrier, assuming it could be sterilized to a very high sterility assurance level (SAL), would be a perfect germ-free environment. As of the publication of this book these systems do not actually exist. However, absolute barriers represent the holy grail of aseptic pharmaceutical production, and there can be little doubt that in the near future they will be a reality. **2.** Obsolete term sometimes used to describe currently available isolators.

Active Isolator—An isolator employing managed airflow or air pressure as one of the elements of barrier technology used.

Aerosol—A dispersion of very small particles and/or droplets in the air. Aerosols can carry microbial contamination.

Air Lock—An enclosed space with two or more doors located between the controlled work space and the outside environment.

The purpose of the air lock is to control the airflow between the two areas to protect the controlled area during the transfer of material from one area to another. Air locks are usually present in clean rooms. Air lock-like spaces can be used in isolation facilities in the production environment to connect "mouse hole"-type openings to the outside environment.

At Rest—Describes an isolator that is fully functioning *without* process operational, and *without* process interface or material transfer.

Background Environment—The environment outside the isolator. Usually a controlled environment where the isolator is located. The background environment does not need to be classified as to the Std. 209 classification.

Bar—To obstruct or prevent passage, progress or action.

Barrier—**1.** In the context of aseptic processing systems, a barrier is a device which prevents contact between operators and the aseptic field enclosed within the barrier. These systems are used in hospital pharmacies, laboratories, and animal care facilities as well as in aseptic filling. Barriers may not be sterilized and do not have sterile transfer systems that allow passage of materials into or out of the system without a loss of sterility. Some pharmaceutical filling and bottling equipment is equipped with shrouds or covers that are in fact barriers. Some of these shrouds are equipped with HEPA-filtered air supply systems. Blow/fill/seal systems for example are equipped with barriers of this type. **2.** A material object which separates, demarcates, or serves as a barricade. Any physical obstacle to contamination. In pharmaceutical processing, any protection apparatus, including curtains in the clean room, goggles, gloves, face masks, biosafety cabinets, etc. are examples of barriers. An isolator is a barrier, but a barrier isn't necessarily an isolator. **3.** An impediment between two different environments that does not have the degree of absoluteness inherent in isolation. **4.** A system that prevents but does not completely exclude the possibility of human borne contamination entering the area of the critical zone.

Barrier Isolator—**1.** Same as isolator. **2.** A mini-clean room that encloses a process and excludes humans. **3.** An isolator is a type of protective barrier, but a barrier is not necessarily an isolator.

Barrier Technology—Specific techniques employed to provide an element of an isolator with a defined degree of containment. (*Note:* may range from absolute segregation to a percentage segregation of a defined challenge to the barrier)

Breach Velocity—The airflow rate through an aperture sufficient to prevent movement of airborne particles in the opposite direction to the airflow. For the purposes of this definition, the aperture should be considered as a glove port or similar size opening.

Buffer Isolator—An isolator connected in series to one or more other isolators. This isolator may enclose one or more processing operations, but its major function is to isolate a containment barrier, thereby enabling the entire system to function as a true isolator. This is accomplished by operating the buffer isolator at a positive air pressure relative to the containment barrier, thereby effectively isolating the work space. If the buffer isolator is an open isolator it must rely on the fail-safe maintenance of internal over pressure relative to the surrounding environment to maintain isolation conditions. (The buffer isolator is also called a dynamic airlock.)

Canopy—Canopy usually refers to the flexible plastic bubble surrounding the work area in an isolator environment. It's the plastic wall, ceiling, and floor unit of the flexible isolator. It's generally the main body of the isolator attached to the rigid framework.

Chemical Decontamination—That part of decontamination which reduces chemical contamination to a defined acceptance level.

Clean Air Device—A clean bench, clean work station, downflow module, or other equipment designed to control air cleanness (particle count) in a localized working area. It incorporates at a minimum a HEPA filter and a fan. Isolators have also been referred to as a Clean Air Device.

Clean Room—A room designed to maintain a defined level of cleanness under operating conditions. Inlet air is cleaned by

HEPA filters. Also referred to as conventional facility or conventional clean room. The term *clean room* is often used to describe the Class 100 area defined in Federal Standard 209b.

Closed Isolator—**1.** An isolator that is, as much as current technology allows, a fully sealed system. The closed isolator has either a HEPA or ULPA filter on both supply and exhaust air. All passages of materials into or out of the isolator are made through special transfer doors which maintain isolation. The interior of these isolators and all contents are sterilizable to a SAL of at least 10^{-6}. Closed isolators are capable of providing both isolation of the work space from external contamination, and containment of dangerous materials within the work space. **2.** Closed isolators comply with the four basic characteristics of the isolator classification and are leaktight. They do not rely on overpressure to maintain sterility or containment. Environment is sterilizable.

Closed System—A system which does not exchange air or contaminants with an adjacent environment, i.e., an isolator system.

Contained Space (Contained Volume)—A building, a building space, room, cell glove box, or other enclosed volume in which air supply and exhaust are controlled.

Containment—**1.** Achieved by completely separating the work area from the outside environment to protect the people and the environment from potent substances. The level of containment usually needs to comply with available guidelines that define the safety level of exposure that ensures a safe workplace for the operator and the environment. **2.** The use of an isolator where the primary objective is to execute the process in a manner that prevents the discharge of contamination to the outside environment, i.e., the handling of a biohazardous material.

Containment Barriers—These systems are not completely closed, but rather rely on the maintenance of a negative air pressure to the surrounding environment to provide containment. These barriers have one or more openings to the outside environment through which transfer systems (i.e., conveyors) pass. These systems may have sealable gates or doors which allow sterilization, but these doors are open during operation. Because these units take in air from the surrounding environment, they cannot be considered isolators. It is unlikely that systems of this type will be widely used since design alternatives exist that make isolation and containment attainable within the same unit (see Containment System).

Containment System—A containment system is designed and operated in a manner which prevents dangerous materials from being dispersed into the surrounding environment. Containment systems may be closed isolators in which both isolation and containment are possible simultaneously. Containment systems may alternatively be barrier systems which have one or more openings to the external environment for the passage of conveyor belts or other transfer devices. Containment systems may be considered isolators only if, through the use of buffer isolators or another design feature, they completely isolate the work space from the surrounding environment. Paramount is the requirement that air exchanges with the surrounding environment be accomplished only through HEPA, ULPA, or other microbial retentive filtration systems.

Contamination—Unwanted material in the air, in process fluids or on surfaces. For the purpose of this book, contamination can be microbial or particulate.

Controlled Work Space—A work space to which access is restricted.

Critical Work Area—The area immediately surrounding the critical (sterile or contained) process area. For example, in the clean room this is the Class 100 area where the filling process takes place. In the isolator it is the area inside the isolator, which has shrunk to a more manageable size.

Decontamination—1. The removal of unwanted substances from personnel, rooms, surfaces, equipment, etc. The process used to reduce contamination to a defined acceptable level. It diminishes the bioburden or particulate levels. For example, in isolation technology, this process can be used to reduce bioburden before sterilization or reduce the particulate levels to a predefined acceptable level. **2.** A process which reduces contaminating substances to a defined acceptance level. 3. A process that renders an object safe to handle.

Disinfection—A process that eliminates virtually all recognized pathogens on inanimate objects, but not necessarily bacterial spores.

Docking Device—A contained chamber that can be connected to an isolator to transfer materials in and out without breaking the integrity of the sterile or contained enclosure.

Docking Transfer Device—An item of barrier technology purposely designed to effect connection of one isolator or container to another without allowing external contamination to enter or internal contamination to escape.

Doors (Air Locks)—At least four different types of doors can be used with isolator systems:

1. **Rapid Transfer Door or Port**—These doors (sometimes called RTPs) enable the operator to link two isolators, an isolator and a container, or an isolator to a piece of equipment. The RTP doors consist of two flanges which can be linked together in a manner that allows the nonsterile surfaces of the flange faces to be positively locked together. A sealing gasket is compressed between the two flanges resulting in an airtight seal. Several design variants of this system are presently available commercially. (A narrow ring typically exists at the apex of the seal that is not sterilized; this ring has been suggested by some as a potential source of contamination.)

2. **Sterilizable Rapid Transfer Ports**—Several different types of these systems have been studied. The objective of these transfer doors is to eliminate the potentially contaminated ring described in number 1.

3. **Ultraviolet Light Equipped Transfer Tunnel**—These units use ultraviolet light (UV) to kill microorganisms on the manufacturing system.

4. **Conventional Doors**—These doors, also referred to as *jam-pot* doors, have no provisions for preventing the

introduction of outside air into the enclosure. Doors of this type preclude the maintenance of an enclosure at a condition of high sterility assurance. Enclosures that utilize this type of door during normal operation are not isolators. At the very best these units are barriers.

DOP Aerosol—A dispersion of dioctyl phthalate (DOP) droplets in air. The DOP test is used with alternative methods to test for the integrity of ULPA and HEPA filters in the isolator.

Double Filtration—An arrangement of two filters in series with the second filter providing backup protection against leakage or failure of the first filter. Most if not all isolation systems are built with a pre-filter and HEPA filter. Some use double HEPA filters for extra protection.

D.P.T.E.—Acronym for *Double Porte de Transfert Etanche.* D.P.T.E. was the first rapid transfer port patented to be used in isolators and it was first used in the nuclear industry to contain the transfer of potent materials.

Enclosure—The isolator sterile work space. Also referred to as Isolator enclosure. All isolators are enclosures, but not necessarily vice versa.

Equipment Barrier—An enclosed processing area, such as a clean room, laminar airflow workbench, or other protective equipment that can be decontaminated to help prevent contamination, but are not built to prevent external contamination from entering the work area.

Flexible Isolator System—An isolator system having flexible components (for example, gloves, flexible isolators, half-suits, and similar systems).

Full-suit (with D.P.T.E.)—Allows the operator to penetrate the work area within the isolator, without exposing the process or the product to human-borne contamination. Full-suits add flexibility to the operator's interaction with the process while keeping the operator isolated from the sterile environment. Full-suits are not very common but are a feasible alternative when the process requires the handling of heavy equipment or other physically demanding tasks.

Glove—A device that allows the arms and hands of an operator to enter the enclosed volume of an isolator whilst maintaining an effective barrier.

Glove Box—A sealed enclosure in which all handling of items inside the box is carried out through long rubber or neoprene gloves sealed to ports in the walls of the enclosure. Glove boxes differ from isolators in the design. They do not have specialized rapid transfer ports and cannot be maintained sterile during transfer of materials in and out.

Half-suit—1. A device that enables the head and trunk of an operator to enter the working volume of an isolator whilst maintaining an effective barrier. **2.** A flexible partial-body suit that allows an operator to conduct manipulations within the isolator or barrier. These suits typically mount at approximately waist level, and the operator enters from beneath the table to which the suit is mounted. In essence, these suits comprise a portion of the isolator wall. Half-suits have their own air supply system, and incoming air is HEPA filtered. **3.** Also called half-body suits. They allow half of the body of an operator to be physically inside the controlled and isolated environment, facilitating reaching and access of a broad area within the isolator.

HEPA Filters—High efficiency particulate air filter. These are filters used to filter the air that enters and exits the isolator. Particle level profile: 99.998 percent efficient for particle size 0.3 μm and larger.

Interface Isolator—An isolator typically attached via a bioseal or plenum to a piece of equipment such as an autoclave, lyophilizer, or dry heat oven. The interface isolator and bioseal/plenum must be sterilizable as a unit. The door and associated hardware to which the interface isolator is linked must also be sterilized to a satisfactory SAL. This must include any and all parts of the system that could be exposed to the isolated (sterile) work area during normal operations.

Isolate—To set apart from others.

Isolation—1. Is achieved by completely separating the work area from the outside environment to protect the product, the operator, and/or the environment. Isolation can be used to maintain sterility or containment. Sterility is not a necessary component of containment. **2.** The use of an isolator where the primary objective is to execute the process in an isolated environment free of contamination, i.e., maintaining a sterile environment through the exclusion of personnel. **3.** Total separation of two different environments.

Isolator—**1.** Any unit that is sterilizable to a high SAL (typically 10^{-6} or less). All air that enters the isolator passes through microbial retentive filters. An isolator must never exchange air with the surrounding environment unless that air is treated by a microbial retentive filter. The surrounding environment must have no impact on the operation of the system for an enclosure to be considered a true isolator. Isolators must also prevent any direct contact between human operators and the product being manufactured or tested. Any manipulation done by operators must be conducted using gloves or partial suit assemblies. **2.** A barrier system that exchanges air with the outside environment only through HEPA or equivalent filters, completely separates process from the operator or the environment, contains specialized transfer devices, and can be sterilized to a high degree of sterility assurance. Isolators can be subdivided into Opened and Closed Isolators. **3.** A device employing barrier technology to achieve a defined degree of segregation of an internal environment from a surrounding or adjacent external environment. **4.** A piece of equipment which provides for complete and total separation between one environment and another.

Isolator System—A system with a positive barrier between the sterile area and the nonsterile surrounding area.

Laminar Airflow—Airflow in which the whole body of air moves with uniform velocity in parallel flow lines. Laminar airflow is hard to achieve in an isolator environment. The term unidirectional flow is preferred. In this book, the two terms should be seen as synonyms.

Laminar Flow Isolator—An isolator designed to provide unidirectional airflow to the work surface. These units may be oriented either vertically or horizontally. It is important to note that *laminar flow,* although widely used to describe airflow in the pharmaceutical industry, is technically incorrect. In actual practice laminar airflow rarely if ever exists. It is more technically correct to call these isolators unidirectional airflow isolators.

Leaktightness—The condition of a system, unit, or component where leakage is eliminated by the nature of the design. Leaktightness of an isolator is a relative term, usually defined by its leak rate (volume per unit time) at a given pressure.

Locally Controlled Environment—Terminology first used by Merck & Co. to define the type of microenvironments being developed at Merck's facilities, using isolators to create high quality environments for aseptic processing.

Media Fill—A process simulation in which microbiological growth media are used instead of the product or test samples.

Minienvironment—Sometimes used as a synonym to isolator. A minienvironment is a type of barrier that doesn't always fit the isolator category.

Nozzle—A fixed connection point in the envelope of an isolator for connecting pipes or ducts.

Opened Isolator—These isolators comply with the four basic characteristics of the isolator classification, but have "mouse holes," or small openings to help the entering and exiting of vials or others types of containers from the filling line. They generally rely on differential pressure to maintain sterility or containment. The enclosure is usually sterilizable.

Open Isolator—An isolator that has one or more openings to the surrounding environment such as holes for conveyor systems to pass through. These isolators must have a positive air over pressurization system that prevents any unfiltered air from entering the enclosure.

Open System—A system which can exchange air or contaminants with an adjacent environment (i.e., a barrier system).

Operating Pressure—The desired pressure corresponding to any single condition of operation. Isolators can be classified into negative and positive pressure isolators depending on the operating pressure required during their operation. Opened isolators depend on overpressure to maintain the sterility of the enclosure.

Operational—Describes an isolator that is fully functioning with a defined process operation, operator interfacing, and material transfer.

Overpressure—Pressure in excess of the design or operating pressure.

Particulate Decontamination—That part of decontamination which reduces visible and sub-visible particle levels to a defined acceptance level.

Passive/As Built—Describes an isolator that is physically complete, but without operation of any air treatment system.

Passive Isolator—An isolator employing only physical barrier elements of barrier technology.

Personal Protective Barrier—Goggles, gloves, face shields, and face masks can be defined as partial barriers. Partial barriers offer minimum protection against contamination.

Prefilter—A filter unit installed ahead of another filter unit to protect the second filter. The prefilter usually has a lower efficiency for the finest particles in order to remove the coarsest particles.

Rigid Barrier Isolator System—A barrier isolator system having rigid walls to maintain overpressures for an integrity control system.

Roughing Filter—A prefilter with high efficiency for large particles and fibers but low efficiency for small particles. They are usually of the panel type.

RTPs (Rapid Transfer Ports)—The American term used to describe the specialized transfer ports that allow for the transfer of materials in and out of isolators without breaking the integrity of the inside work area. Synonym with D.P.T.E.

RTS (Rapid Transfer Systems)—Synonym with RTPs.

Sanitization—**1.** That part of decontamination which reduces viable microorganisms to a defined acceptance level. **2.** The act of applying a sanitizer to effectively maintain the microbial control of an area or specific material. 3. A process that renders an object safe to handle by reducing viable contamination to a defined acceptance level.

Sterile—The condition of being free of viable microorganisms.

Sterility Assurance Level (SAL)—The probability that a sterilized product may contain viable microorganisms that may have survived the process of sterilization. For aseptic processing the accepted SAL is 10^{-3} and for terminal sterilization the expected SAL is 10^{-6} or better.

Sterility Confidence Level (SCL)—A verifiable contamination rate.

Sterilization—1. The process applied to a specified field which inactivates viable microorganisms, thereby transforming the nonsterile field into a sterile one. 2. The method used to render a surface, environment, or material completely free of microbial contamination. No microbial growth should be detectable in a sterile isolator. Sterilization applies agents that destroy or eliminate all forms of microbial life in the inanimate environment. 3. A physical or chemical process capable of destroying all microbial life, including bacterial spores.

Sterilization Isolator—An isolator used to sterilize production materials using a gas sterilization method. The sterilization isolator is typically part of a manufacturing system consisting of one or more other isolators. These isolators may function in either a continuous or semicontinuous manner.

Transfer Chamber—A chamber, usually with entry and exit doors, used to facilitate the transfer of materials into or out of an isolator while minimizing the transfer of contaminants.

Transfer Container—A container, commonly steam sterilizable, equipped with an RTP to allow sterilized goods to be transferred into an isolator. These containers are generally small enough to allow hand carrying and attachment.

Transfer Isolator—1. A system that can be used to transfer sterile goods from one isolator to another. The transfer is generally effected using an RTP or some variation of a port transfer system. 2. A specific example of an active or passive isolator used to transfer materials to and from another fixed or static isolator.

Transfer Units—Synonym with Transfer Isolators. They are isolators that can be fixed or mobile, being used to attach to other operational units to act as a transfer device to move materials in and out of isolators.

Transport Container—A specific example of a small passive isolator used to transport materials to and from an isolator. (*Note:* may be flexible or rigid and will be designed to interface with a docking transfer device)

Turbulent Flow—Flow of air that is nonlaminar or not unidirectional. This type of airflow is used in sterility testing isolators and other applications that do not require unidirectional or laminar airflow.

Turbulent Flow Isolator—An isolator with a mixing airflow rather than unidirectional or *laminar* airflow. Isolators of this design can be useful for a variety of applications including sterility testing and some pharmaceutical production activities.

ULPA Filters—Ultra low particulate air filters. ULPA filters have also been used in isolators. Most users to not find it necessary to use ULPA filters in isolators, but they can be used in certain applications to enhance the filtration/ventilation system. Particle level profile: 99.9999 percent efficient for particle size 0.3 μm and larger.

Appendix

List of Resources

BARRIER/ISOLATOR MANUFACTURERS

AEA Technology (Commercial Div. of the UK Atomic Energy Authority)
Chadwick House
Risley, Warrington
Cheshire WA36AT, United Kingdom
Phone: (0)1925-252158
FAX: 0925-252089

The Baker Company
Custom Products Division
P.O. Drawer E
Sanford, ME 04073
Phone: (207) 324-8773
FAX: (207) 324-2632

B.O.C. Edwards Calumatic

Netherlands
Steenstratt 7
P.O. Box 111
NL-5100 AL
Dongen
The Netherlands
Phone: 31 1623 13454
FAX: 31 1623 12552

United States
2175 Military Rd.
Tonawanda, NY 14150
Phone: (716) 695-6354
FAX: (716) 695-6367

Containment Technologies Group, Inc.
10329 Vandergriff Rd.
Indianapolis, IN 46239
Phone: (317) 862-5945
FAX: (317) 862-9135

Despatch Industries Inc.
63 St. Anthony Pkwy
Minneapolis, MN 55418
Phone: (612) 781-5363
FAX: (612) 781-5353

Envair Ltd.
York Avenue
Maslingden, Lancashire,
 England BR4 4HX
Phone: (0)1706 228416
FAX: (0706) 831957

Flanders Filters Inc.
531 Flanders Filters Rd.
Washington, NC 27889
Phone: (919) 946-8081
FAX: (919) 946-3425

Isolation Technologies
3231 South Platte River Dr.
Englewood, CO 80110
Phone: (303) 762-8282;
 (800) 886-1878
FAX: (303) 762-1888

ISO Tech Design
2947 Autoroute Laval Ouest
Technologies, Inc.
Laval (Québec), CANADA
 H7L 3w3
Phone: (514) 973-3520
FAX: (514) 973-2051

Kuhlman Technology
10512 NE 68 St.
Kirkland, WA 98033
Phone: (206) 822-8282
FAX: (206) 827-9055

La Calhène

France
BP184
78142 Vélizy CEDEX
Phone: (1) 46-306600
FAX: (1) 46-8730

United States
1325 Field Avenue South
Rush City, MN 55069
Phone: (612) 358-3091
FAX: (612) 358-3549

Laminar Flow, Inc.
102 Richard Rd.
Ivyland, PA 18974
Phone: (215) 672-0232
FAX: (215) 441-0426

Liberty Industries
133 Commerce St.
East Berlin, CT 06023
Phone: (800) 828-5656;
(203) 828-6361
FAX: (203) 828-8879

MDH Limited
Walworth Road
Andover, Hampshire
SP10 5AA
Phone: (01264)3621
FAX: (01264)35645

METALL + PLASTIC GmbH
D-78315 Radolfzell-
Stahringen
Bodmaner Strasse 2
Germany
Phone: (0 77 38) 92 80-0
FAX: (0 77 38) 92 80-10

Total Process Containment Ltd.
Tanshire House
Shackleford Rd.
Elstead, Surrey GU86LB, UK
Phone: +44(0)1252 703663
FAX: +44(0)1252 703684
In the U.S.: Don Stollen-
maier: (201) 540-9836

FILLING MACHINE MANUFACTURERS

Bausch & Strobel Machinenfabrik-GMBH
Bunderstrasse Postfach #20
D-74530 Iishofen, Germany
Phone: 49-7904-701218
FAX: 49-7904-701222

B.O.C. Edwards Calumatic
Netherlands

Steenstratt 7
P.O. Box 111
NL-5100 AL
Dongen
The Netherlands
Phone: 31 1623 13454
FAX: 31 1623 12552

United States

2175 Military Rd.
Tonawanda, NY 14150
Phone: (716) 695-6354
FAX: (716) 695-6367

Robert Bosch GmbH
Germany

P.O. Box 1454
D-74554 Crailsheim
Germany
Phone: 49 (0) 7951 402-453
FAX: 49 (0) 795 402-252

North America

See TL Systems Corporation

Chase-Logeman Corp.
303 Friendship Dr.
Greensboro, NC 27409
Phone: (910) 665-0754
FAX: (910) 665-0723

Filamatic—National Instrument Company, Inc.
4119-27 Fordleigh Rd.
Baltimore, MD 21215
Phone: (410) 764-0900
FAX: (410) 764-7719

Groninger and Co. GmbH
Hofäckerstrasse 9
D-7180 Crailsheim
Germany
Phone: 49 (0) 7951 495 13
FAX: 49 (0) 7951 495 38

IMA (Pharmaceutical Division)
Italy
via Emilia 428/442
40064 Ozzano Emilia
Bologna, Italy
Phone: 051-6514111
FAX: 051-6514666

United States
418 Meadow St.
Fairfield, CT 06430
Phone: (203) 331-0331
FAX: (203) 384-2555

M&O Perry Industries, Inc.
591 North Smith Ave.
Corona, CA 91720
Phone: (909) 734-9838
FAX: (909) 734-2454

Shibuya Kogyo Co. Ltd.
Chemi and Pharmatech Division
KO-58, Mameda Honmachi
Kanazawa, Japan
Phone: 762-62-1203
FAX: 762-65-6800

TL Systems Corporation —Bosch Group
8700 Wyoming Ave., N.
Minneapolis, MN 55445-1840
Phone: (612) 493-6770
FAX: (612) 493-6776

Vetter Pharma Fertigung
P.O. Box 2380
D-7980 Ravensburg
Germany
Phone: 497513700-0

VALIDATION SUPPORT AND CONSULTING SERVICES

Advanced Barrier Concepts
115 Disraeli Dr.
Cary, NC 27513
Phone: (919) 469-8876
FAX: (919) 469-4665

Advanced Aseptic Technologies
725 Morningside Drive
Lake Forest, IL 60045
Phone: (708) 234-2180
FAX: (708) 234-6685

Agalloco & Associates
216 US Hwy. 26, Suite 21
Sommerville, NJ 08876
Phone: (908) 874-7558
FAX: (908) 874-8161;
 (908) 874-8968

Akers Kennedy & Associates, Inc.
P.O. Box 22562
Kansas City, MO 64113-0562
Phone: (816) 822-7444
FAX: (816) 822-7555

Ardien Consulting Services
3330 Walnut Creek Parkway, Suite I
Raleigh, NC 27606
Phone: (919) 859-0386
FAX: (919) 859-0386

I+C Technology
29-31 Bessborough Avenue
North Strand, Dublin 3
Ireland
Phone: 353(0) 1 8363495
FAX: 353(0) 1 8366931

Kemper Masterson and Associates
375 Concord Ave.
Belmont, MA 02178
Phone: (617) 484-9920
FAX: (617) 484-9068

Performance Solutions
2410 Executive Dr.
Indianapolis, IN 46241
Phone: (317) 248-8848;
 (800) 875-8897
FAX: (317) 248-0464

R&D Scientific
272 Route 206
Flanders, NJ 07836
Phone: (201) 252-8700
FAX: (201) 927-1443

Seiberling and Associates
11415 Main St.
Roscoe, IL 61073
Phone: (815) 623-7311
FAX: (815) 623-2029

Shibuya Kogyo Co. Ltd.
Chemi and Pharmatech
 Division
KO-58, Mameda Honmachi
Kanazawa, Japan
Phone: 762-62-1203
FAX: 762-65-6800

Steril (Subsidiary of Foster Wheeler US)
Società per Azioni
via Carlo Farini 81
20159 Milano, Italy
Phone: 66891-1
FAX: 6888404

Validation Services
272 Route 206
Flanders, NJ 07836
Phone: (201) 927-1489
FAX: (201) 927-1443

Vechtech. Inc.
24543 Indoplex Circle
Farmington Hills, MI 48335
Phone: (313) 478-5820;
 (800) 966-VTEC

ENGINEERING COMPANIES AND CONSULTING SERVICES

Some of these companies also have experience with validation of isolation systems.

Advanced Barrier Concepts
115 Disraeli Dr.
Cary, NC 27513
Phone: (919) 469-4665
FAX: (919) 469-8876

John Brown Engineers and Constructors Ltd.
1 Buckingham St.
Portsmouth PO11HN
UK
Phone: (01483) 751-133
FAX: (01483) 750-598

Contain-Tech
10329 Vandergriff Rd.
Indianapolis, IN 46239
Phone: (317) 862-4552
FAX: (317) 862-9135

Fluor Daniel
301 Lippincott Center
Marlton, NJ 08053
Phone: (609) 985-6500
FAX: (609) 985-6997

Foster Wheeler
Perryville Corporate Park
Clinton, NJ 08809-4000
Phone: (908) 730-4000
FAX: (908) 730-5315

Haremead Ltd.
Tanshire House
Shackleford Road
Elstead GU86LB
Surrey
UK
Phone: 44 (0) 1252 703663
FAX: 44 (0) 1252 703684

Jacobs-Sigel-Triad
101 Centerpoint Blvd.
New Castle, DE 19720
Phone: (302) 323-1550
FAX: (302) 323-1557

The Kenny Lindquist Partnership
2301 Chestnut St.
Philadelphia, PA 19103
Phone: (215) 569-5911
FAX: (215) 569-5963

Life Sciences International
1818 Market St.
Philadelphia, PA 19103
Phone: (215) 299-8700
FAX: (215) 299-2273

Lockwood Greene
1500 International Drive
Box 491
Spartanburg, SC 29304
Phone: (803) 578-2000
FAX: (803) 599-0436

Pharmaceutical Engineering and Design Limited
Tanshire House
Shackleford Road
Elstead
Surrey GU8 6LB
UK
Phone: 44 (0) 1252 703663
FAX: 44 (0) 1252 703684

Raytheon Engineers & Constructors
30 S. 17 St.
P.O. Box 8223
Philadelphia, PA 19101-8223
Phone: (215) 422-3000
FAX: (215) 422-4034;
  (215) 422-4648

Shibuya Kogyo Co. Ltd.
Chemi and Pharmatech
  Division
KO-58, Mameda Honmachi
Kanazawa, Japan
Phone: 762-62-1203
FAX: 762-65-6800

STERILIZATION EQUIPMENT

AMSCO
1002 Lufkin Rd.
P.O. Box 747
Apex, NC 27502
Phone: (800) 444-9009
FAX: (919) 387-1817

Despatch Industries Inc.
P.O. Box 1320
Minneapolis, MN 55440
Phone: (612) 781-5363
FAX: (612) 781-5353

La Calhène
France
BP184
78142 Vélizy CEDEX
Phone: (1) 46-306600
FAX: (1) 46-8730

United States
1325 Field Avenue South
Rush City, MN 55069
Phone: (612) 358-3091
FAX: (612) 358-3549

MicroFLOW
MDH Limited
Walworth Rd.
Andover, Hampshire
SP10 5AA
UK
Phone: (01264) 362111
FAX: (01264) 356452

MANUFACTURERS OF ACCESSORY EQUIPMENT OR SERVICES

BGI Incorporated
(Dräger tubes)
58 Guinan St.
Waltham, MA 02154
Phone: (617) 891-9380
FAX: (617) 891-8151

BIOCON
(contamination control specialists, testing)
8100 Brownleigh Dr.
Raleigh, NC 27612
Phone: (919) 781-9777 ext. 14
FAX: (919) 781-9793

Biotest Diagnostics Corp.
(environmental monitoring equipment—RCS and RCS-Plus)
66 Ford Rd., Suite 131
Denville, NJ 07834
Phone: (201) 625-1300;
   (800) 522-0090
FAX: (201) 625-9454

Central Research Laboratories
(transfer devices/ports)
250 Hwy. 19
Red Wing, MN 55066
Phone: (612) 385-2142
FAX: (612) 388-1232

Appendix—List of Resources

Charcoal Service Corporation
Glove Box Division
P.O. Box 3
Bath, NC
Phone: (919) 923-2911
FAX: (919) 923-6931

Edwards/Calumatic
(lyophilizers)
Manor Royal
Crawley
West Sussex BH·102LW
UK
Phone: 44-1293-28844

Intelligent Enclosures Corp.
Norcross, GA
Phone: (404) 564-5640
FAX: (404) 564-5548

In vitro Scientific Products, Inc.
823 Hanley Industrial Ct.
St. Louis, MO 63144
Phone: (314) 963-1993

Millipore Corporation
(sterility testing equipment)
80 Ashby Rd.
Bedford, MA 01730
Phone: (617) 275-9200
FAX: (617) 275-5550

R&D Scientific
(data collection—Compliance Computer System)
31 Fairmount Avenue
P.O. Box 733
Chester, NJ 07930
Phone: (908) 879-2400
FAX: (908) 879-8009

Sartorius
Postfach 19
D-3400 Gottingen
Germany
Phone: 49-7171-82091

Serail Division SGD North America
(lyophilizers)
680 Hollow Rd.
Phoenixville, PA 19460
Phone: (215) 983-0260
FAX: (215) 983 0268

Walker Stainless Equipment Co., Inc.
625 State St.
New Lisbon, WI 53950
Phone: (608) 385-2142
FAX: (608) 562-3178

ASSOCIATIONS, INSTITUTES, AND LABORATORIES—INFORMATION RESOURCES

American Association of Pharmaceutical Scientists (AAPS)
1650 King Street
Alexandria, VA 22314-2747
Phone: (703) 548-3000
FAX: (703) 684-7349

American Society for Pharmacology
1325 Massachusetts Ave., NW
Washington, DC 20005
Phone: (301) 530-7060

European Committee for Standardization (CEN)
2 Rue Brederode, Boite 5
B-1000 Brussels, Belgium
Phone: 2-5196811

Glove Box Society
P.O. Box 9099
Santa Rosa, CA 95405-1099
Phone: (800) 530-1022

Institute for Applied Technology (IAT)/ Interpharm Press, Inc.
1358 Busch Parkway
Buffalo Grove, IL 60089
Phone: (708) 459-8480
FAX: (708) 459-6644

Institute for Environmental Sciences (IES)
940 East Northwest Highway
Mt. Prospect, IL 60056
Phone: (708) 255-1561
FAX: (708) 255-1699

International Society for Pharmaceutical Engineering (ISPE)
3816 West Linebaugh Ave., Suite 412
Tampa, FL 33624
Phone: (813) 960-2105
FAX: (813) 264-2816

Japanese Pharmaceutical Society
Kyoto University
Sakyo-ku
Kyoto, 606 Japan

Parenteral Drug Association (PDA)

7500 Old Georgetown Rd.,
   Suite 620
Bethesda, MD 20814
Phone: (301) 986-0293
FAX: (301) 986-0296

Parenteral Society

6 Frankton Gardens
Stratton St. Margaret
Swindon
Wiltshire
SN3 4LU
Phone: +44 (0) 1793 824254
Fax: +44 (0) 1793 832551

Society for Industrial Microbiology

3929 Old Lee Hwy
Suite 92A
Fairfax, VA 22030
Phone: (703) 691-3367

U.S. Pharmacopeia Convention (USP)

12601 Twinbrook Parkway
Rockville, MD 20852
Phone: (800) 227-8772

Name/Company Index

AAPS, 366
ACGIH, 167
Adams, R., 170
Advanced Aseptic
   Technologies, 361
Advanced Barrier Concepts, 13,
   361, 362
AEA Technology, 357
Agalloco, J., 8, 60, 169, 228, 277
Agalloco & Associates, 361
Akers, J. E., 8, 29, 31, 33, 60, 157,
   169, 214, 228, 277, 321
Akers Kennedy & Associates,
   Inc., 361
Alcide Corp., 151
American Association of Pharmaceutical Scientists. *See* AAPS
American Conference of
   Governmental Industrial
   Hygienists. *See* ACGIH
American Society for
   Pharmacology, 366

AMSCO International, Inc., 136,
   139, 144, 153, 156, 157, 218,
   219, 225, 316, 364
API, 68, 69, 90, 283–292
Aquitaine Pharm International.
   See API
Ardien Consulting Services, 361
Avallone, H., 49
Ayres, J. C., 280

Baker Company, The, 357
Baldry, M. G. C., 151, 169
Bausch & Strobel Machinenfabrik-
   GMBH, 359
Baxter, 90
Becton Dickinson, 295
BGI Inc., 167, 227, 364
BIOCON, 364
Biotest Diagnostics, Inc., 177, 178, 364
Block, S. S., 150, 169, 277
B.O.C. Edwards Calumatic, 357,
   359, 365

Bosch, Robert, GmbH, 32, 159, 359
Bradley, A., 277
Brandys, R. C., 169
B. Braun Medical, 106
Bristol Meyers Squibb, 107
British Standards Institute, 28, 67
Brown, John, Engineers and Constructors Ltd., 362
BSI. *See* British Standards Institute
Buck, A., 187
Burroughs Wellcome, 291, 303–306

Cabot Corp., 255
Carroll, M., 187
Casamassina, F. J., 277
CBER, 26, 65, 70
CDER, 26, 65, 69
CEN, 28, 67, 73, 83, 86, 90, 366
Center for Biological Evaluation and Research. *See* CBER
Center for Drug Evaluation and Research. *See* CDER
Center for Veterinary Medicine, 70
Central Research Laboratories, 143, 164, 257, 258, 364
Charcoal Service Corporation, 365
Chase-Logeman Corp., 360
Cilag, 90
Clintec, 106
Containment Technologies Group, Inc., 358
Contain-Tech, 362
Cooper, M. S., 194
Curran, H. R., 277
Czander, W., 117, 121

Davenport, S. M., 151, 153, 163, 164, 169, 217, 218, 228
Desjardins, C., 220, 228
Despatch Industries, 159, 271, 358, 364
Dixon, A. M., 195
Dodd, J., 172
E.I. du Pont de Nemours & Co., 255

Edwards, L. M., 15, 16, 31, 170
Eli Lilly, 107, 243

EMEA, 65
Envair Ltd., 358
Environmental Protection Agency. *See* EPA
EPA, 167, 168, 169
Escher, F. E., 280
European Committee for Standardization. *See* CEN
European Medicines Evaluation Agency. *See* EMEA
Evans, R. R., 277
Evans Medical, 68, 69, 90, 293–301

Farquharson, G., 8, 29, 277
Fasonut, 106
FDA, 35, 60–61, 64–65. *See also* CBER; CDER
  aseptic processing, 47, 195, 203, 300, 304, 307, 328, 334
  background environment, 69, 70
  containment, 55
  definitions by, 66
  enabling legislation for, 72
  filling in isolators, 26–27
  finished pharmaceuticals, 195, 283, 291–292
  industrial isolators, 66
  inspections by, 228
  isolator configuration, 68–69
  location of isolators, 33
  process validation, 202
  retesting of lots, 12, 211, 303, 304
  skepticism of, 327, 330–331
  standards recognition by, 73
  terminal sterilization, 45, 48–49, 70–71, 74, 190, 195
  USP and, 72
Federal Standard 209b, 346
Federal Standard 209D, 277
Federal Standard 209E, 91, 195, 202
Filamatic—National Instrument Company, Inc., 360
Flanders Filters Inc., 358
Fluor Daniel, 362
Food and Drug Administration. *See* FDA
Foster Wheeler, 362, 363
Frieben, W. R., 195, 277

General Electric Co., 255
Glove Box Society, 366
Goethe, J. W. von, 60
Gonzalez, J. P., 108, 122, 152, 170, 187
Griego, V., 61, 187, 318, 321
Groninger and Co. GmbH, 360
Groves, M. J., 98, 122, 228

Haas, P. J., 61, 170, 277, 278, 279, 322
Harbord, P. E., 206, 228
Haremead Ltd., 363
Hargreaves, P., 43, 61, 66, 69, 71
Hoffman, G., 277
Hoffman, R. K., 151, 171
Howmedica, 90
Hulse, J. W., 277

I+C Technology, 361
IAT, 366
IES, 366
IMA, 360
Institute for Applied Technology. *See* IAT
Institute for Environmental Sciences. *See* IES
Intelligent Enclosures Corp., 365
International Organization for Standardization. *See* ISO
International Society for Pharmaceutical Engineering. *See* ISPE
In vitro Scientific Products, Inc., 365
ISO, 75
   aseptic processing standard, 72–73, 195, 203
   cleanroom standard, 73
   pharmaceutical isolators, 28, 67
Isolation Technologies, 24, 358
Isolation Technology Users Group. *See* ITUG
ISO-TC 198, 47, 63, 72
ISO-TC 209, 73, 86, 89, 90
ISO Tech Design, 358
Isotech Designs, 14
ISPE, 49, 83, 86, 220, 366
ITUG, 26, 49

Jacobs-Sigel-Triad, 363
Japanese Pharmaceutical Society, 366
Jeng, D. K., 153, 170
Jennrich, C., 170
Johnson, R., 31
Jorkasky, J. F., 171

KabiPharmacia, 106
Kemper Masterson and Associates, 361
Kennedy, C. M., 169, 228
Killick, P. F., 278
Klapes, N. A., 61, 278, 318, 322
Knapp, J. E., 171
Kochansky, 48
Koseisho, 65
Kuhlman Technology, 358

la Calhène, 4, 15, 19, 21–22, 23, 104, 105, 110, 213, 214, 289, 358, 364
Laminar Flow, Inc., 108, 358
Larson, A. B., 279
Lauer, J., 150, 167
Leaper, S., 278
Lee, G. M., 28, 35, 61, 67, 75, 187
Levchuk, J. W., 98, 121
Leviton, A., 277
Lewis, J. S., 278
Lhoest, W., 232
Liberty Industries, 359
Life Sciences International, 363
Lindquist Partnership, The Kenny, 363
Lockwood Greene, 363
Lord, A. J., 98, 121
Loy, L. H., 278
Luna, C. J., 98, 122
Lyda, J., 29, 33
Lysfjord, J., 16, 29, 61, 170, 277, 278, 322

M&O Perry Industries, Inc., 360
Marohl, R., 164, 170
MCA, 65, 74, 90, 182, 331
   definitions by, 67–68
   environment for isolator, 330

isolator configurations, 68, 299
isolator effectiveness, 71
isolator mishaps, 66
isolator monitoring, 70
location of isolators, 69
pharmaceutical isolators, 28, 83–86
sterility failures, 43
MDA Scientific, 167
M.D.H. Limited, 221, 225, 359, 364
Meadows, C. A., 170, 279
Medicines Control Agency. See MCA
Melanhn, J. F., 278
Melgaard, H. L., 164, 170, 195, 277, 278, 279
Merck & Co., 234, 243, 281–282, 352
METALL + PLASTIC GmbH, 359
Meyer, D., 108, 122, 152, 187
Micro Diagnostics, 177
MicroFLOW, 364
Midcalf, B., 28, 35, 61, 67, 75, 187
Millett, M., 172
Millipore Corporation, 214, 215, 365
Ministry of Health and Welfare (Japan), 65
Morrissey, R. F., 169, 228
Muhvich, K., 61, 70, 71

NASA, 278
National Aeronautics and Space Administration. See NASA
National Institute of Occupational Safety and Health. See NIOSH
NIOSH, 167, 168
Northwest Regional Health Authority, 28
Norton Co., 255

Occupational Health and Safety Administration. See OSHA
Olson, W. P., 98, 122, 206, 228
Orelski, P. A., 61, 203, 279, 322
Organon, 90
OSHA, 145

Parental Drug Association. See PDA
Parenteral Society, 47, 367

PDA, 63, 64, 83, 309, 367
acceptance criteria, 49
aseptic processing, 195
industrial isolators, 66
USP and, 72
Peck, R. D., 279
Pennwalt Corp., 255
Performance Solutions, 361
Peterson, A., 279
Pflug, I. J., 61, 159, 170, 203, 277, 278, 279, 322
Pharmaceutical Engineering and Design Limited, 363
Phillips, G. B., 169
Phillips Petroleum Co., 255
PIC, 65
Pierre Fabre Laboratories, 283, 291
Porter, M. E., 159, 170
Portner, D. M., 151, 171
Probert, S. P., 277

R&D Scientific, 34, 361, 365
Raytheon Engineers & Constructors, 363
Regional Quality Control Sub-Committee of Regional Pharmaceutical Officers, 28, 203
Reyniers, J. A., 4, 35
Reynolds, L. I., 35
Rickloff, J. R., 31, 61, 155, 157, 171, 187, 203, 278, 279, 318, 322
Roussel-Uclaf, 107
Rosenblatt, A. A., 171

Sandia Laboratories, 231
Sandoz Pharm, 108, 152
Sartorius, 365
Schafer, A., 161, 171
Schaffer, S. M., 279
Seiberling and Associates, 362
Serail Division SGD North America, 365
Sheldon, B. W., 168, 172
Shibuya Kogyo Co. Ltd., 360, 362, 363
Sinclair, C. S., 277, 279
Smithkline Beecham, 232, 233

Name/Company Index

Society for Industrial
 Microbiology, 367
Steril, 362

Tallentire, A., 277
Thorogood, D., 61, 151, 171, 322
3M Co., 255
TL Systems, 243, 282, 360
Toledo, R. T., 280
Tomaselli, R. P., 277
Total Process Containment, 25,
 107, 293, 359. *See also*
 Evans Medical
TPC. *See* Total Process
 Containment
Trexler, P. C., 4, 35

UKAEA, 77
UK Pharmaceutical Isolator
 Group, 28
United Kingdom Atomic Energy
 Authority. *See* UKAEA
United States Pharmacopeia, 75,
 195, 203, 228, 367
 BIs, 157
 documents of, 27
 drug regulation by, 72
 growth promotion test, 290
 manipulation controls, 209
 sterility testing, 205–206, 207,
  303–304

Upjohn Company, 151, 153, 164,
 232, 234, 243
U.S. National Formulary, 206
USP. *See* United States
 Pharmacopeia

Validation Services, 362
Vechtech. Inc., 362
Veltek Associates, Inc., 177
Vesley, D., 61, 150, 171, 278, 322
Vetter Pharma Fertigung, 360

Wagner, C., 61, 187, 277, 322
Walker, N., 157, 159, 171
Walker Stainless Equipment Co.,
 Inc., 365
Wallace, J., 153, 172
Whistler, P. E., 168, 172
Whyte, W., 18, 36, 98, 122, 280
Wilke, B., 159, 160, 172
Wilkins, J., 157, 159, 171
Wood, R. T., 16, 71, 187, 213, 228
Woodworth, A. G., 153, 170

Yon-sen, W., 228

Subject Index

absolute barrier, 38–39, 66, 343
acceptance criteria, 38, 46, 47, 48, 49, 50, 190
acetic acid, 167, 168
active isolator, 86, 343, 354
adenovirus, 156
aerosol, 343
agar plate, 174, 176, 178, 180
air lock, 21, 40, 113, 295, 297–299, 343–344, 348
air sampler, 201
air velocity monitor, 58
Alcide (sterilant), 100
alcohol, 31, 184
alpha/beta system, 92–93, 102, 142, 194, 338–339
Andersen sampler, 175, 177
anthropometrics, 297
antiserum, 97
APA, 324, 325. *See also* aseptic manufacturing
aseptic manufacturing. *See also* isolators (isolation technology)
    control of, 3, 18

    environmental monitoring in, 55
    human contamination in, 18, 43, 46, 57
    isolators in, 26, 328–329
    sterility in, 12, 29
    validation of, 73 (*see also* validation)
aseptic processing area. *See* APA
aseptic processing isolator, 83
Aspergillus niger, 156
Aspergillus terreus, 156
atomizer, 152
at rest, 344
atrium sampler, 177, 178
ATV, 22, 24
autoclave isolator, 17, 100, 212, 214, 220, 282, 305
automatic transfer value. *See* ATV

Bacillus cereus, 156
Bacillus circulans, 151
Bacillus macerans, 156
Bacillus pumilus, 156

Subject Index

Bacillus stearothermophilus, 155, 156, 202, 221, 226, 264, 266, 268, 290, 318
Bacillus subtilis, 217, 320
Bacillus subtilis (globigii), 156, 218
Bacillus subtilis var. *niger,* 152, 153, 163–164, 217
Bacillus thuringensis, 156
background environment, 18, 68, 69, 193, 344
bacteriostasis, 320, 321
bar, 325, 344
"Barr" decision, 64
barrier, 38, 67, 284
   acceptance criteria for, 48
   decontamination of, 53
   definition of, 5–6, 39, 66, 325, 344
   examples of, 7
   key concepts of, 6
   production/manufacturing, 185–186
   terminal sterilization and, 49
   vs. isolator, 325–326, 330, 344
barrier technology, 86, 345
batch processes, 106–107
Bernoulli equation, 261–262
BI, 157, 161, 162–163, 191, 202, 221, 226, 305, 318–319
bioburden testing, 30, 33, 201, 233
biohazard hood, 209. *See also* biosafety cabinet
biological indicator. *See* BI
biosafety cabinet, 7, 44, 344
blow/fill/seal, 34, 39, 48, 49, 344
Bosch MLF 3002, 159, 161–163
bovine viral diarrhea, 156
B-propiolactone, 31
breach velocity, 87, 345
Brevibacterium acetylicum, 156
buffer isolator, 39, 40, 54, 345
bunny suit, 237

calibration, 30
Candida parapsilosis, 156
canopy, 345. *See also* flexible (film) isolator
centrifugal air sampler, 176

cephalosporin, 54
cGMP, 69, 145
challenge testing, 19, 90, 92, 93, 157, 193, 201, 206, 318–319
checkweighing, 194, 243, 246, 273
chemical decontamination. *See* decontamination
chemical indicator. *See* CI
Chemdi-VHP®, 157
chlorine dioxide, 31, 151–153, 165, 167, 168, 208, 216, 224
CI, 221, 317
CIP
   constraints of, 133
   floor drains for, 111
   mechanical interfaces and, 135
   OQ of, 200
   product sterility and, 285
   rubber/plastic and, 242
   use in barrier system, 131, 243, 247
   use in isolator system, 262–263, 340
   validation of, 239, 271
clean air device, 345
clean-in-place. *See* CIP
clean room, 74, 94, 231, 281, 293, 295, 345–346
   barriers in, 7, 344
   classification of, 37, 53, 347
   control in, 78
   costs for, 79, 132
   entry into, 295
   HEPA filtration in, 90, 346
   media fills in, 290
   monitoring in, 70
   origination of, 231
   particulates in, 97, 98, 193
   SAL for, 30
   sampling in, 57
   standards, 73, 89
   vendors and, 114
   vs. isolator, 234, 235, 236, 303, 327, 329, 331, 333
clinical manufacturing, 83, 329
closed barrier, 8, 9
closed isolator, 7, 8, 10, 21, 39, 40, 43, 346, 351

closed system, 325, 346
Clostridium sporogenes, 156
compatibility
　　material, 111, 113, 136–138, 147, 164–166
　　VHP, 108, 179
contact plate, 57
contact swab, 57, 180, 181, 201
contained space (volume), 346
containment, 66, 234, 237
　　closed isolator and, 10, 16, 39
　　cost, 234
　　definition of, 326, 346
　　hazard/toxic, 54–55, 83, 327, 328
　　high-level, 133
　　maintenance of, 16–17, 101
　　operator protection, 101–102
　　product recovery in, 102
containment barrier, 40, 346–347
containment cabinet, 80
containment device, 67
containment system, 40, 347
continuous processes, 107–108, 242
controlled work space, 67, 347
CQ Trans Plus®, 22–24
critical work area, 347
cytotoxic compounds, 4, 54–55, 79, 84, 97, 183, 284, 286, 335, 336

decontamination, 87, 150, 345, 347–348. *See also* sterilization
depyrogenation
　　in-line, 192
　　oven, 183
　　/sterilization tunnel, 110
　　tunnel, 132, 141, 142, 200, 242, 251, 285, 289
　　vial/ampoule, 100, 339
destructive sampling, 189
dioctyl phthalate, 19, 237, 349
disinfection, 150, 163, 295, 348
dispensing isolator, 82
docking device, 348. *See also* transfer isolator
docking transfer device, 87, 88, 348. *See also* transfer isolator
DOP. *See* dioctyl phthalate
DOP aerosol, 349

double-porte de transfert etanche. *See* DPTE
downstream processing, 80
DPTE, 21–22, 35, 110, 306, 349, 353
　　principles of, 22
　　specifications of, 23
　　sterile transfer through, 4, 22
Dräger tube, 167, 227, 320
dry heat sterilization, 192, 256, 257. *See also* sterilization
D-value, 136, 217, 221, 226, 264, 265, 266, 318
dynamic airlock, 39, 54, 345

Eagle 3000 SL series, 139, 158
ELA, 128, 132
electron beam radiation, 191
electronic particle counting, 37
enclosure, 349
end product testing, 79, 81, 205
engineered turbulent flow. *See* ETF; *see also* turbulent flow isolator
environmental monitoring, 45, 119, 186, 200, 211, 223, 227, 313, 327, 332
　　continuous, 48, 233, 291
　　requirements for
　　　　surrounding isolator, 51–53, 91–96, 120, 182–184
　　　　within isolator, 55–59, 69–70
equipment barrier, 349
ergonomics, 243
　　design, 131, 241, 245, 251, 298, 324, 338
　　evaluation of, 253
　　glove box, 98
　　modeling, 128, 297
　　studies in, 296–297
erythropoietin, 103
Escherichia coli, 156
establishment license application. *See* ELA
ETF, 113
ethanol, 184
EtO. *See* ethylene oxide
ethylene oxide, 31, 32, 80, 101, 183, 201

fermentation, 80
fermenter, 31
filler, design of, 240–243
filling isolator, 100, 104, 105, 110, 328
flexible (film) isolator, 80–81, 209, 237, 349
   autoclave connection to, 285
   background particulate counts in, 52
   BI locations in, 161, 162–163
   clinical manufacturing, 83
   design of, 102
   end product testing in, 79
   standards/guidelines for, 78, 90
   sterilization of, 157
   transfer and, 289
   turbulent flow, 159
   versatility of, 4
formaldehyde, 6, 31, 94, 168, 295–296, 315, 336
freeze-dryer isolator, 100
full-suit, 20, 349
fumigation, 295, 296
fungistasis, 320, 321
Fusarium oxysporum, 156

gamma irradiation, 147
gamma radiation, 101, 191
germicidal lamp, 164
glove box, 350
   barriers, 6, 9, 43
   clean room vs., 44
   disposability in, 184
   ergonomics of, 98
   limitations of, 324
   radioactive containment, 80
   research in, 77–78, 153
   RTPs and, 209, 350
glove port, 134, 208, 243, 245, 263, 297
gloves, 7, 87, 237, 333, 344, 350
   composition of, 148
   cost of, 306
   displacement effect of, 93
   faults in, 57
   heavy, 179
   in filler isolator, 100
   in flexible isolator, 349
   inspection of, 225
   in workstation isolator, 101, 102
   leaks in, 13
   manipulation via, 19–20, 52, 194, 208, 227
   monitoring of, 57–58, 120, 332
   sterilization of, 180, 181
   susceptibility of, 136, 137, 210
GMPs, 300
   European, 28, 63
   harmonization of, 55
gray-side maintenance system, 126, 131, 135, 232, 276
guided wave technology, 157

half-suit, 41, 88, 237, 333, 350
   absorption by, 137
   aeration of, 134
   blowers for, 321
   composition of, 148
   disinfection of, 184
   fragility of, 210
   HEPA filtration for, 18–19, 350
   in filler isolator, 100
   in flexible isolator, 349
   in interface isolator, 312
   inspection of, 225
   in workstation isolator, 13, 99, 101, 102
   limitations of, 210
   manipulation via, 19, 20, 194, 208, 227
   monitoring of, 57–58, 319, 332
   personnel comfort in, 211
   schematic of, 21
   sterilization of, 180, 181
HCT, 25–26
heat sink, 202
HEPA filtration, 345, 350
   as part of monitoring process, 33, 120, 198, 201, 332
   certification for, 27, 314
   double vs. single, 90
   in background environment, 18, 193
   in barrier, 6, 178, 344
   in clean room, 90, 324

in containment system, 40, 347
in half-suit, 19, 41, 350
in isolator, 7, 16, 39, 50, 103, 183, 184, 208, 237, 238, 260, 261, 285, 310, 312, 346, 351
in laminar flow system, 98
inspection of, 114
integrity of, 211, 349 (*see also* integrity)
in transfer device, 111, 174
maintenance of, 185
material selection and, 137, 227
validation of, 239
VHP and, 319
wetting in, 263
herpes simplex virus, 156
high containment port. *See* HCT
high-volume sampling, 175
hormones, 54
HVAC, 183
hydrogen peroxide. *See also* VHP
disinfection with, 100
material compatibility, 165–166, 247, 249, 254–255
sanitization with, 298–299
SIP cycle with, 13, 340
sterilization with, 125, 151, 264–270, 289–290, 329–330, 336
biodecontamination, 94
design considerations, 135–147
hazards of, 224
method comparisons, 32
microorganism elimination by, 208
product sterility and, 285
project management, 126–130
qualification of, 225–227
retrofitting vs. new equipment, 130–135
VHP®1000 (*see* VHP®1000)
vial filling and, 282
venting of, 183, 311
hypochlorites, 31

IDLH, 168
immediately dangerous to life or health. *See* IDLH
incline manometer, 223
incubation, 13, 56, 212, 223, 282, 306, 311
influenza virus, 156
infrared spectroscopy, 157
installation qualification. *See* IQ
integrity
confirmation of, 324
container, 191, 201, 305, 320
enclosure, 18, 86, 210, 271
filter, 30, 198, 200, 211, 349
glove, 33, 137, 225
half-suit, 225
isolator, 21, 90, 91–92, 99, 201, 239
maintenance of, 201
physical, 38, 314
system, 200
transfer port, 33, 85
interface isolator, 17, 41, 139, 311–312, 315, 319, 337, 350
IQ, 29, 114, 129, 199, 224–225, 314
isolate, 325, 350
isolators (isolation technology), 38, 41–42
acceptance criteria for, 48, 49
advantages of, 326–327
applications of, 79–83, 327–329
benefits of, 300–301
challenges to users/designers, 26–33
classification of, 95, 111, 135, 182, 259, 272, 289, 339
construction materials for, 17–18
costs of, 95–96, 115–118, 130, 131, 234, 326, 331
design of, 8, 11, 13, 15–16, 133–135, 243, 245, 247 (*see also* sterility testing isolator)
aeration and, 145–147
air handling, 138–139
automation, 144–145
customizing, 103–109

Subject Index 379

documentation of, 145
gas distribution, 138
interface, 139–142, 251, 255–257
internal monitoring and, 261–262
material selection, 136–138, 247, 249, 311
particulate control and, 259–261
product handling and, 257, 259
retrofit vs. new, 130–135, 331
transfer, 142–144
definition of, 7, 66, 67, 88, 237, 310, 325, 326, 344–345, 350–351
documentation for, 118–119
efficacy of, 70–71
engineering considerations for, 109–112, 335–340
environmental monitoring (*see* environmental monitoring)
equipment considerations for, 112–113
functional requirements of, 11–17
future of, 33–35, 147–148, 333–334
history of, 4, 77–78, 232–233, 304–305, 323–324
installation of, 299–300
integrity of, 21 (*see also* integrity)
key concepts of, 6
market stimulus for, 78–79
microbiological monitoring, 173–174, 186
 air, 174–180
 surface, 180–181
operational features of, 18–26
operator training for, 199–120
purpose of, 3, 121
regulatory issues for, 323, 330–331
 background environment, 69

compliance, 26–27, 120–121, 193
containment, 54–55
environmental monitoring, 51–53, 55–59, 69–70, 94–95
European GMP/Guidelines, 28
isolator siting, 109
key issues, 44–45
media fills, 71
safety, 167–169
sterility assurance, 45–48
terminal sterilization, 48–51, 70–71
standards for (*see also in name/company index for* FDA, ISO, USP)
 FDA, 73
 European, 73, 83, 86, 89–91
 ISO, 72–73, 83
 USP, 72
sterilization of, 30–31, 32 (*see also* sterility testing isolator; sterilization)
terminal sterilization and, 49–51 (*see also* terminal sterilization)
today, 64
types of (*see under different isolator names*)
validation of (*see* validation)
vendor coordination for, 113–115
weaknesses in, 71, 327
working conditions for, 89
isopropanol, 184

jam-pot, 21, 41, 92, 348

Lactobacillus casei, 156
LAF, 113, 207, 297, 300, 333, 351, 355
laminar airflow. *See* LAF; *see also* laminar flow isolator
laminar flow isolator, 42, 108, 113, 134, 135, 138, 313, 351–352
LCE. *See* locally controlled environment

leaktightness, 120, 352
lecithin, 320
limulus amebocyte assay, 37
line intervention, 46, 47
liquid impingement sampler, 176
localized control environment, 5
locally controlled environment, 66, 131, 352
lyophilizer, 20, 197

MAFS™, 248, 249, 250
Material Safety Data Sheet. See MSDS
media fill, 30, 45–46, 47, 48, 71, 182, 190, 234, 352. See also MFT
membrane filtration, 206, 214, 216, 226
MFT, 290–291
microbial retentive filter, 42
microbiological monitoring, 173–181, 201–202, 210, 223, 330
microbiological safety cabinet, 78, 80, 86, 90, 92. See also biosafety cabinet
MICROFLOW HyPer-Phase™ 31000, 221, 222
minienvironment, 5, 66, 352
mobile ancillary isolator, 100
mobile isolator, 17, 103, 355
moist heat sterilization, 71. See also sterilization
monoblock machine, 336
MSDS, 167
Mycobacterium smegmatis, 156

Nacconal, 153, 217
Navelbine, 283, 291–292
needs assessment, 127
negative pressure isolator, 101–102, 107
Norcardia lactamdurans, 156
nozzle, 88, 352

OEL, 100
open-broth tube, 174, 223
open isolator, 8, 10, 39, 42, 345, 351, 352
opened isolator, 352, 353
open-manual production, 231, 232
open system, 325
operating pressure, 352–353
operational, 353
operational qualification. See OQ
operational unit, 17
operator exposure level. See OEL
OQ, 29, 129, 200, 224, 225–226, 314
outgassing, 134, 139, 146, 165
output isolator, 101
oven isolator, 100
overkill, 191, 318
overpressure, 353

PAA. See peracetic acid
partial barrier, 5, 7, 8, 9, 133
particle counter, 179–180
particulate decontamination, 353. See also decontamination
passive/as built, 353
passive isolator, 88, 353, 354
Passport™, 24–25
pass-through chamber, 164
pass-through hatch, 92
pass-through lock, 4
pass-through tunnel, 256, 258. See also ultraviolet light equipped transfer tunnel
PBS, 5, 8, 9–10
penicillin, 54
Penicillium chrysogenum, 156
peracetic acid, 151, 216–218, 310, 314, 330, 332, 336
 apparatus for, 152, 305
 barriers and, 6
 biocontamination via, 94, 208
 combined with other sterilants, 163
 compatibility of, 31
 corrosiveness of, 165
 dilution required for, 167
 disposal of, 183
 Dräger tubes and, 167, 227
 exposure limits for, 168
 media growth and, 180
 safety and, 167, 224
 stability of, 30
performance qualification. See PQ
personal protective barrier, 353
petri dish, 180, 320

phenolics, 31
photohelic gauge, 223
PLC, 144
plenum, 319, 350
PNSU, 47, 49, 50, 55
polio virus, 156
positive pressure isolator, 98–101, 107
powder handling isolators, 82–83
PQ, 29, 129, 200–202, 224, 226–227
prefilter, 52, 353
probability of a nonsterile unit. See PNSU
process validation. See validation
production isolator, 10, 12, 179, 185–186
profile door, 142
project management, 126–130
protective barrier system. See PBS
Proteus vulgaris, 156
Pseudomonas aeruginosa, 156
Pseudomonas cepacia, 156

qualification. See IQ; OQ; PQ
quality assurance, 79, 95, 119, 305
quality control laboratory, 12, 13, 99, 103, 106
quality control testing, 147
quaternary ammonium compounds, 31

RAB, 133, 164
rapid transfer port. See RTP
rapid transfer system. See RTS
RCS®, 176, 177, 178, 291
recommended exposure limit. See REL
REL, 168
remote counting, 179
request for proposal. See RFP
restricted access barrier. See RAB
restrictive access barrier, 9. See also RAB
Reuter Centrifugal Sampler. See RCS
revalidation, 202
RFP, 127
rhinovirus, 156
Rhodotorula glutinis, 156

rigid isolator, 237, 353
  aseptic filling in, 84, 104
  background particulate counts in, 52
  clinical manufacturing in, 83
  construction of, 15–16, 102, 243, 245
  durability of, 209
  equipment in, 289
  laminar vs. turbulent flow in, 313
  powder handling in, 82
  RTPs in, 284
  standards/guidelines for, 78, 90
  sterility testing in, 81
risk assessment, 91
RODAC plate, 176, 178, 180, 201
roughing filter, 353
RTP, 40–41, 256, 257, 258, 348, 353
  barriers and, 7
  effectiveness of, 58
  glove box and, 350
  in filler isolator, 101
  in rigid isolator, 284
  in transfer container, 42
  in transfer isolator, 99, 101
  inspection of, 224
  key design for isolators, 16
  profile door and, 142
  purpose of, 101–102, 209, 255
  sterilization and, 144, 147, 208
  types of, 22–26
RTS, 353

Saccharomyces cervisiae, 156
SAL, 45–48, 346, 354
  absolute barrier, 38, 343
  claims of, 18, 151, 190, 197, 297, 310
  improvement in, 79, 132, 326, 329, 351
  interface isolator, 41, 350
  isolator vs. clean room, 30
  limitations of, 206–207
  terminal sterilization and, 49–51
  TPN and, 43
  validation of, 192, 200, 314
sanitization, 68, 87, 94, 150, 157, 298–299, 326, 353–354

SAS®, 176, 177
SCL, 131, 132, 163, 189, 191, 233, 234, 354
    continuous process, 242
    filler speed and, 241
    improving, 272
    validating to, 234, 237, 238–239
S. epidermitis, 320
Serratia marcescens, 156
setting plate, 174, 291
short-term exposure limit. See STEL
SIP, 263–264
    barrier system and, 131
    constraints on, 133
    control of, 271
    filler and, 242, 247
    hydrogen peroxide cycle, 13, 146 (see also hydrogen peroxide)
    mechanical interfaces and, 135
    OQ of, 200
    product sterility and, 285
    RTP and, 144
    temperature for, 129
    timing of, 262
slit-to-agar sampler. See STA sampler
SMA, 177
SMIF, 259
sodium chlorite, 151, 153
SOPs, 119, 120, 131, 184, 225
spectrophotometric assay, 146
Spordex-VHP®, 156–157, 162–163
SPRAM, 289
spray atomization, 163. See also atomizer
Standard Mechanical Interface. See SMIF
standard operating procedures. See SOPs
Staphylococcus aureus, 156
STA sampler, 176, 178
steam-in-place. See SIP
steam sterilization, 191, 192, 198, 310. See also hydrogen peroxide; sterilization
STEL, 168
sterile, 354
sterility assurance. See SAL

sterility assurance level. See SAL
sterility confidence level. See SCL
sterility hold, 184–186
sterility testing isolator, 81–82, 184, 208–209, 227, 310, 321, 328, 335
    advantages of, 209–210
    centrifugal samplers for, 178
    classification of, 312–313
    components of, 208
    design of
        integrated, 214–215, 311–312
        location, 211–212
        material flow in, 213–214, 311
        size, 212–213, 310–311
        sterilization of, 216–221, 222
        utilities, 215–216, 311, 312
    disadvantages of, 210–211
    hydrogen peroxide parameters for, 157
    installation of, 109
    monitoring in and around, 183, 221, 223
    particle counting in, 179
    peracetic acid parameters for, 153
    SOPs for, 119
    validation of, 223–227, 319–321 (see also validation)
sterilizable microbiological atrium sampler. See SMA
sterilization, 30–32, 198, 314–315, 329–330. See also terminal sterilization
    antimicrobial action, 150–151
    chlorine dioxide (see chlorine dioxide)
    cycle development, 315–316
    definition of, 67, 88, 150, 354
    depyrogenation and, 100, 113 (see also depyrogenation)
    design and, 13
    effectiveness of, 94, 209, 312, 332
    ethylene oxide, 80 (see also ethylene oxide)
    hydrogen peroxide (see hydrogen peroxide)
    improvement in, 336
    lack of, 98

leaktightness and, 120
maintenance of, 197
material compatibility with, 111, 113, 164–166
parameters for, 173
peracetic acid (*see* peracetic acid)
regulations for, 167–169
sanitization vs., 326
trends in, 149–150
validation of, 29–30, 192–193, 201–202
sterilization isolator, 17, 42, 354
sterilize-in-place. *See* SIP
Steritest™ System, 214–215, 223
Streptococcus faecalis, 156
Streptococcus faecium, 156
surface swabbing, 94. *See also* contact swab
swab. *See* contact swab
swipe, 180, 181

terminal sterilization
 aseptic processing vs., 70–71, 90, 97
 debates on, 37–38
 eliminating, 192
 isolator equivalency to, 45, 48–51
 pharmaceutical, 189, 190–191
 regulations for, 74
 SCL for, 189
 sterility testing for, 205
thermal imaging, 267
thermocouple, 316, 317
threshold limit valve. *See* TLV
throughput, 102–103, 185
time weighted average. *See* TWA
TLV, 167
total barrier, 133
total parenteral nutrition, 43, 84
TPN. *See* total parenteral nutrition
transfer chamber, 88, 354
transfer container, 42
transfer device, 92, 111
transfer isolator
 definition of, 42, 88, 354
 docking of, 212, 224, 311
 in QC laboratory, 13
 need for RTP, 101, 208

 reduction of *B. subtilis* in, 217, 218
 sterilization of/in, 185, 315, 316, 317
 temperature mapping in, 316
 validation of, 318
 VHP®1000 attached to, 219, 220
 with autoclave isolator, 305, 310
 with workstation isolator, 174, 178, 213, 282
transfer port, 33, 82, 143, 181, 310, 332
transfer unit, 17, 355
transport container, 88, 355
trypticase soy agar, 320
turbulent flow, 355
turbulent flow isolator, 43, 52, 106, 108, 113, 138, 159, 355
TWA, 145, 168
Tween 80, 320

ULPA filtration, 16, 18, 39, 40, 237, 238, 239, 261, 346, 347, 349, 355
ultraviolet light equipped transfer tunnel, 41, 147, 348
unidirectional airflow isolator, 42, 52, 135, 138, 351, 355
UV radiation, 191

vaccines, 97, 282, 293, 295
vaccinia, 156
validation, 73, 189–191, 199, 271–272, 309, 314. *See also* IQ; OQ; PQ
 design and, 135, 193–194
 dividends of, 130
 documentation of, 119, 129
 integrated approach to, 29–30
 methods for, 155
 need for, 31, 44, 197–198
 process, 181–182, 332–333
 program for, 115, 289–291
 SCL, 234, 237, 238–239
 sterility hold, 185–186
validation plan, 128
vapor-phase hydrogen peroxide. *See* VHP
vendors
 coordination with, 113–115
 education of, 127–128

project management with, 130
selection of, 127
VHP, 6, 26, 30, 31, 82, 180, 211, 293, 309, 310, 314–315
   B. stearothermophilus and, 202
   challenge studies, 318–319
   compatibility with, 108, 179
   concentration of, 317–318, 320–321
   control of, 313, 332
   cycle development, 315–316
   impact of, 300, 320
   success of, 306
   temperature mapping, 316–317
   TPC patent of, 296
VHP®1000, 99, 153–155, 218–221
   abort cycle, 167
   cycle parameters for, 158
   modifications in, 113
   qualification of, 224–225
   recirculation in, 138
   signal capability, 144
   sterilization results, 162–163

WFI, 311
workstation isolator
   access to, 212
   half-suit, 99, 101, 103, 212
   in QC laboratory, 13, 99
   installation of, 224
   maintenance of, 174
   size of, 212
   sterility testing in, 184
   storage in, 100
   with autoclave isolator, 210, 212
   with interface isolator, 315
   with output isolator, 101
   with transfer isolator, 174, 178, 213, 282

X-ray radiation, 191
xylenol orange assay, 146